Manual of Practical Anatomy

Volume – I
UPPER AND LOWER LIMBS

Manual of Practical Anatomy

Volume – I
UPPER AND LOWER LIMBS

Second Edition

Dr. Nafis Ahmad Faruqi

MBBS, MS, MNYAS

Professor
Department of Anatomy
J.N. Medical College
AMU, Aligarh-202002, India

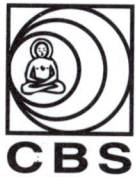

CBS

CBS Publishers & Distributors Pvt. Ltd.

New Delhi • Bengaluru • Chennai • Kochi • Kolkata • Mumbai
Hyderabad • Nagpur • Patna • Pune • Vijayawada

ISBN: 978-81-239-2271-3

First Edition: 2006
Reprint: 2008
Second Edition: 2013
Reprint: 2014, 2017

Published by **Satish Kumar Jain** and produced by **Varun Jain** for
CBS Publishers & Distributors Pvt. Ltd.,
4819/XI Prahlad Street, 24 Ansari Road, Daryaganj, New Delhi - 110002
delhi@cbspd.com, cbspubs@airtelmail.in • www.cbspd.com
Ph.: 23289259, 23266861, 23266867 • Fax: 011-23243014

Corporate Office: 204 FIE, Industrial Area, Patparganj, Delhi - 110 092
Ph: 49344934 • Fax: 011-49344935
E-mail: publishing@cbspd.com • publicity@cbspd.com

Branches:
• *Bengaluru:* 2975, 17th Cross, K.R. Road, Bansankari 2nd Stage,
  Bengaluru - 70 • Ph: +91-80-26771678/79 • Fax: +91-80-26771680
  E-mail: cbsbng@gmail.com, bangalore@cbspd.com
• *Chennai:* No. 7, Subbaraya Street, Shenoy Nagar, Chennai - 600030
  Ph: +91-44-26681266, 26680620 • Fax: +91-44-42032115
  E-mail: chennai@cbspd.com
• *Kochi:* Ashana House, 39/1904, A.M. Thomas Road, Valanjambalam,
  Ernakulum, Kochi • Ph: +91-484-4059061-65
  Fax: +91-484-4059065 • E-mail: cochin@cbspd.com
• *Kolkata:* 6-B, Ground Floor, Rameshwar Shaw Road, Kolkata - 700014
  Ph: +91-33-22891126/7/8 • E-mail: kolkata@cbspd.com
• *Mumbai:* 83-C, Dr. E. Moses Road, Worli, Mumbai - 400018
  Ph: +91-9833017933, 022-24902340/41 • E-mail: mumbai@cbspd.com

Representatives:

• Hyderabad: 0-9885175004	• Nagpur: 0-9021734563
• Patna: 0-9334159340	• Pune: 0-9623451994
• Vijayawada: 0-9000660880	

Printed at :
Swastik Packagings, Delhi

Preface to the Second Edition

The new edition begins with a new chapter called "Naming Bones of Limbs" which reminds students the names of the bones forming the particular region. Some of the mistakes encountered by the students in previous edition, have been corrected to make the book more accurate.

I am highly obliged to respected Dr. Krishna Garg, whom I admire for her simplicity and loving attitude towards everyone. I don't find words to thank Mr. Chand S. Naagar and Ms. Nishi Verma of Limited Colours for their friendly help whenever I needed.

Shri Satish K. Jain and Shri Vinod K. Jain always encouraged me in bringing about new editions of my books.

The help rendered by Brij Mohan Singh specially during critical stage of its publication is highly appreciated.

I always request my readers to provide me feedback about this edition because there is always scope of further improvement in all the books.

NAFIS AHMAD FARUQI

Contents

PART-III: LOWER LIMB

Naming Bones of Limbs

Following bones constitute the upper limb:

1. **Clavicle:** Bone of pectoral region
2. **Scapula:** Bone of scapular region
3. **Humerus:** Bone of arm
4. **Radius:** Lateral bone of forearm
5. **Ulna:** Medial bone of forearm
6. **Corpus:**
   - Eight carpal bones together constitute the corpus
   - These are bones of proximal part of hand
   - These are arranged in two rows, proximal and distal
   - Each row has 4 carpal bones
   - Carpal bones of proximal row are from lateral to medial:
     (i) Scaphoid   (ii) Lunate   (iii) Triquetral   (iv) Pisiform
   - Carpal bones of distal row are from lateral to medial:
     (i) Trapezium   (ii) Trapezoid   (iii) Capitate   (iv) Hamate
7. **Metacarpus:**
   - Five metacarpal bones together constitute the metacarpus
   - These are bones of middle part of the hand
   - These are named from lateral to medial
     (i) First metacarpal bone: It lies in the line of thumb
     (ii) Second metacarpal bone: It lies in the line of index finger
     (iii) Third metacarpal bone: It lies in ths line of central finger
     (iv) Fourth metacarpal bone: It lies in the line of ring finger
     (v) Fifth metacarpal bone: It lies in the line of little finger
8. **Phalanges:**
   - Fourteen phalanges occupy the distal part of the hand i.e. digits
   - There are two phalanges in thumb:

(i) Proximal phalanx   (ii) Distal phalanx

- There are three phalanges in each of the rest of the four digits:

(i) Proximal phalanx   (ii) Middle phalanx   (iii) Distal phalanx

Following bones constitute the lower limb:

1. **Hip bone:** Bone of gluteal region and pelvis
2. **Femur:** Bone of thigh
3. **Patella:** Sesamoid bone in the tendon of quadriceps
4. **Tibia:** Medial bone of leg
5. **Fibula:** Lateral bone of leg
6. **Tarsus:**
   - Seven torsal bones together constitute the tarsus
   - These are the bones of hind-foot
   - These are named as:

   (i) Talus   (ii) Calcaneus   (iii) Navicular   (iv) Cuboid

   (v) Medial cuneiform   (vi) Intermediate cuneiform   (vii) Lateral cuneiform

7. **Metatarsus:**
   - Five metatarsal bones together constitute metatarsus
   - These are named from medial to lateral:
     (i) First metatarsal: It lies in the line of great toe
     (ii) Second metatarsal: It lies in the line of second toe
     (iii) Third metatarsal: It lies in the line of third toe
     (iv) Fourth metatarsal: It lies in the line of 4th toe
     (v) Fifth metatarsal: It lies in the line of 5th toe

8. **Phalanges:**
   - Fourteen phalanges occupy the toes of the foot
   - Metatarsus and phalanges constitute the skeleton of fore-foot
   - Great toe has got only two phalanges
     (i) Proximal phalanx   (ii) Distal phalanx
   - There are three pharanges in each of the rest of the toes:
     (i) Proximal phalanx   (ii) Middle phalanx
     (iii) Distal phalanx

Total number of bones in the limbs of both sides are as follows:

(i) Upper limbs – 64   (ii) Lower limbs – 62

General Introduction

It is unfortunate that the study of anatomy has to be carried out on the cadavers (dead and preserved bodies) in which the texture and appearance of the organs has been altered. Dissection can become a meaningless exercise unless the student approaches it with an enquiring mind and avoids assuming that it is simply a method of learning a number of dead facts. Dissection is only a means for fuller understanding of function. It deals, for example, with simple concepts such as arrangements of valves in the veins and the more complex structure of the heart, without which normal and abnormal circulation of the blood could not be understood properly.

GENERAL INSTRUCTIONS FOR DISSECTION

Instruments

The dissector requires: one scalpel with solid blade (for cutting skin and dense deep fascia), two pairs of forceps, preferably with rounded points, a strong blunt hook or seeker (for blunt dissection to free the organs from the surrounding connective tissue matrix in which the structures are embedded) and a hand lens to partially bridge the gap between gross and microscopic anatomy.

Removal of the skin

After making appropriate skin incision suitable for particular region the skin and superficial fascia can be removed in one layer or in separate layers. Since small nerves and vessels run together in the superficial fascia, knowledge about cutaneous nerves is important before dissection. This can be achieved through diagrams. Most of the time tracing of small nerves and vessels in the superficial fascia is not a very rewarding task. In certain regions, especially in the limbs, some large veins also run in the superficial fascia. These superficial large veins possess valves to prevent reflux at the sites where they pierce the deep fascia to join the deep veins.

Deep dissection

Identification and removal of deep fascia is important. At places it is easily removed but quite often it is difficult to separate it from the underlying muscles because it is intimately associated with the outer covering of the muscles and it also sends septa between the muscles. Each muscle must be mobilized from its bed to find out its attachments making the understanding of its functions easy. The neurovascular bundles entering on the surface of the muscles should be identified and traced back to their origins by blunt dissection. So far as the location of nerves and vessels are concerned, the nerves follow most standard course, followed by arteries and then the veins. Deep arteries are commonly associated with multiple interconnecting veins which obscure nerves and vessels and in such situations it advisable to remove such veins to facilitate dissection.

Variations

Like wide variations in the external features among persons there exists variations in the size, position and shapes of various organs of the body in different individuals. Therefore, no single description of the structure of the body exactly fits every individual. Students should avail the opportunity of finding variations among different internal organs by looking into the other bodies being dissected in the dissection room. Some variations especially those of nerves and arteries are of great clinical significance as compared to that of muscles and superficial veins.

Congenital abnormalities arising due to defect in development are less commonly found during dissection. Some milder forms of anomalies which are compatible with life, can be found during dissection. e.g., ectopic kidney and double ureter. For explanation of these structures student should have knowledge about the development of these structures.

Terms of Position and Movement

TERMS OF POSITION

Anatomical position. Body standing upright with upper limb hanging by the side and palms of the hands directed forward.

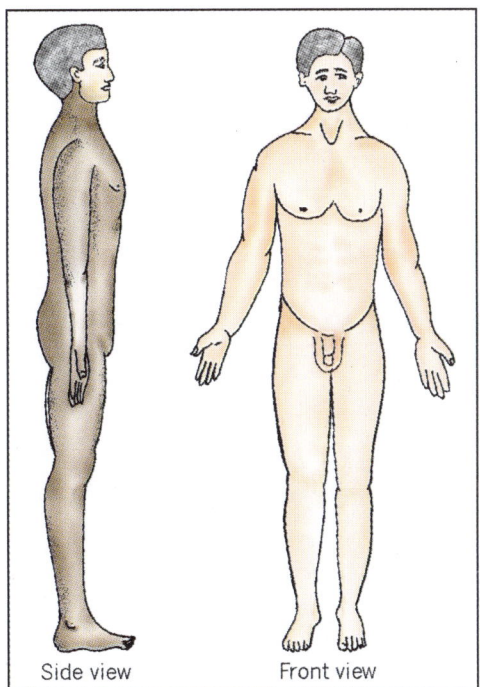

Fig.2.1 Anatomical position

Superior (cephalic) refers to the position of a part nearer the head. **Inferior** (caudal) refers to the position of a part nearer the feet or tail. **Anterior** (ventral): means nearer the front of the body. **Posterior** (dorsal) means nearer the back of the body. **Palmar** and **plantar** replace anterior in hand and foot respectively. **Median** means in the middle. **Median plane** is an imaginary plane that divides the body into equal halves, right and left. **Median lines** (anterior and posterior) are edges of the median plane on the front and back of the body. **Medial** means nearer the median plane. **Lateral** means further away from the median plane. **Ulnar and tibial**: may replace medial in the forearm and leg respectively. **Radial and fibular** may replace lateral in the forearm and leg respectively. **Inner/internal** and **outer/external** cannot be used in place of medial and lateral respectively. **Superficial** means nearer the skin. **Deep** means further from skin and are used when direction is of no importance. **Sagittal plane** is a plane passing through any part of the body parallel to the median plane. **Coronal plane** a vertical plane at right angle to the median plane. **Proximal** (nearer to) **distal** (further from) indicate the relative distance of structures from the root of that structure. **Middle** (medius): indicates a position between superior and inferior or anterior and posterior. **Intermediate** indicates a position between lateral and medial. **Superolateral, inferomedial, antero-inferior and postero-superior** etc are combination of standard terms used to indicate the intermediate positions much the same way as the points of the compass are described.

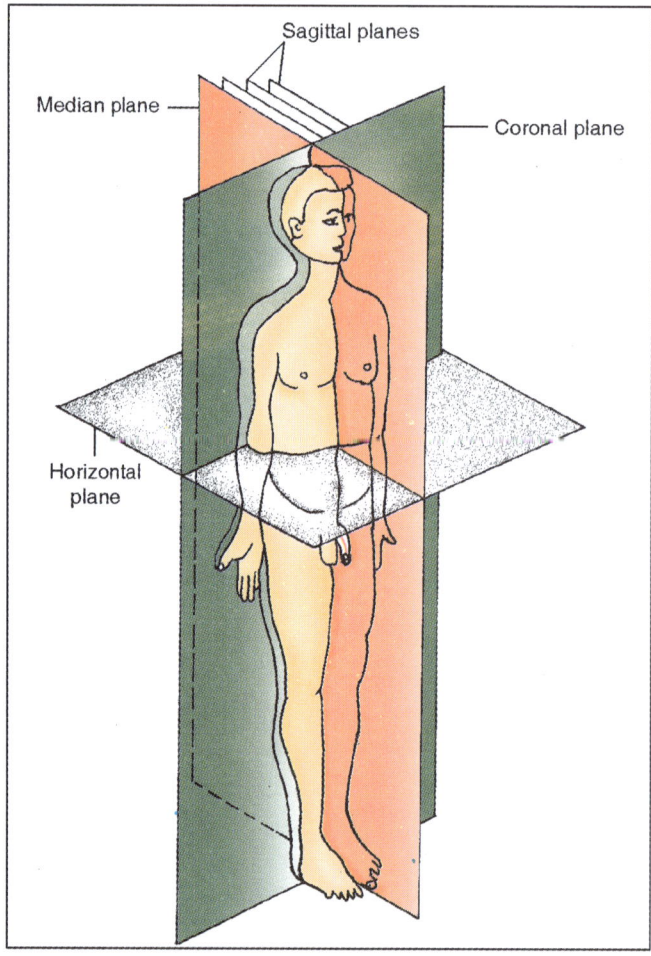

Fig. 2.2 Planes of the body

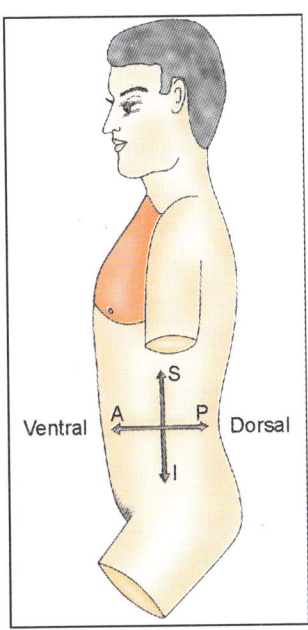

Fig. 2.3 Terms of position (A-Anterior, P-Posterior, S-Superior, I-Inferior)

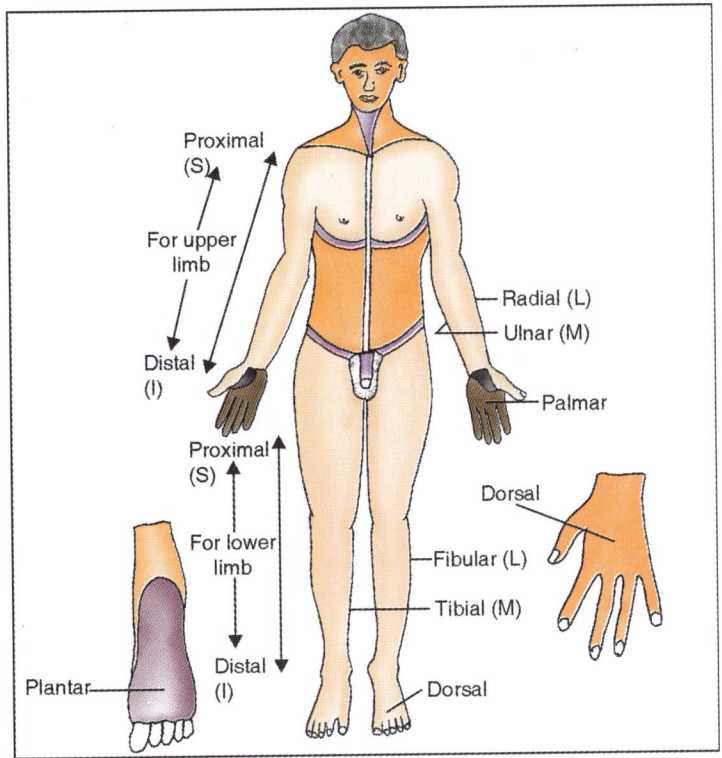

Fig. 2.4 Terms of position (M-Medial, L-Lateral, S-Superior, I-Inferior)

TERMS OF MOVEMENT

Flexion and Extension are the movements of the trunk in the sagittal plane anteriorly and posteriorly respectively. These movements at elbow and knee are angulation and straightening in the same plan respectively.

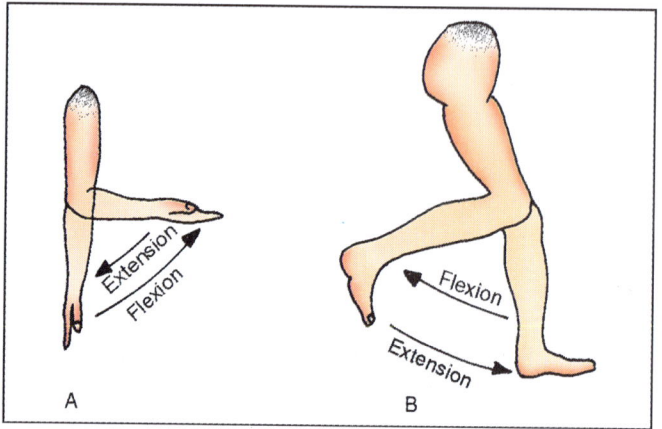

Fig. 2.5 Flexion and extension at elbow (A) and knee (B)

Plantar flexion (movement towards the sole) and **dorsiflexion** (movement towards the dorsum): indicates flexion and extension at the ankle. **Lateral flexion**: movements of the trunk in the coronal plane.

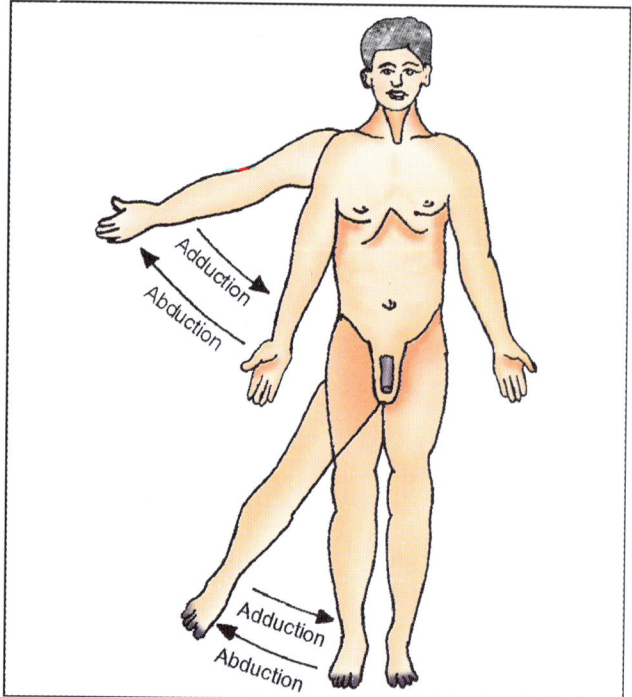

Fig. 2.6 Abduction and adduction

   Abduction and adduction are the movements of the limb in the coronal plane taking it away and towards the median plane respectively. **Radial deviation and ulnar deviation**: indicate abduction and adduction at the wrist. Turning of the part of the body around its own longitudinal axis is called **Rotation. Medial and lateral rotations** indicate the direction of the movement of the anterior surface of the limbs.

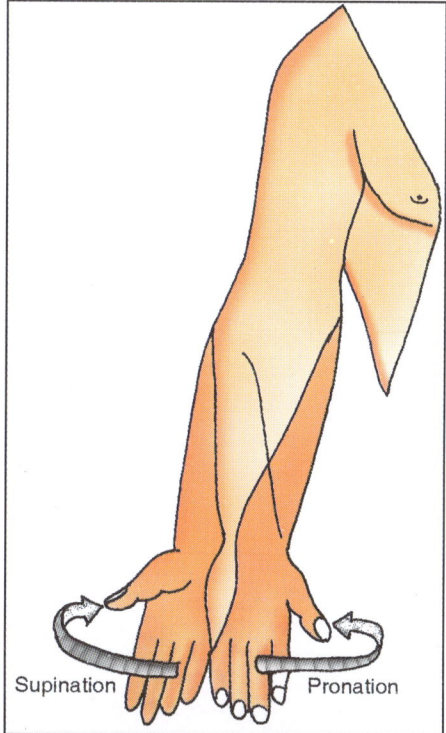

Supination   Pronation

Fig.2.7 Pronation and supination

   Pronation (palm facing posteriorly) and **supination** (palm facing anteriorly) indicate medial and lateral rotation of forearm along with the hand.

3

Structures Met in Dissection

SKIN

Skin covers the whole body. It consists of superficial, avascular , stratified epithelial tissue called epidermis and a deep, vascular, fibrous tissue called dermis. Dermis provides both structural and metabolic support to the epidermis. **The superficial fascia** is the fibrous mesh filled with fat, connecting the dermis with underlying deeper structures. It also contains small arteries, veins, lymph vessels, lymph nodes and cutaneous nerves. The amount of fat (adipose tissue) varies with age, sex and region of the body.

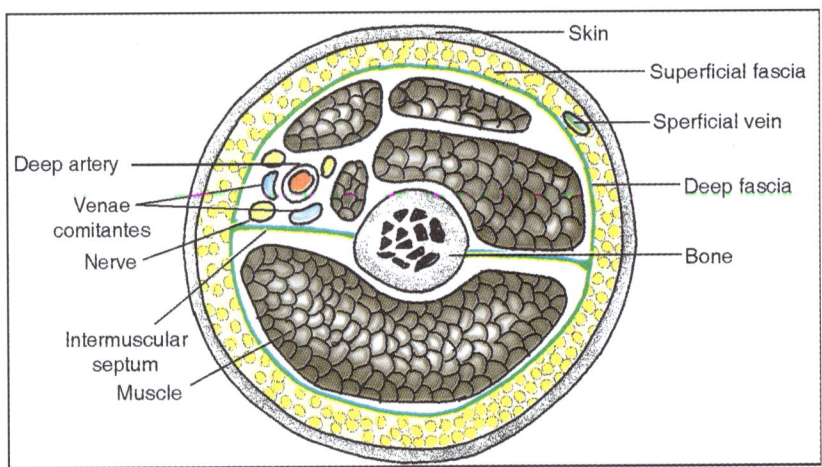

Fig. 3.1 Structures met in dissection

VESSELS

It includes blood vessels and lymph vessels.

Blood vessels

It consists of arteries, capillaries and veins

Arteries

These are tubes that convey blood from heart to the tissues at high pressure.

Elastic/conducting arteries are large arteries like aorta and its main branches. *Muscular* (distributing) arteries are medium sized like brachial and its terminal branches. *Arterioles* (resistance vessels) are smallest muscular arteries (diameter <1mm) that transmit blood into capillaries. *Anastomoses* are tubular loops formed by the union of small arteries. They are important in maintaining the circulation when one of the arteries to the tissue is blocked. It is commonly found around joints, in the gastrointestinal tract and around the base of the brain. *Collateral circulation* is due to enlargement of unblocked vessels in the region of anastomoses. *End arteries* are arteries having such an insufficient degree of anastomoses with the neighbouring vessels that their blockade cannot be compensated by the adjacent vessels resulting into death of the part supplied by the blocked vessel. These are found in the eye, the brain, the lungs, the kidneys and spleen. *Blood capillaries* (exchange vessels) are endothelial cell lined thin-walled narrow tubes (diameter 5-13 micrometer). *Arteriovenous anastomoses* form direct communications between small arteries and veins, thus short-circuiting the capillaries. These vessels are contractile in nature and are located in exposed parts of the skin and some organs like nose and are helpful in greater heat transfer.

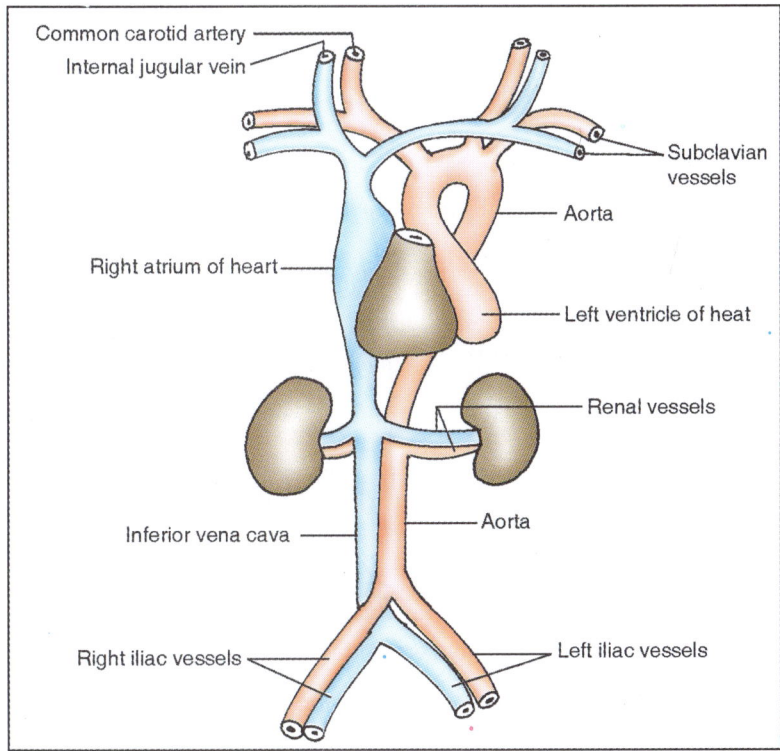

Fig. 3.2 General plan of vascular system

Veins

Veins (*reservoir vessels*) are low pressure, valved vessels with sluggish blood flow. Blood flow is aided by compression produced by the contraction of surrounding muscles and inspiration associated fall of intrathoracic pressure. Back flow of the blood is prevented by the presence of valves. *Venae comitantes* are the deep veins accompanying arteries, an arrangement for heating the venous blood and helping venous return by the contraction of the surrounding muscles.

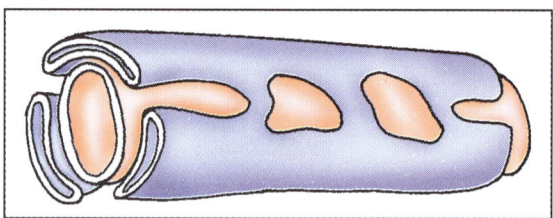

Fig. 3.3 Venae comitantes of an artery

Perforating veins are communications between superficial and deep veins which permit the superficial veins to drain their blood into deep veins.

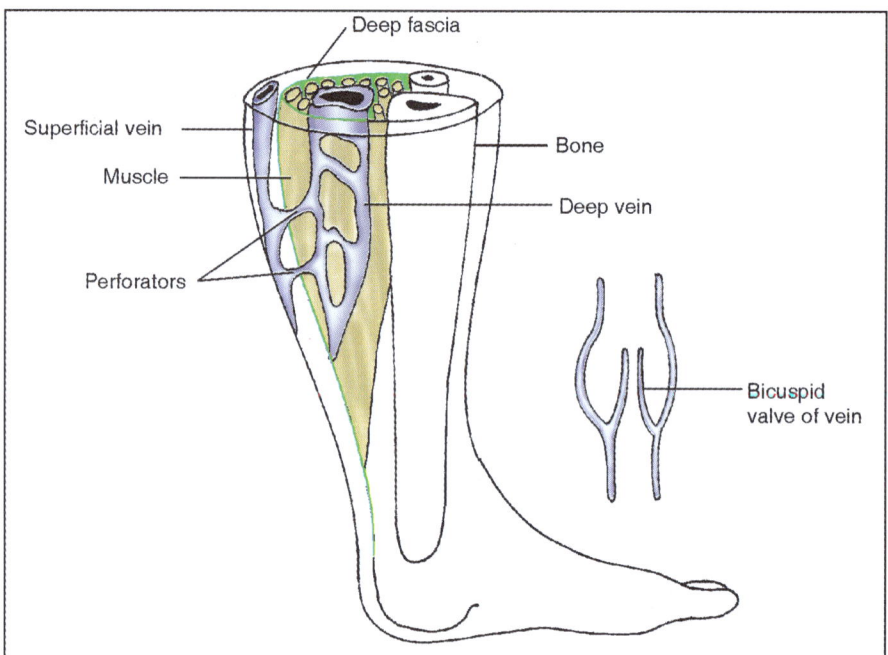

Fig. 3.4 Perforators and venous valves

Lymphatic vessels

These are endothelial lined thin walled tubes filled with clear fluid called lymph. Like veins they possess valves but these are more in number imparting them a beaded appearance. Only the large lymph vessels can be visualized by the naked eye. Their main trunks finally open into veins at the root of the neck. They are numerous near epithelial surface like skin, alimentary canal and respiratory tract but absent in the central nervous system. More lymph is formed in the active tissue and in the inflamed tissues due to excessive permeability of the blood capillary endothelium. *Afferent vessels* carry lymph to a node. *Efferent vessels* carry the lymph away from the node. *Lymph nodes* are encapsulated, firm, gland-like structures involved in production of lymphocytes. They also act as filter for lymph and harbour the phagocytic cells. They vary in size and usually occur in groups. They are numerous in the armpit and groin and are commonly enlarged in inflammatory and cancerous conditions. Knowledge of the primary groups of the lymph nodes is important as it helps in localizing the primary site of the disease.

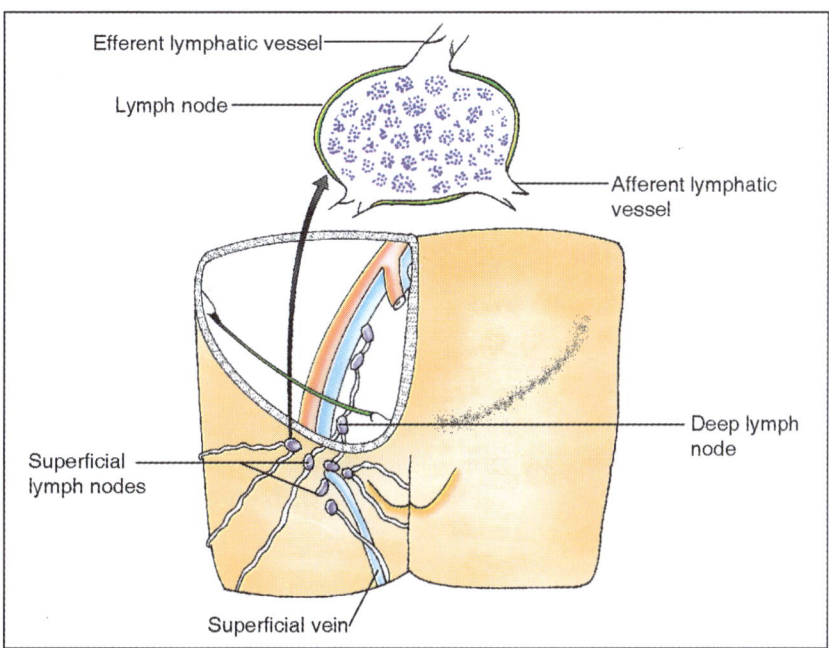

Fig. 3.5 Lymphatic system

NERVES

These are cord-like structures consisting of large number of nerve fibres surrounded by connective tissue sheath. They have considerable tensile strength and can be stretched to a certain degree without damage. **Endoneurium** is delicate connective tissue sheath around each nerve fibre. **Perineurium** is cellular and fibrous connective tissue sheath around individual bundle of nerve fibres. **Epineurium** is dense fibrous sheath binding together many bundles of nerve fibres. **Myelin sheath** consists of a discontinuous, laminated, fatty structure surrounding nerve processes of large diameter, imparting them **white** appearance. Such fibres are called **myelinated** fibres. Thinner nerve fibres devoid of laminated myelin but enclosed only by the sheath cells, **grey** in colour, are called **non-myelinated** nerve fibres.

Efferent (motor) fibres. These carry impulses from the central nervous system to the other parts or organs of the body. **Afferent (sensory) fibres** carry impulses from the different organs to the central nervous system. Most of the peripheral nerves are **mixed** in nature that is they contain both sets of fibres. **Cranial nerves** are attached to the brain and emerge from the cranium. These are 12 pairs. **Spinal nerves** are attached to the spinal medulla and emerge from the intervertebral foramina. They are 31 pairs-8 cervical, 12 thoracic, 5 lumbar, 5 sacral and 1 coccygeal. Spinal nerves are attached to the spinal cord by two roots – ventral and dorsal. **Ventral roots** consist of efferent fibres (axons) arising

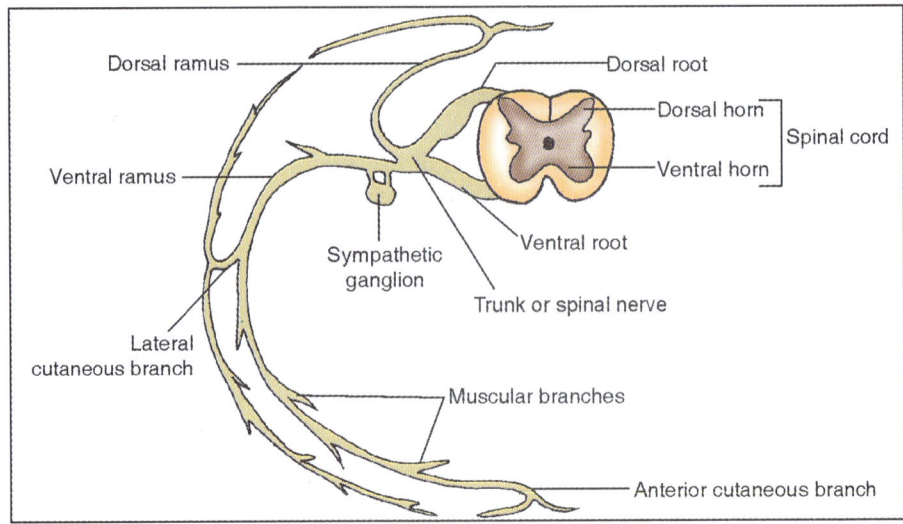

Fig. 3.6 Typical spinal nerve

from the motor neurons located in the ventral grey horn of the spinal cord. **Dorsal roots** consist of bundles of afferent fibres (central processes of the pseudo-unipolar neurons of the dorsal root ganglia or spinal or sensory ganglia located on each of the dorsal root). **Trunk of the spinal nerve** is short and formed in the intervertebral foramen by the union of the dorsal and the ventral roots and thus containing both afferent and efferent nerve fibres.

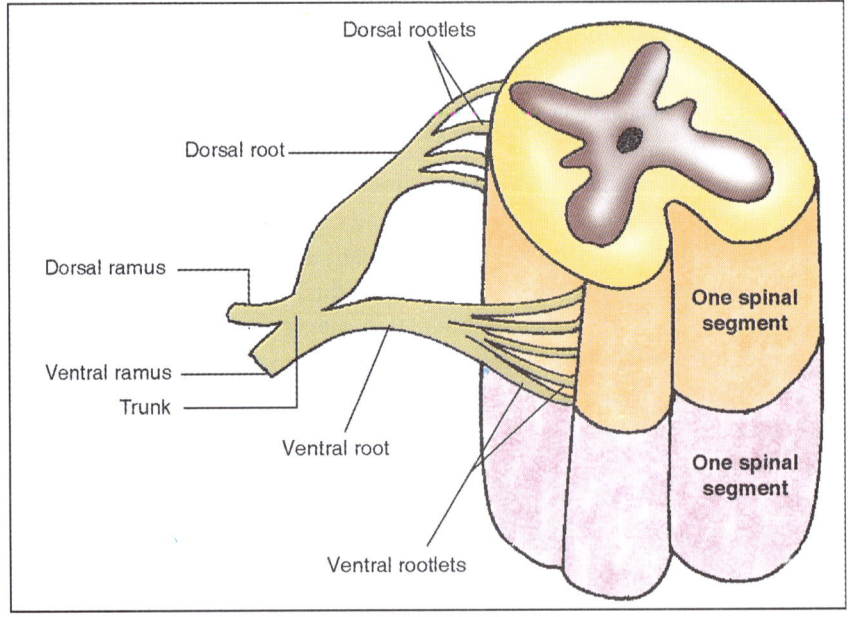

Fig. 3.7 Spinal segment

Ventral and dorsal rami are divisions of the nerve trunk emerging out of the intervertebral foramen. Both rami contain sensory and motor nerve fibres and therefore mixed in nature. The ventral rami of the thoracic region constitute the intercostal and subcostal nerves. **Nerve plexuses.** The ventral rami of cervical, lumbar, sacral and coccygeal nerves (that is except thoracic) unite and divide and thus forming a network.

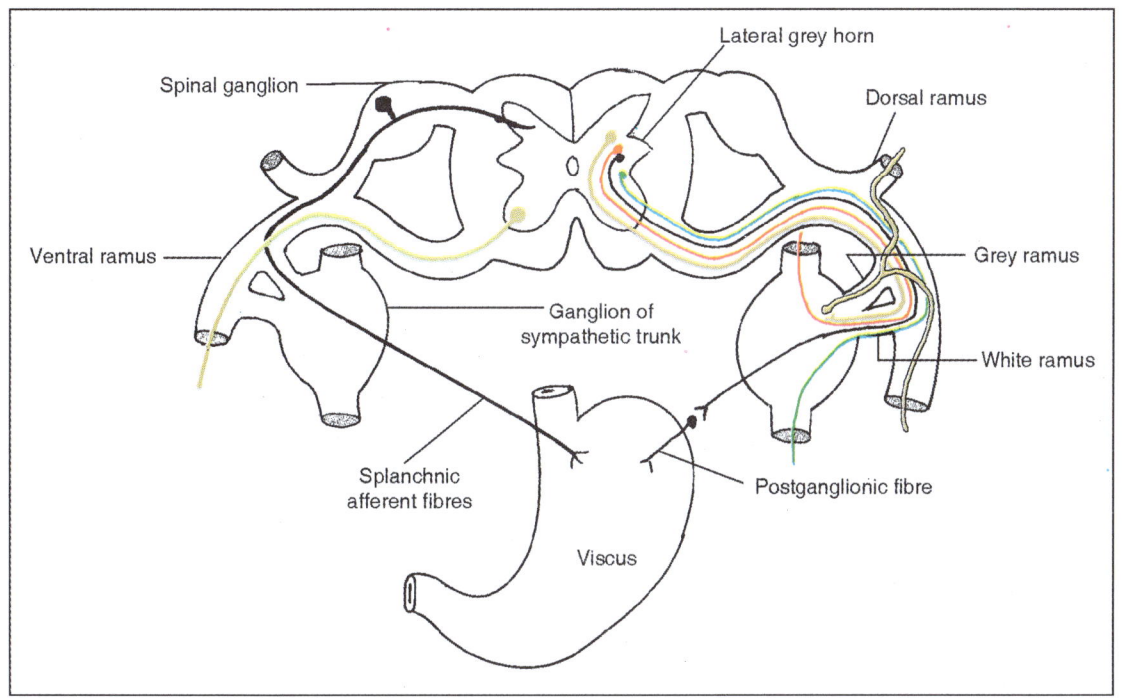

Fig. 3.8 Relation of sympathetic nerve to spinal nerve

Grey rami communicantes. These are slender non-myelinated nerve fibres connecting each ganglion of the sympathetic trunk to the corresponding ventral ramus. Each consists of processes of the neurons in the sympathetic ganglion itself (**post-ganglionic fibres**). Fibres enter both ventral and dorsal rami and their branches. In addition, they also run along vessels (periarterial plexuses) to reach their destination. The sympathetic fibres supply the muscles of the blood vessels, arrector pilorum and sweat glands. **White rami communicantes** are fine, myelinated nerve fibres arising from the thoracic and upper two or three lumbar ventral rami and enter the sympathetic trunk. That is why sympathetic nervous system is also called the thoracolumbar part of the autonomic nervous system. It consists of **pre-ganglionic fibres** having neuronal cell bodies located in the lateral grey horn of the spinal cord. Through these nerve fibres central nervous system controls the activity of all the neurons of the sympathetic trunk. **Ganglion** consists of group of nerve cells outside the central nervous system. **Sympathetic trunk** is a row of ganglia united by nerve fibres, one on each side of the vertebral column and extending from the base of the skull to the coccyx. **Splanchnic or visceral ganglia** are located in close association with the arteries supplying viscera. **Splanchnic nerves** are pre-ganglionic fibres arising from ventral rami and passing through the sympathetic ganglia (without synapse) and apparently emerging as branches of the ganglia to join the splanchnic ganglia. **Parasympathetic nervous system** (craniosacral part of the autonomic nervous system). Like sympathetic nervous system its preganglionic neurons are located in the central nervous system. Its pre-ganglionic fibres emerge through some of the cranial nerves and second, third and fourth sacral nerves and join peripheral ganglia in small groups or scattered in or near the viscera. They innervate viscera and are not primarily associated with their arterial supply. They affect the smooth muscles and glands. The short **post-ganglionic fibres** are cholinergic in nature.

DERMATOMES

The strip of skin supplied by single spinal nerve (by both rami) is known as dermatome. Usually there is overlap between adjacent dermatomes.

MYOTOMES

The total mass of muscle supplied by single spinal nerve is called myotome. Muscles receive afferent as well as efferent nerve fibres.

DEEP FASCIA

It is dense, inelastic membrane which separates the superficial fascia from the structures lying deep. It surrounds the muscles and sends septa from its deep surface which enclose vessels and nerves in it. It sends intermuscular septa between the adjacent muscles of different functions. It is also helpful in the venous return from the lower limb. **Retinacula** are the restraining bands formed by the thickening of the deep fascia that hold the tendons in position and form pulley within which the tendons slide where they change direction, for example at wrist and ankle. **Aponeurosis** is the thickening of the deep fascia parallel to the force applied by the muscle attached to it. **Ligaments** are strong bands of inelastic, white, fibrous tissue which connect bones. Like tendons they are classified as regular, dense connective tissue but their margins are less well defined.

MUSCLES

Muscles are contractile tissue responsible for movements of different parts of the body. Action of a muscle can be predicted from the knowledge of its attachments. Though most muscles play a key role in some movements they are often used in complex grouping. Muscles are used in a number of different ways. **Concentric action**, muscles shorten and thus produce a movement. **Isometric contraction**, tension generated in the muscle equals the load against which it is acting and thus fixing a part of the body. **Excentric action**, tension generated in the muscle is less than the load against which it is acting, thus lengthening of muscle occurs while it is active. It helps to control the speed and force of movement in the direction opposite to that normally produced the concentric action. It should be remembered, however, that any muscle may act concentrically, isometrically or excentrically.

The **origin of muscle** is one of the attachments of a muscle, generally fixed during contraction. **The insertion of muscle** is the other site of attachments of a muscle normally considered to move during contraction. Which attachment moves is determined by other forces in action at that time and is not an intrinsic property of the muscle. These terms are interchangeable for the muscles in the lower limb depending whether the foot is off or on the ground. **Muscle belly** is the fleshy part of a muscle. It is composed of bundles of muscle fibres and is contractile. **Tendons** (sinews) are fibrous, inelastic cords at the ends of a muscle through which it finds attachment to the bone. **Aponeurosis** is a thin, wide, fibrous sheet through which a muscle finds its attachment to the bone. **Sesamoid bone** is cartilage-covered bone that develops in some tendons. It is said to protect the tendon from friction injury, its blood supply from compression and also acts as pulley. **Raphe** is linear, tendinous, stretchable strip where two flat sheet of muscles meet each other, like linea alba of the anterior abdominal wall. **Power of a muscle** depends on the number and diameter of its muscle fibres. In multipennate muscles the obliquity of the fibres reduces the power of each but not proportionately to the increase in number of fibres. The diameter and power of individual muscle fibre is increased by exercise because of an increase in the number of contractile elements (myofibrils) in each fibre. Muscle fibres can only contract to **40%** of their fully stretched length. Thus the short fibres of pinnate muscles are more suitable where power rather than range of contraction is required. The manner in which a muscle acts on a joint depends on its position relative to the joint. Most muscles are attached to the bones close to the joints on which they act. Thus they loose mechanical advantage over the fulcrum (joint) but gain in speed

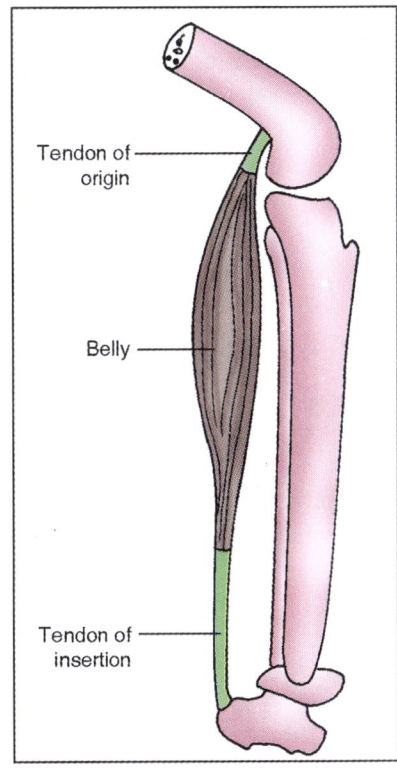

Fig. 3.9 Parts of a muscle

and rage of movement through the levers (bones) on which they act. **Active insufficiency**-Those muscles which act over several joints may be unable to shorten sufficiently to produce full range of movement at all of them simultaneously, e.g., fingers cannot be fully flexed when the wrist is also flexed. **Passive insufficiency**-Here opposing muscles are unable to stretch sufficiently to allow such movements to take place. **Synergists** (fixators) are muscles which fix certain joint so that the other can be moved effectively, e.g. fixation of the wrist during the full flexion of the fingers in clenching the fist.

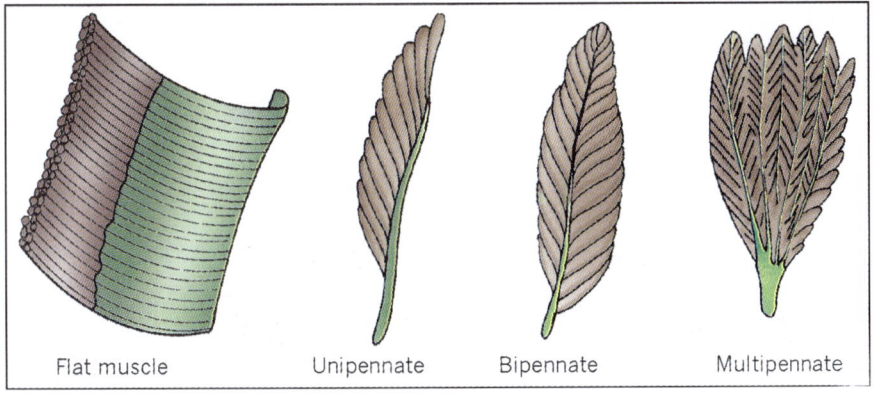

Flat muscle   Unipennate   Bipennate   Multipennate

Fig. 3.10 Morpholgical types of muscles

Bipennate muscles have muscle fibres which converge on a central tendon like barbs of a feather. **Multipennate muscles** have a series of intramuscular tendinous sheets. **Neurovascular hilum** is a distinct site where the main artery and nerve enter the most limb muscles. **Flexors** are groups of muscles of limb that develop from ventral sheet of muscle and are supplied by the ventral rami of the spinal nerves. **Extensors** are groups of muscles of the limb that develop from the dorsal sheet of muscle and are innervated by the dorsal rami of the spinal nerves. **Bursa** is a closed sac lined by smooth synovial membrane which secretes small amount of glutinous fluid into the sac. Its presence reduces the friction where two structures slide freely over each other; e.g., muscle, tendon, or skin over bone or fascia. **Synovial sheath** is a closed sac lined by synovial membrane which encloses a long tendon; e.g., tendons sliding in the fingers.

JOINTS

A **joint** is present where two or more bones and or cartilages come together (bone-to-bone, bone-to-cartilage, cartilage-to-cartilage). Joints may or may not allow movements. **Sutures** are immovable joints, e.g., sutures of the skull bones. **Synovial joint** exhibits maximum mobility. Bearing surfaces are covered

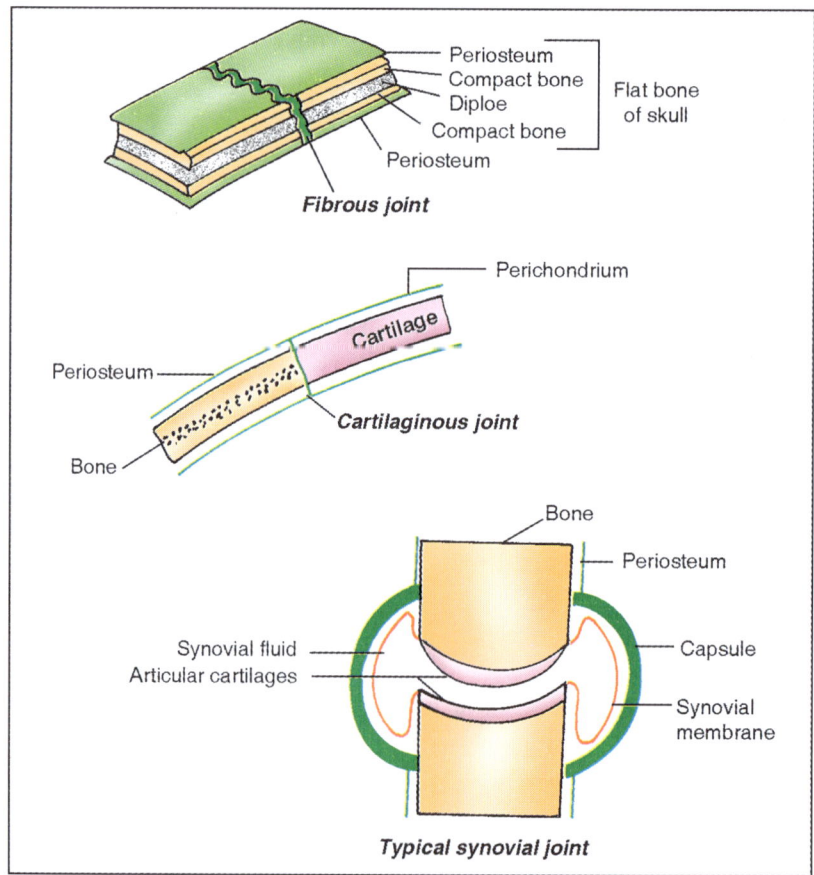

Fig. 3.11 Joints

with firm, slippery **articular cartilages** and slide on each other in a narrow cavity containing lubricant **synovial fluid**. Outside cavity, the bones are held together by fibrous capsule. All structures which immediately surround the joint cavity, except the articular cartilage, are separated from that cavity by **synovial membrane**. **Ligaments of the joint** are in addition to capsular ligament placed suitably around the joint either to strengthen the joint or limit the movement.

Types of synovial joints (depending on the shape of the articulating surfaces). **Plane joint**, articulating surfaces of the bone are flat; permit slight gliding movements; e.g. joints between bones of the hand and foot. **Ball-and-socket type of joint** (multi-axial): articulating surfaces of the bone are curved and permit great number and range of movements; e.g. shoulder joint. **Condyloid joint** (bi-axial), e.g. joint of the knuckles (metacarpo-phalangeal joints). **Ellipsoid joint** (bi-axial), e.g., wrist joint. **Saddle type of joint**: e.g. carpo-metacarpal joint at the base of the thumb. **Hinge joint** (uni-axial): e.g. interphalangeal joints of the fingers and ankle joint. **Pivot joint** (uni-axial), e.g., proximal radio-ulnar joint and atlanto-axial joint. Here only rotational movements are possible. Many joints are used to achieve a single movement and that their combined actions are necessary for normal activity. Therefore, damage of one joint may affect many movements. **Intra-articular disc**, a fibro-cartilaginous disc placed between the articulating bones increasing the stability and complexity of the joint. It acts as shock absorber and helps in spreading the synovial fluid.

BONES

Bone is a specialized and mineralized form of tissue. It is highly vascular. The fibrous tissue imparts resilience to the bone, while the calcium salts resist compression forces. Bones occur in two form.

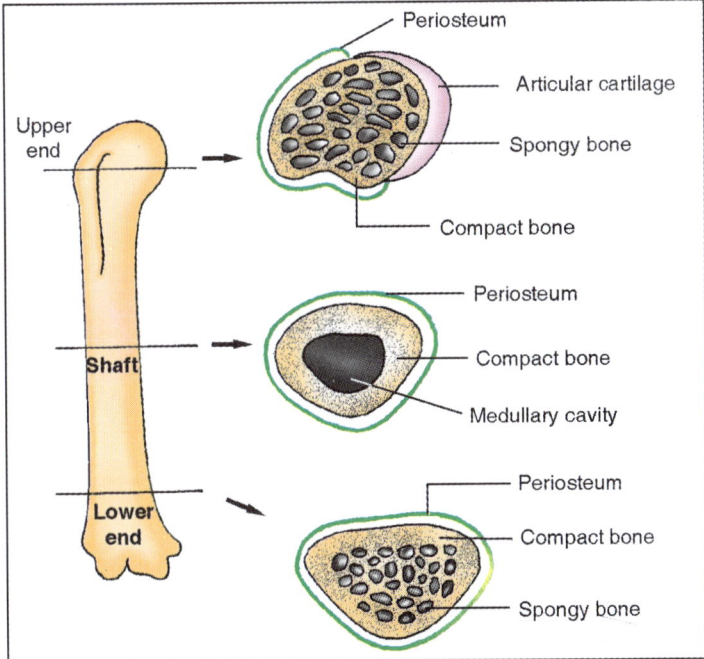

Fig. 3.12 A typical long bone

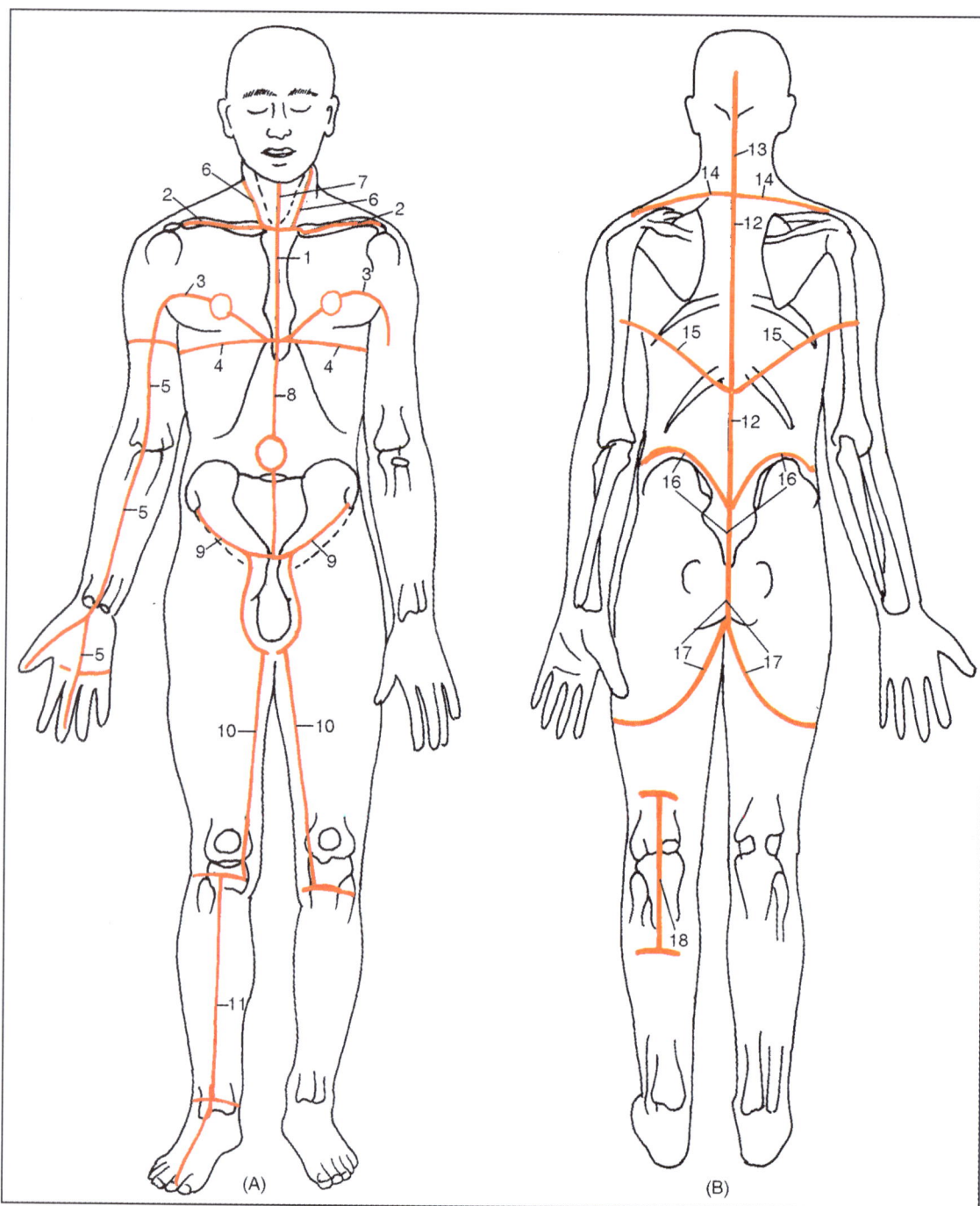

Fig. 3.13 Landmarks and incisions for dissection of human body
(A) Ventral incisions (B) Dorsal incisions

(1) **Compact bone.** It is dense and forms the outer tubular bodies of the long bones. It consists of longitudinal, laminated tubules of bones- Haversian systems. (2) **Cancellous bone.** It is a lattice of bone spicules. It occurs at the ends of the long bones. The spaces between the spicules are filled with highly vascular bone marrow engaged in haemopoiesis.**The periosteum.**, It forms the outer covering of the bones consisting of dense fibrous tissue. It is absent where the bone takes part in the formation of synovial joints. Bones are usually classified according to their shape,

1. The long bones – bones of the limbs e.g., humerus.
2. The short bones – bones of wrist and foot e.g., carpals and tarsals.
3. The flat bones, e.g., sternum and vault of the skull.
4. The irregular bones, e.g., vertebrae.
5. The pneumatic bones, e.g., skull bones with air sinuses.

On the basis of mode of development the bones are of two types,

1. The **cartilage bones**, develop by ossification in the preformed cartilage model, e.g., limb bones.
2. The **membrane bones**, are formed by ossification of connective tissue without intervention of the cartilaginous stage. e.g., vault of the skull.

4

Subdivisions of Human Body into Six Regions

1. Upper limb (right and left)
2. Lower limb (right and left)
3. Head and neck
4. Brain
5. Thorax
6. Abdomen and pelvis

Thorax, abdomen and pelvis together constitute the trunk.

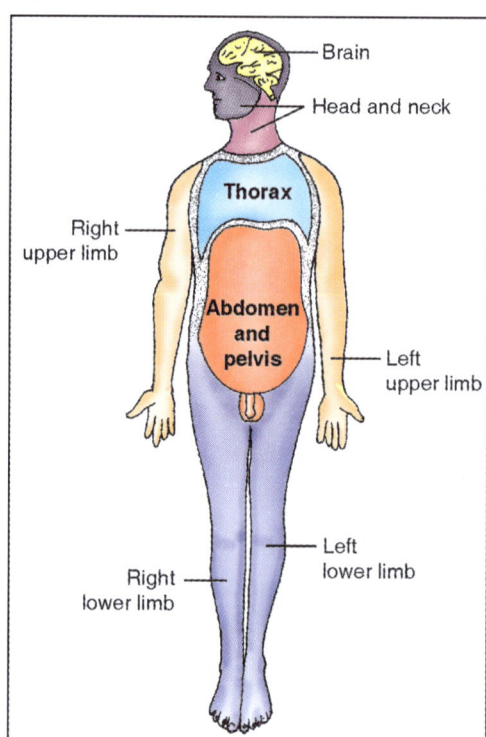

Fig. 4.1 Subdivisions of human body

22

Part-II
Upper Limb

Functions and Subdivisions

FUNCTIONS OF THE UPPER LIMB

1. Prehension (act of grasping).
2. Tactile function (blind man's eyes).

SUBDIVISIONS OF THE UPPER LIMB

1. **Shoulder region:** pectoral region, axilla and scapular region
2. **Arm or brachium**
3. **Forearm or antebrachium**
4. **Hand**

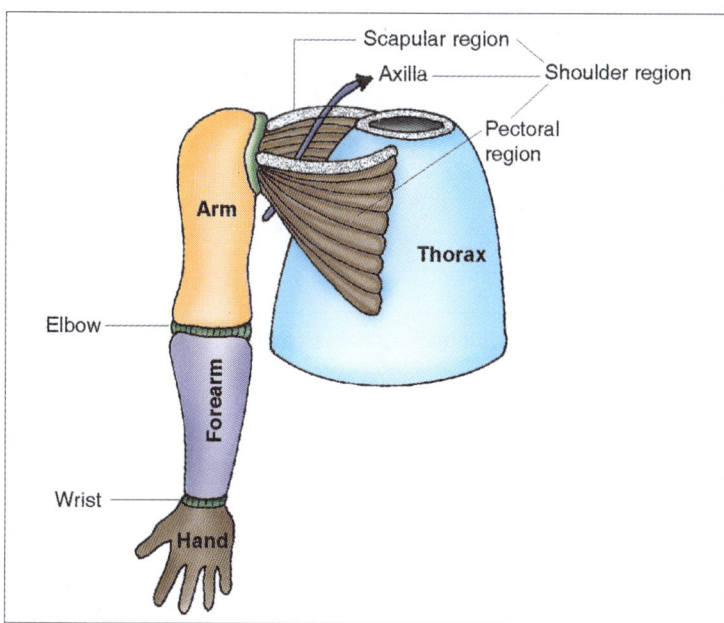

Fig. 5.1 Subdivisions of the upper limb – Front view

6

Pectoral Region

CUTANEOUS NERVES

Nerves supplying the skin of the pectoral region converge from three sides. Supraclavicular nerves $(C_{3,4})$ descend from cervical plexus in the neck, cross the clavicle and supply the skin upto the level of sternal angle (of Louis). Anterior and lateral cutaneous branches of 2nd to 6th intercostal nerves converge from medial and lateral aspects respectively. Lateral cutaneous branch of second intercostal nerve supplies upper part of the medial arm and it is therefore called the intercostobarchial nerve.

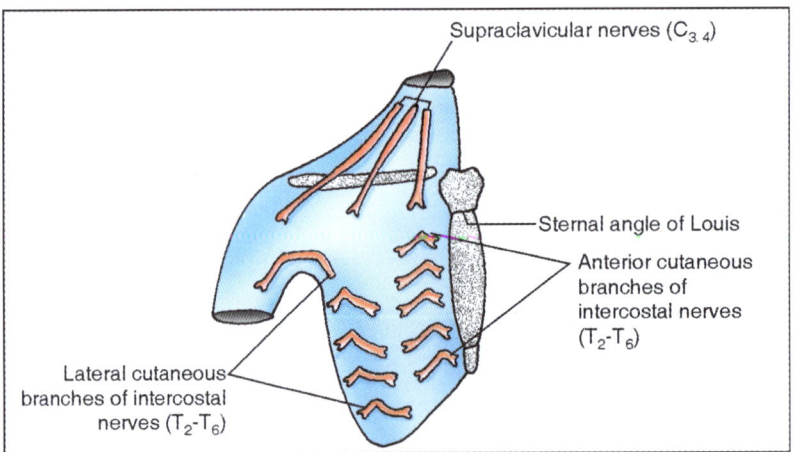

Fig. 6.1 Cutaneous nerves of pectoral region

DISSECTION STEPS

Pectoral region and mammary gland

Make incisions 1–4 (Fig. 3.13). Reflect the skin flap laterally leaving the nipple and surrounding skin in position. Define the extent of breast in female. Follow an extension of breast (axillary tail) from its lateral aspect to deep fascia of arm pit. Try to identify one of the lobes of breast by blunt dissection. Note the fibrous strands connecting the deep fascia to the skin especially prominent in the deeper part of the breast. Find out cuaneous nerves in the fatty connective tissues converging to pectoral region from above (supraclavicular nerves), medial side (anterior cutaneous branches of intercoastal nerves) and lateral side (lateral cutaneous branches of intercostal nerves). Divide the deep fascia in the deltopectoral groove. Remove the fascia from the anterior part of the pectoralis major and deltoid and define their attachments. Detach the clavicular and sternal heads of pectoralis major and reflect it towards its insertion. While reflecting the pectoralis major identify the medial pectoral nerve piercing pectoralis minor and supplying pectoralis major.

BREAST

It is modified sweat gland. In male throughout and in female before puberty, it is rudimentary. A well developed female breast after puberty is described here.

Extent

Breast extends from 2nd to 6th ribs vertically and side of the sternum to midaxillary line horizontally. An extension from its lateral part (axillary tail of Spence) enters the axilla by passing through a passage in the axillary fascia (foramen of Langer).

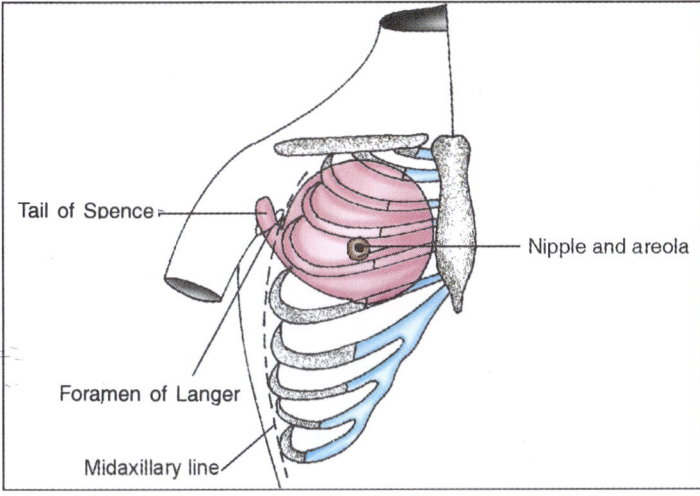

Fig. 6.2 Extent of the breast

Architecture

Nipple is a conical projection located in the 4th intercostal space and approximately 4 inches (10 cm) from the midline. The pigmented area around the nipple is called areola which is pink in colour before pregnancy but becomes permanently brown after pregnancy. Superficial fascia is marked by abundant fat but the latter is lacking under nipple and areola. Main glandular mass is comprised of 15-20 lobes which radiate from nipple. Each lobe consists of secretory units called acini which ultimately drain into central duct called lactiferous duct. The duct dilates (lactiferous sinus) before opening on the surface of nipple. Large number of fibrous bands (Ligaments of Astley Cooper), connect the adjacent lobes, lobes with skin and deep fascia and support the breast.

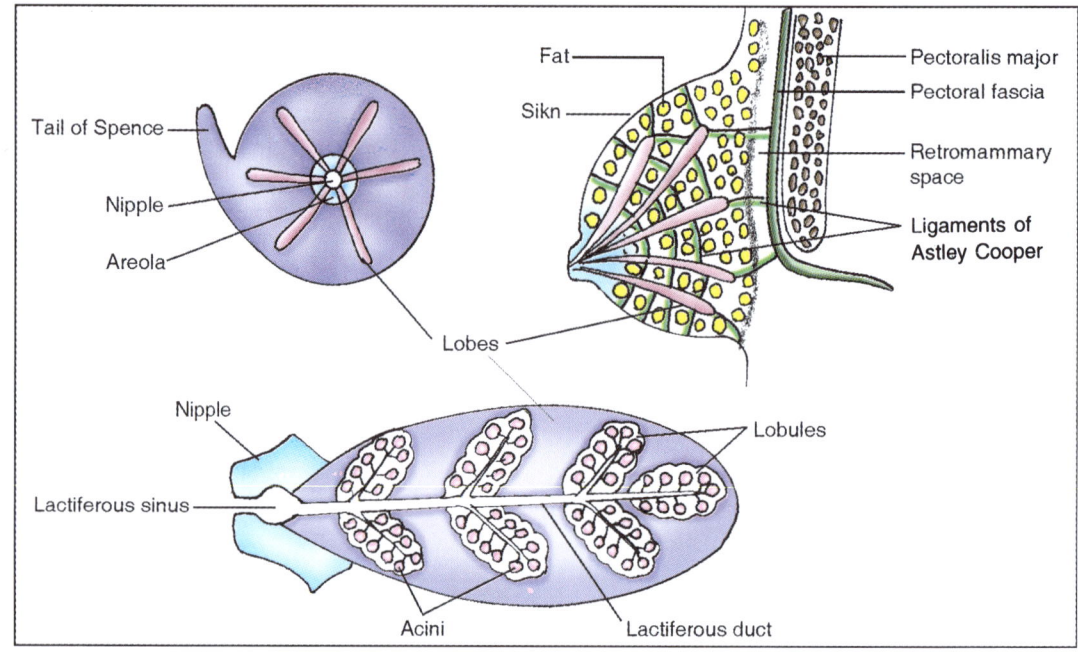

Fig. 6.3 Architecture of the breast

Blood supply

Arteries and veins concerned with breast are internal thoracic, lateral thoracic, thoracoacromial and intercostal.

Lymphatic drainage

Superficial lymphatics drain skin but exclude nipple and areola. Majority of them drain laterally into the pectoral lymph nodes. Some of them from upper part drain into infraclavicular lymph nodes. Lymphatics from the medial part drain into parasternal lymph nodes located by the side of sternum.

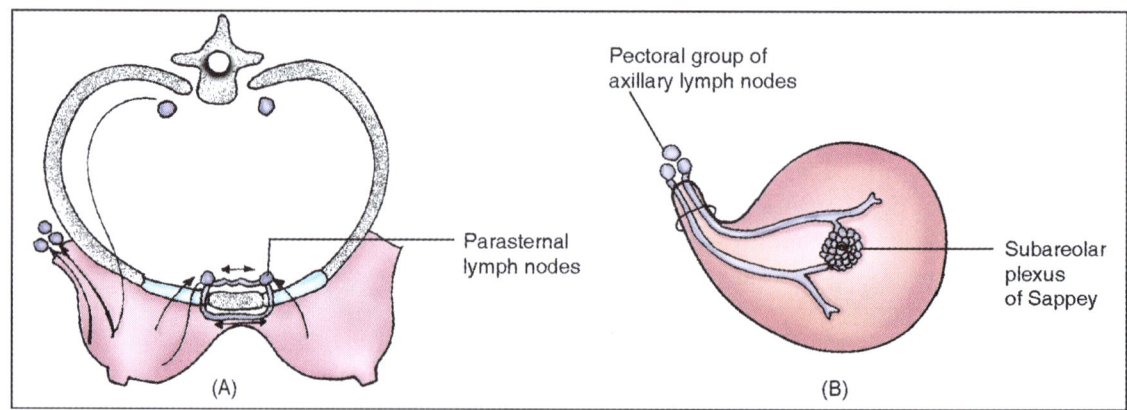

Fig. 6.4 Lymphatic drainage of the breast

Deep lymphatics drain glands, nipple and areola. A lymphatic plexus deep to the areola (subareolar plexus of Sappey) is a constant feature. Lymphatics from the lateral part mostly drain into the pectoral lymph nodes but some also drain into the posterior intercostal lymph nodes.

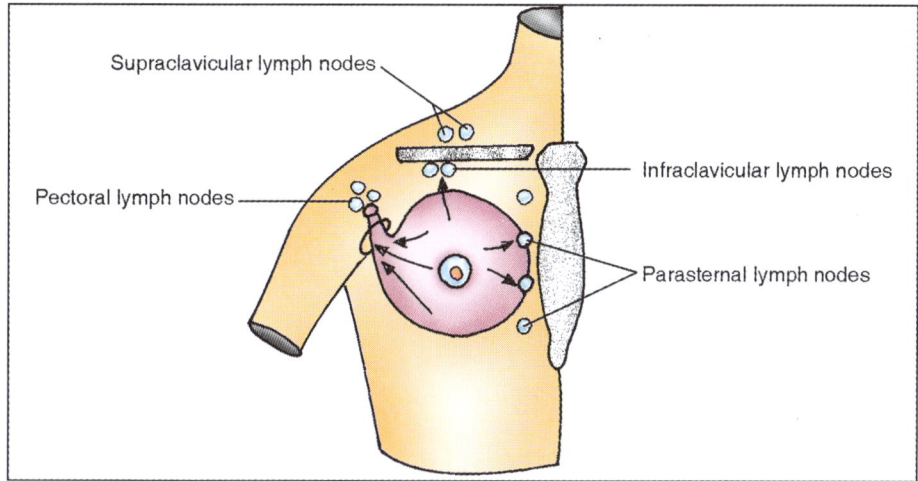

Fig. 6.5 Superficial lymphatics of the breast

Medial part of the breast drains into parasternal lymph nodes. The latter of the two sides are interconnected with each other through lymphatics which run both superficial and deep to the sternum. Some of the lymphatics from the deeper part may pierce the pectoral and clavipectoral fascia and end into the apical axillary lymph nodes. Lymphatics from the lower part also communicate with subperitoneal lymphatic plexus of the abdomen.

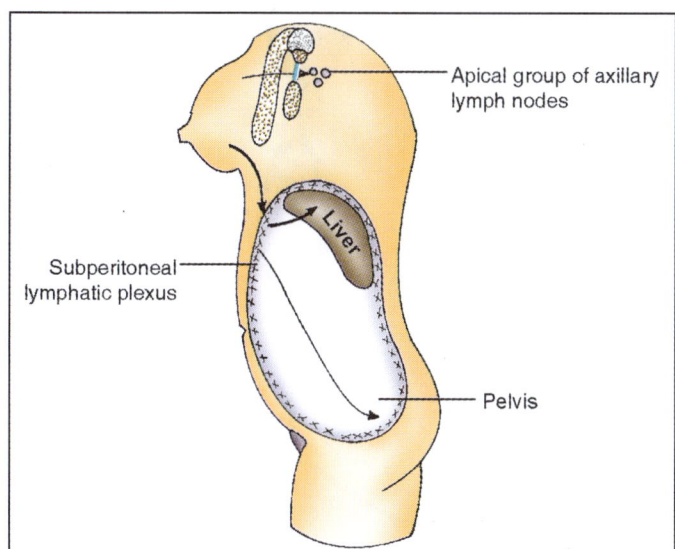

Fig. 6.6 Deep lymphatics of the breast
(Malignant growth from the lower breast can spread to liver or pelvic viscera)

Applied anatomy

- *Malignancy* (cancer)

  Female breast is common site of malignancy. Involvement of the opposite breast is due to the communication between parasternal lymph nodes. Secondaries (involvement of orther organs) of the abdominal viscera are explained on the basis of the communication with subperitoneal lymphatic plexus. Retraction of nipple is due to involvement of glands. Puckering of skin of breast surface is because of infilteration of cancer in the fibrous bands. Orange peel like appearance (*Peau d' orange*) is due to oedema resulting from the blockage of lymphatics by the cancerous cells.

DEEP FASCIA

Pectoral fascia covers the pectoralis major. It gets attached supriorly to the clavicle and medially to the sternum. At the lower border of the pectoralis major it continues backwards as axillary fascia.

Clavipectoral fascia is another fascia deep and parallel to the pectoralis major. It extends from the clavicle to the axillary fascia. It is divisible into four parts, 1. Uppermost part enclosing subclavius, 2. Part between subclavius and pectoralis minor, 3. Part enclosing pectoralis minor, and 4. Part between pectoralis minor and axillary fascia. This part is also called the suspensory ligament. The second part of the clavipectoral fascia is pierced by, 1. Lateral pectoral nerve, 2. Thoracoacromial artery, 3. Cephalic vein and 4. lymphatics.

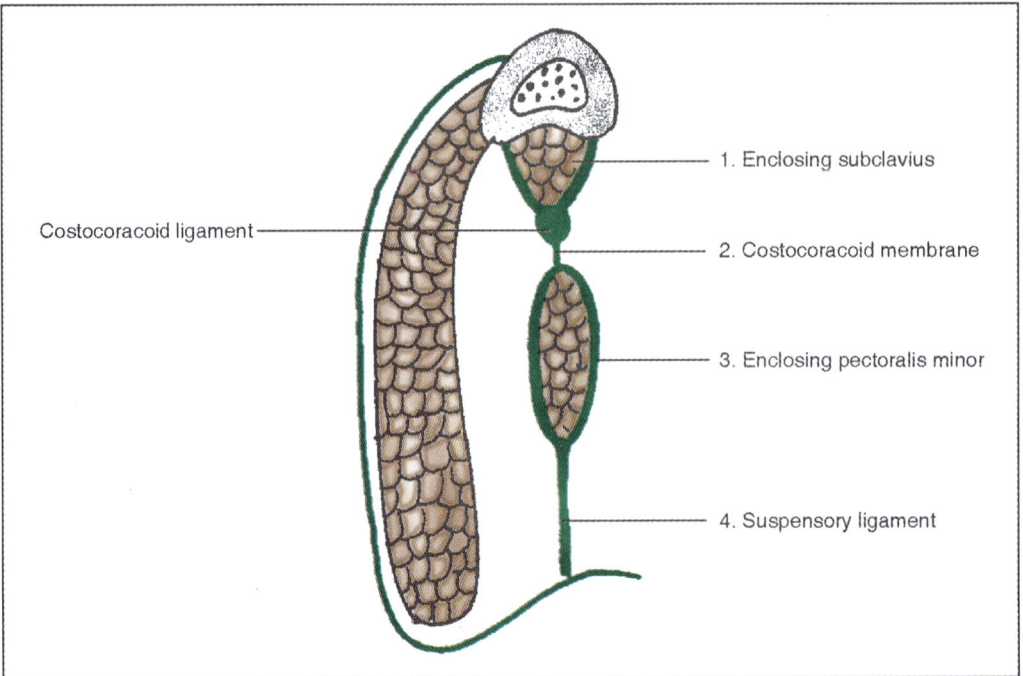

Fig. 6.7 Parts of the clavipectoral fascia

MUSCLES

Pectoralis major

Origin. Clavicle (front of medial half), sternum (corresponding part), upper six costal cartilages and aponeurosis of the external oblique muscle of abdomen.

Insertion. Tendon is trilaminar in nature and gets attached to the lateral lip of intertubercular sulcus.

Nerve supply.   Lateral pectoral nerve ($C_{5, 6}$)

Medial pectoral nerve ($C_{7,8}$,T_1)

Actions. Adduction, medial rotation and flexion (clavicular head) of arm at shoulder joint.

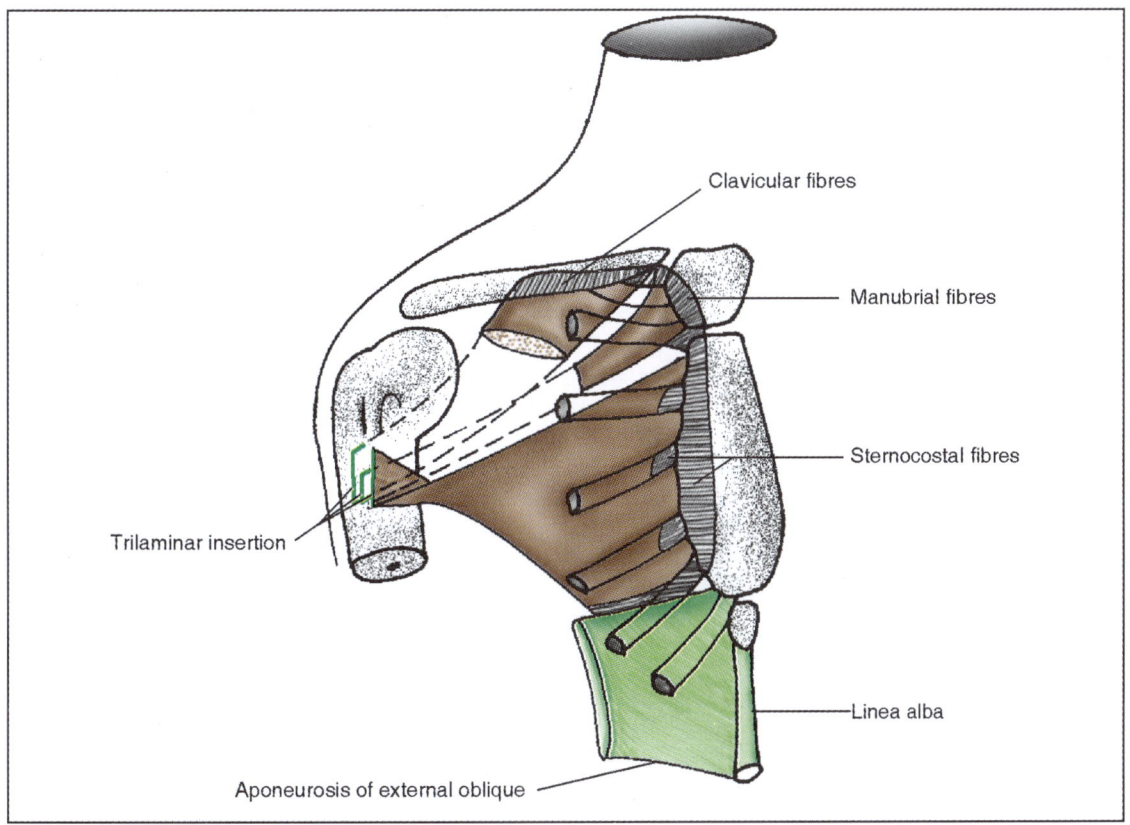

Clavicular fibres

Manubrial fibres

Sternocostal fibres

Trilaminar insertion

Linea alba

Aponeurosis of external oblique

Fig. 6.8 Pectoralis major

Pectoralis minor

Origin. Ribs 3 to 5

Insertion. Coracoid process (medial border)

Nerve supply. Medial pectoral nerve ($C_{7,8}$,T_1)

Actions. To help serratus anterior during protraction, and depression of shoulder

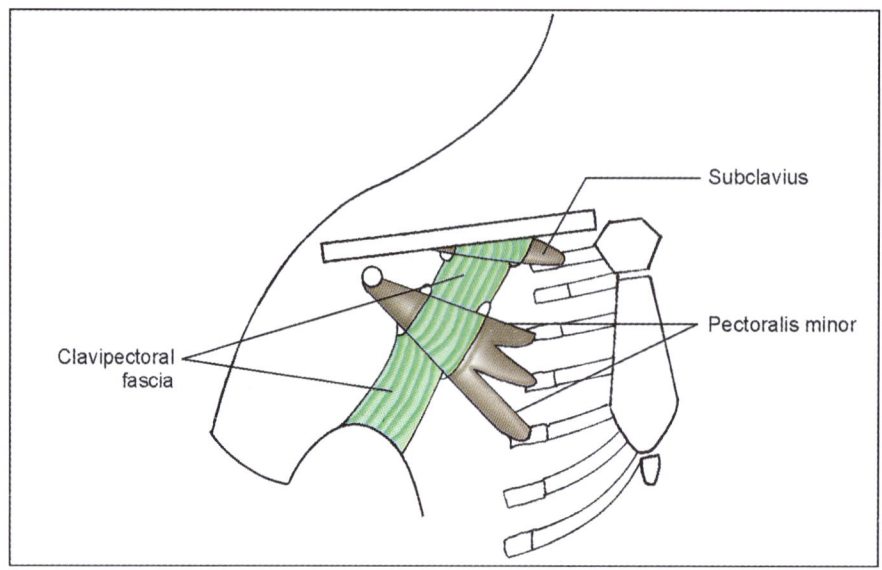

Fig. 6.9 Pectoralis minor and subclavius

Subclavius

Origin. Ist costochondral junction

Insertion. Middle third of the clavicle (inferior surface)

Nerve supply. Nerve to subclavius ($C_{5, 6}$)

Actions. To steady clavicle during movement of shoulder

7

Axilla

DISSECTION STEPS

Clean and define the boundaries of the axilla. Remove the loose connective tissue and lymph nodes from the axilla. Expose its contents.

AXILLA

Axilla is a four sided pyramidal space with truncated triangular apex located between upper arm and side of thorax.

Boundaries

Apex (triangular)

Anterior	—	Clavicle
Posterior	—	Superior border of scapula
Medial	—	Outer border of Ist rib

Base. Axillary fascia

Anterior wall. Pectoralis major, pectoralis minor, subclavius, pectoral and clavi-pectoral fasciae.

Posterior wall. Scapula, subscapularis, teres major, latissimus dorsi.

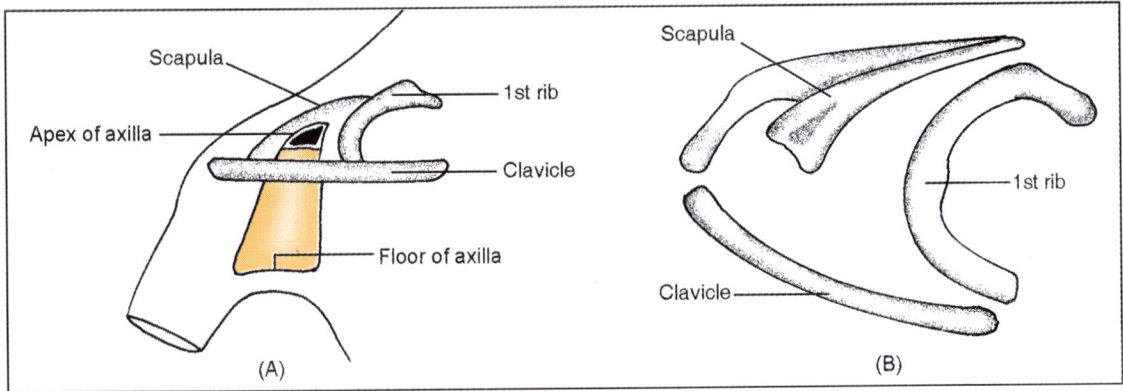

Fig. 7.1 Apex of axilla: (A) Anterior view, (B) Superior view

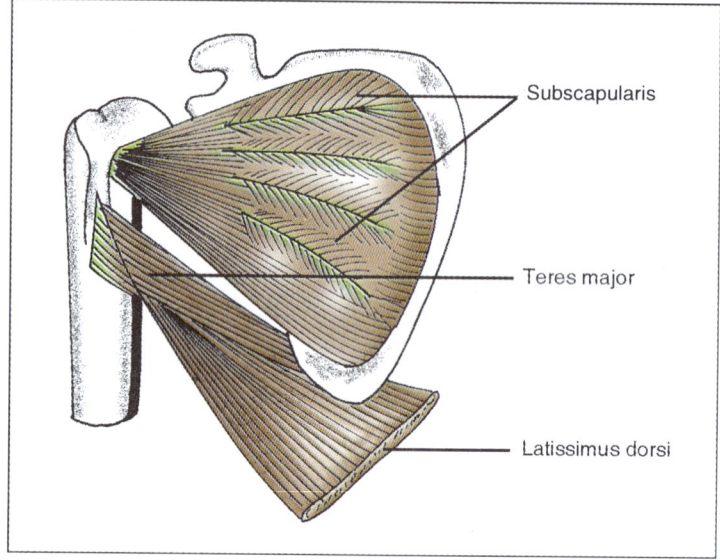

Fig. 7.2 Posterior wall of axilla

Medial wall. Upper 5 ribs and intercostal spaces with serratus anterior.
Lateral wall. Intertubercular sulcus with biceps heads and coracobrachialis.

Contents

Axillary artery, axillary vein, axillary lymph nodes, brachial plexus and fat. Axillary artery and brachial plexus are enclosed in a tubular sheath (axillary sheath) derived from the prevertebral fascia of neck.

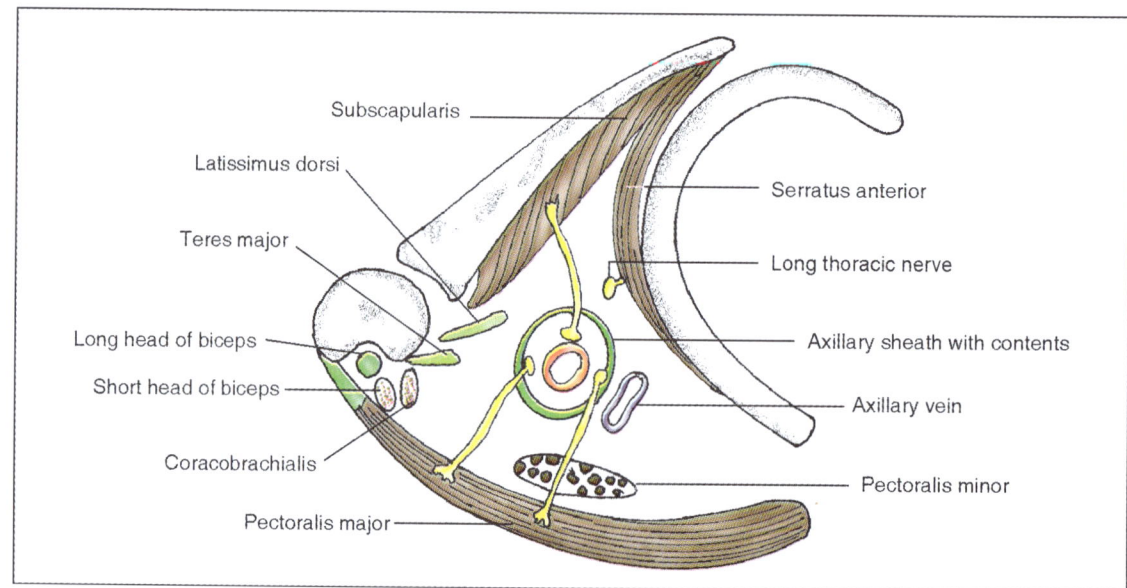

Fig. 7.3 Boundaries and contents of the axilla

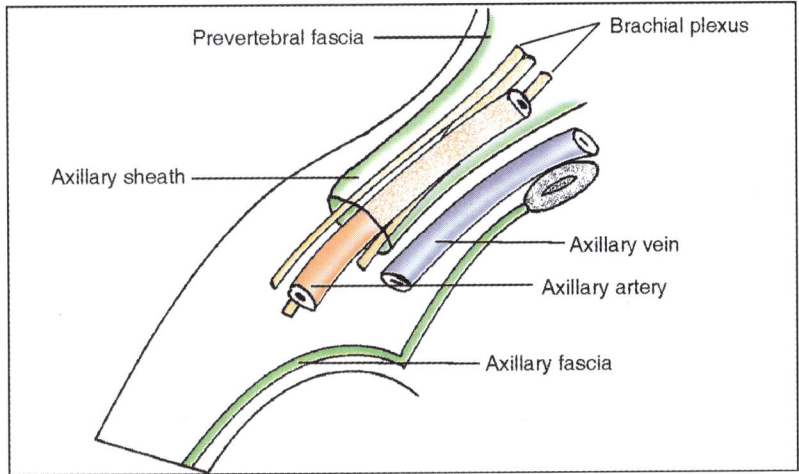

Fig. 7.4 Formation of axillary sheath

AXILLARY ARTERY

Origin. It is continuation of subclavian artery at the outer border of the first rib.

Extent. It extends from the outer border of the first rib to the lower border of the teres major.

Termination. It continues as the brachial artery at the lower border of teres major.

Parts. It has 3 parts with respect to the pectoralis minor, i.e., 1st part—proximal; 2nd part—behind; 3rd part—distal, to pectoralis minor.

Relations. It is closely related to the cords and branches of the brachial plexus (as showen below). Axillary vein is medial throughout. Pectoralis minor crosses the front of its 2nd part.

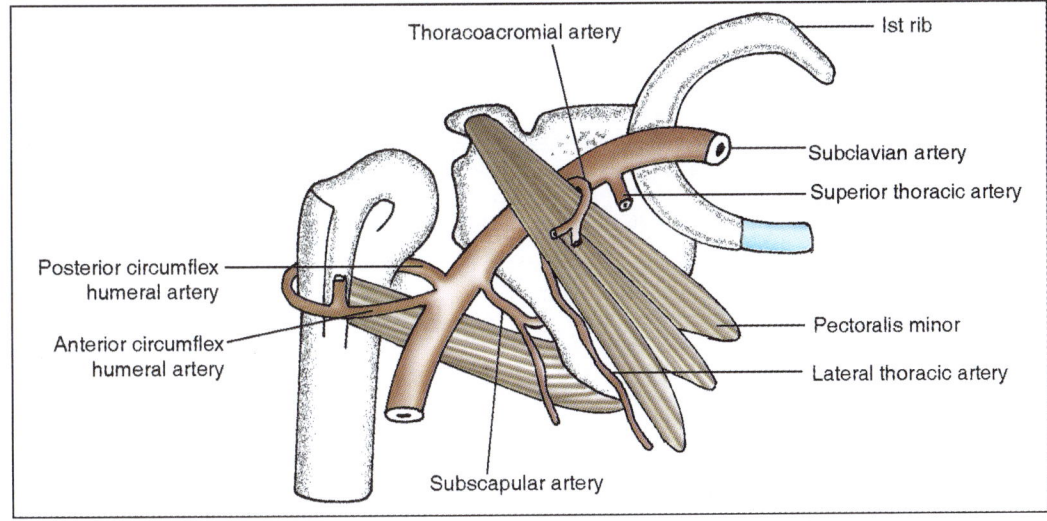

Fig. 7.5 Axillary artery

Branches

Part	No. of branches	Name of branches
1st	1	• Superior thoracic artery.
2nd	2	• Thoracoacromial artery. It splits into four branches, clavicular, humeral, acromial and pectoral.
		• Lateral thoracic artery.
3rd	3	• Subscapular artery which splits into, circumflex scapular and throracodorsal artery.
		• Anterior circumflex humeral artery.
		• Posterior circumflex humeral artery.

Applied anatomy

- Branches may arise from abnormal sites.
- Localized dilataion of the artery (axillary aneurysm) may produce swelling below the clavicle or in the armpit depending upon its location.
- Subscapular artery participates in the anastomoses around the scapula and it is therefore important in providing collateral circulation in cases of obstruction of the main artery.
- Laceration of axillary artery is common (second to the popliteal artery).

AXILLARY VEIN

It is continuation of basilic vein at the lower border of teres major. Beyond the outer border of the first rib it continues as subclavian vein. It receives cephalic vein and venae comitantes of brachial artery (brachial veins) in addition to the veins accompanying the branches of the axillary artery.

Applied anatomy

- Damage to the vein results into profuse bleeding (as the vein is unable to retract due to fibrous bands connecting its wall to the clavipectoral fascia) and possibly entry of air into it (air embolism).
- *Cardiac catheterization.* A catheter can be introduced into the heart through the axillary vein. Following pathway is followed, Cephalic vein → Axillary vein → Subclavian vein → Brachiocephalic vein → Superior vena cava → Heart

AXILLARY LYMPH NODES

Lymph nodes in the axilla are arranged in five groups.

1. **Anterior or pectoral group**. These are located along lateral thoracic vessels and drain pectoral region and skin of the front of abdomen above the level of umbilicus.
2. **Posterior or subscapular group**. These are located along the subscapular vessels and drain scapular region and skin of the back of trunk above the level of umbilicus.

3. **Lateral group.** These are associated with axillary vessels and drain arm, forearm and hand.

4. **Central group**. It is located in the axillary fat and receives lymphatics from upper three groups. Their efferents form subclavian lymph trunk in relation to the subclavian vein.

5. **Apical group.**It is located in the upper part of axilla and receives afferents from the central group.

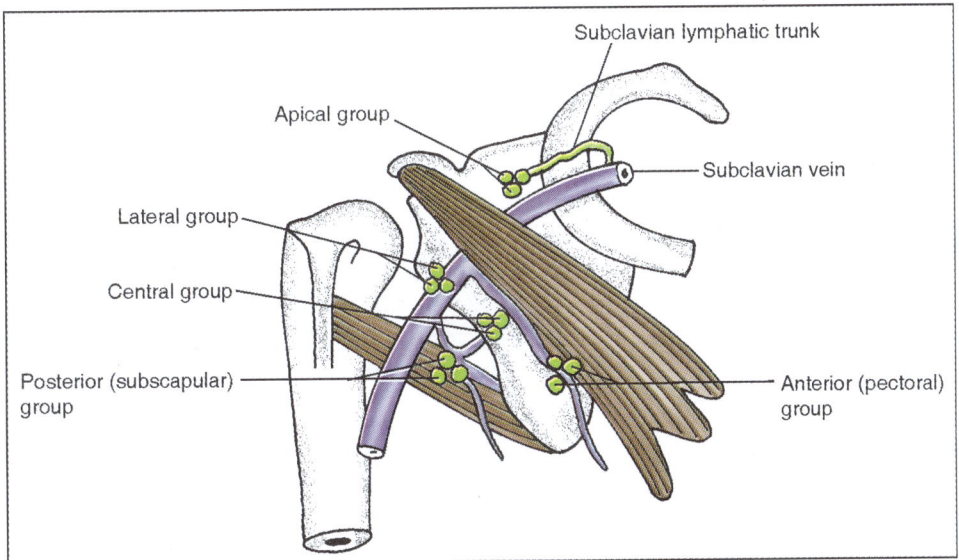

Fig. 7.6 Axillary lymph nodes

BRACHIAL PLEXUS

Origin. Ventral rami of 5th, 6th, 7th and 8th cervical and 1st thoracic nerves participate in the formation of brachial plexus. The root value of the plexus therefore is $C_{5, 6, 7, 8}$ and T_1.

Formation. There are five components of brachial plexus.

1. *Roots*. 5 Ventral rami constitute the 5 roots of the brachial plexus.
2. *Trunks*. Upper two roots (C_5 and $_6$) unite to form upper trunk. Middle root (C_7) continues as the middle trunk. Lower two roots (C_8 and T_1) unite to form the lower trunk.
3. *Divisions*. Each trunk divides into a ventral and a dorsal divisions.
4. *Cords*. All three posterior divisions unite to form the posterior cord. Ventral divisions of upper and middle trunk unite to form lateral cord. Ventral division of lower trunk continues as the medial cord.

Location

Part of the plexus	Location
Roots and trunks	Neck
Divisions	Behind the clavicle
Cords and branches	Axilla

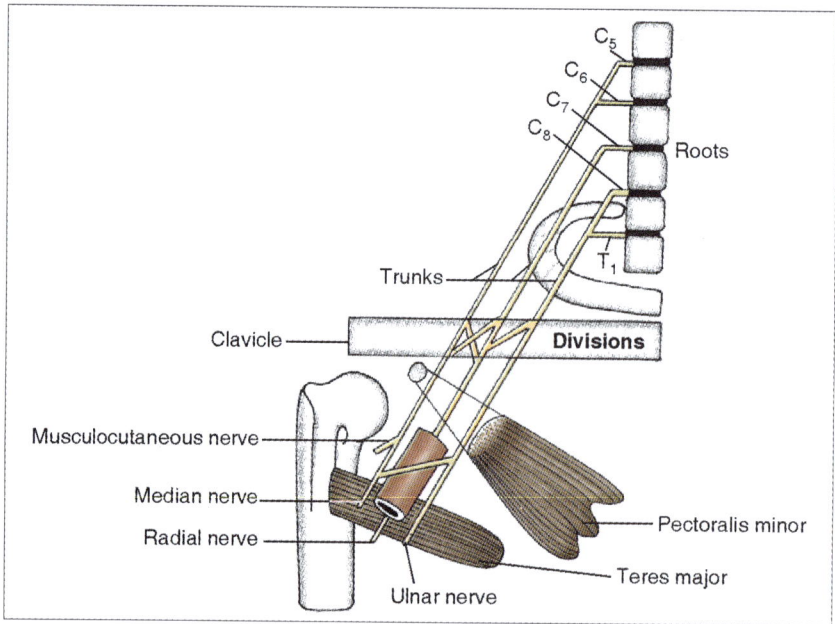

Fig. 7.7 Formation of brachial plexus

Branches – Numbers

Part of the plexus	No. of branches
Roots	2
Uper trunk	2
Lateral cord	3
Medial cord	5
Posterior cord	5

Named branches

FROM ROOTS

1. *Dorsal scapular nerve*. It arises from C_5 root and supplies levator scapulae, rhomboid minor and rhomboid major.
2. *Long thoracic nerve*. It arises from upper three roots ($C_{5, 6, 7}$) and descends behind the roots to reach the lateral aspect of the thorax where it runs over the digitations of serratus anterior and supplies it.

FROM UPPER TRUNK

1. *Nerve to subclavius* ($C_{5, 6}$). It supplies subclavius muscle.
2. *Suprascapular nerve* ($C_{5, 6}$). It passes through suprascapular notch and supplies both supraspinatus and infraspinatus muscles.

FROM CORDS

Lateral cord

1. *Lateral pectoral nerve* ($C_{5, 6, 7}$). It supplies pectoralis major.
2. *Musculocutaneous nerve* ($C_{5, 6, 7}$). It supplies muscles of flexor compartment of arm and continues as lateral cutaneous nerve of forearm.
3. *Lateral root of median nerve* ($C_{5, 6, 7}$). It joins medial root to form median nerve. Median nerve supplies most of the muscles of flexor compartment of forearm, few muscles of hand and some skin of hand.

Medial cord

1. *Medial pectoral nerve* (C_8, T_1). It supplies both pectoralis major and pectoralis minor.
2. *Medial root of median nerve* (C_8, T_1). It crosses the axillary artery to join the lateral root to form the median nerve.
3. *Medial cutaneous nerve of arm* (C_8, T_1). It supplies most of the skin on the medial aspect of arm.
4. *Medial cutaneuos nerve of forearm* (C_8, T_1). It supplies most of the skin on the medial aspect of forearm.
5. *Ulanar nerve* (C_8, T_1). It supplies few muscles of flexor compartment of forearm, most of the muscles of hand and some skin of the hand.

Posterior cord

1. *Axillary nerve* ($C_{5, 6}$). It supplies deltoid and teres minor.
2. *Upper subscapular nerve* ($C_{5, 6}$). It supplies upper part of subscapularis

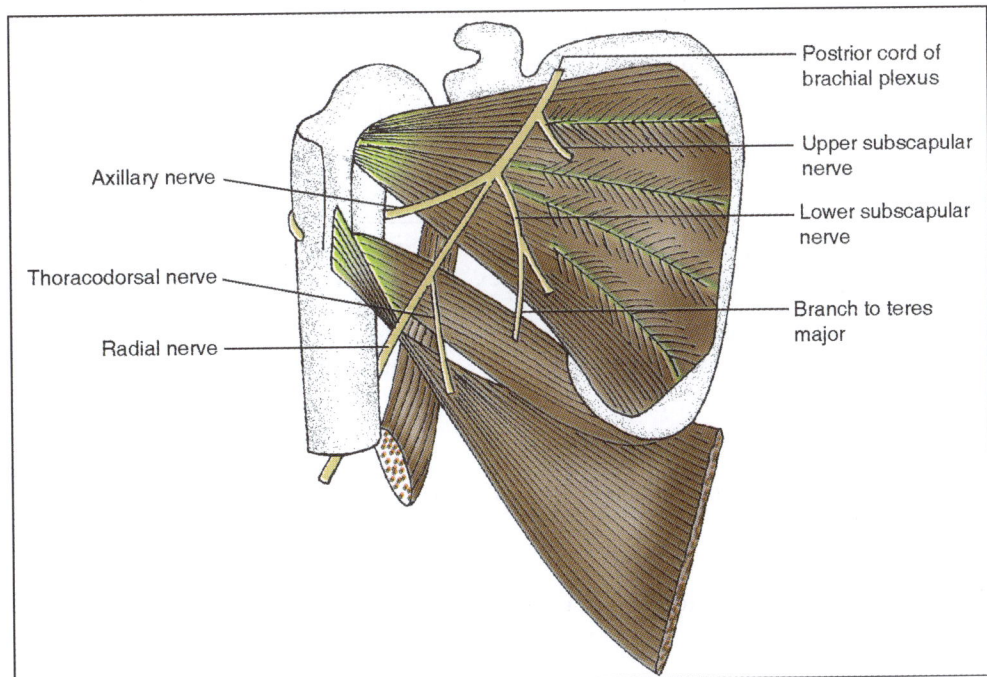

Fig. 7.8 Posterior cord of brachial plexus

3. *Lower subscapular nerve* ($C_{5, 6}$). It supplies lower part of subscapularis and teres major.
4. *Thoracodorsal nerve* ($C_{6, 7, 8}$). This is also called nerve to latissimus dorsi.
5. *Radial nerve* ($C_{5, 6, 7, 8}$, T_1). It supplies all the muscles of extensor compartments of arm and forearm and some skin of hand.

Relations

Cords and branches are closely associated with the axillary vessels.

Applied anatomy

UPPER LESION

Site	Upper trunk (Erb's point—meeting point of six nerves, upper two roots, two divisions, and two branches of upper trunk).
Cause	Difficult labour.
	Fall of weight on the shoulder.
Mechanism	Increase in the angle between neck and the shoulder.
Paralysis	Erb's Duchenne paralysis.
Deformities	Porter's tip or Policeman tip deformity.
	Due to the paralysis of following muscles the limb is adducted, pronated and medially rotated.
	D...Deltoid,
	B...Brachialis, Biceps, Brachioradialis
	S....Supraspinatus, Supinator
	T...Teres major, Teres minor
	I... Infraspinatus

To remember the names of muscles, remember "Don't Be Sorry, Treat It"

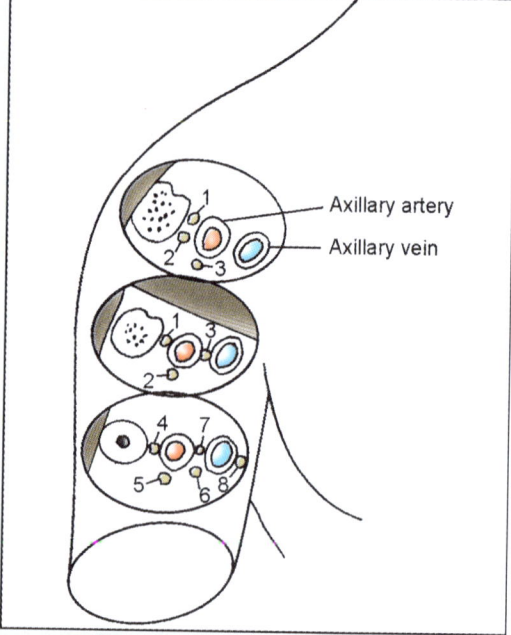

Fig. 7.9 Relations of brachial plexus with axillary vessels. 1. Lateral cord; 2. Posterior cord; 3. Medial cord; 4. Median nerve; 5. Radial nerve; 6. Ulnar nerve; 7. Medial cutaneous nerve of forearm; 8. Medial cutaneous nerve of arm

LOWER LESION

Site	Lower trunk
Cause	Forceful hyperabduction of arm when holding a branch of tree during fall from height.
Paralysis	Klumpke's paralysis
Deformity	Claw-hand deformity. It is due to paralysis of muscles of hand supplied by the ulnar nerve.

Back and Scapular Region

8

CUTANEOUS NERVES OF THE BACK

Skin of the back of the head, neck and trunk is supplied by the dorsal rami of the spinal nerves.

Some interesting facts regarding the dorsal rami of spinal nerves:

1. All divide into medial and lateral branches.
2. Both the branches supply erector spinae.
3. Only one of the two branches become cutaneous.
4. In the upper part of back upto the level of 6th thoracic nerve, it is the medial branch which gives cutaneous nerves. Below the level of T_6, cutaneous nerves arise from the lateral branches of dorsal rami.
5. No cutaneous branches appear from the 1st, 7th and 8th cervical and last two lumbar ($L_{4, 5}$) dorsal rami.

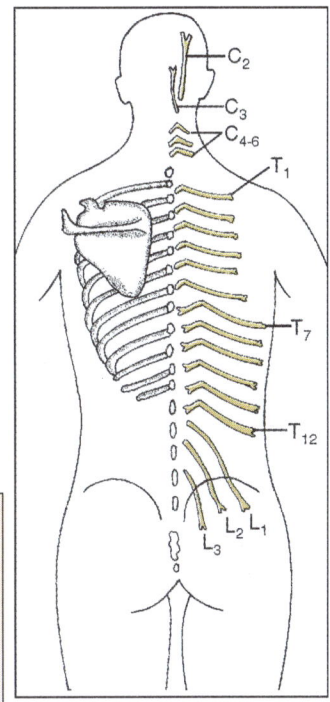

Fig. 8.1 Cutaneous nerves of the back

DISSECTION STEPS: DISSECTION OF BACK

Make incision Nos. 12, 14, 15 and 16 (Fig. 3.13). Reflect skin flaps laterally. Strip the superficial fascia from the deep fascia. Remove the fascia from the surface of the trapezius and define its extent. Define and uncover the latissimus dorsi. Reflect the lower part of the trapezius by dividing it vertically, 5 cm lateral to the median plane and identify the levator scapulae and rhomboideus major and minor.

SUPERFICIAL MUSCLES OF BACK

Trapezius

Origin.   Superior nuchal line, external occipital protuberance, ligamentum nuchae, 7th cervical and all thoracic spines, supraspinous ligaments.

41

Insertion   Upper fibres—posterior border of lateral one third of clavicle.

Middle fibres—acromion process (medial border) and crest of spine (superior border).

Lower fibres—deltoid tubercle of crest of spine.

Nerve   Accessory nerve (XI cranial nerve) — motor supply.

Branches from the cervical plexus ($C_{3, 4}$) — proprioceptive supply.

Actions   Upper fibres, act with levator scapulae to elevate scapula.

Both upper and lower fibres with lower 4 digitations of serratus anterior produce lateral rotation of scapula.

Middle fibres act with rhomboids to retract the scapula.

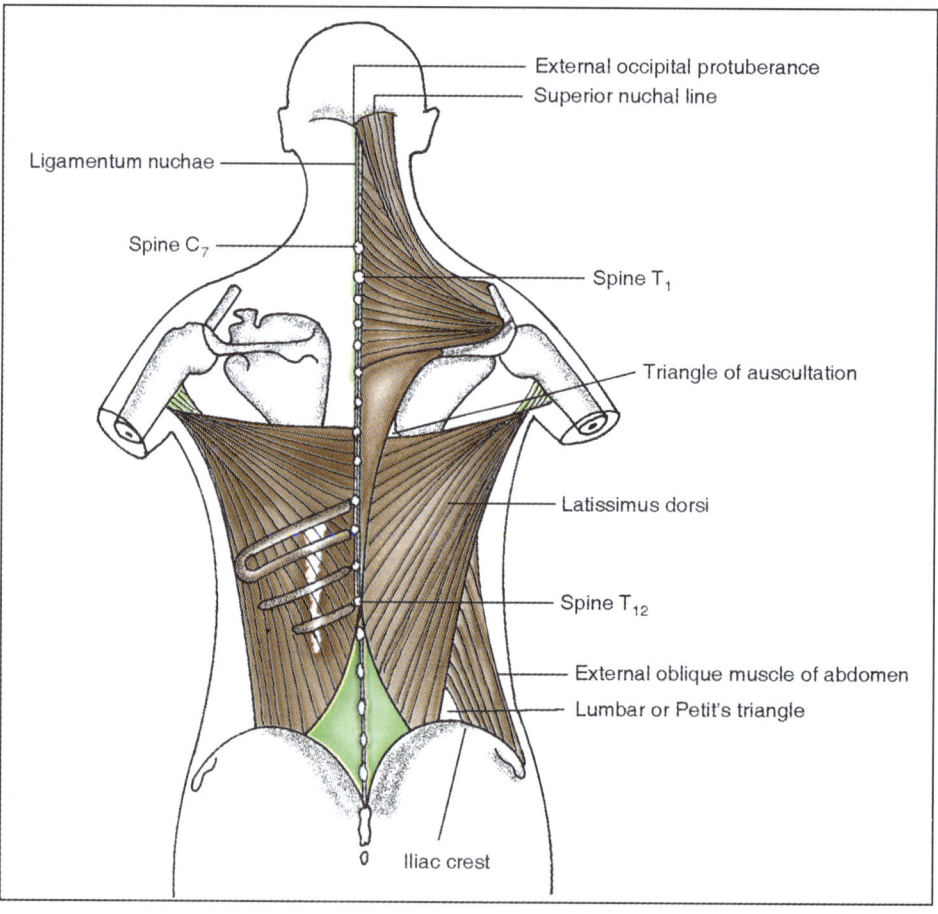

Fig. 8.2 Trapezius and latissimus dorsi

Latissimus dorsi

Origin   7th to 12th thoracic spines with supraspinous ligaments, lumbar fascia, iliac crest, lower 4 ribs, inferior angle of scapula.

Insertion   Intertubercular sulcus of humerus. At the lower border of teres major, the muscle makes a 180° turn so that the fibres of lowest origin become heighest at insersion and vice versa.

Nerve   Thoracodorsal nerve ($C_{6, 7, 8}$).

Actions   Adduction, extension and medial rotation of arm.

Triangle of auscultation

It is bounded by the trapezius, latissimus dorsi and medial border of scapula. Rhomboid major muscle lies in the floor. Deep to this triangle on the left side lies cardiac end of stomach. The patency of this opening can be confirmed by auscultation. The sound produced by the swallowing of fluid entering the stomach can be auscultated, a procedure practiced before the invention of X-ray.

Lumbar triangle of Petit

It is bounded by the iliac crest (base of the triangle), external oblique muscle of abdomen (anteriorly), and latissimus dorsi (posteriorly). It may be a site of hernia called lumbar hernia (hernia is abnormal protrusion of viscera through a weak point).

Three muscles (levator scapulae, rhomboid minor and rhomboid major) lie in the same plane deep to trapezius and latissimus dorsi and connect the scapular medial border with the vertebral column.

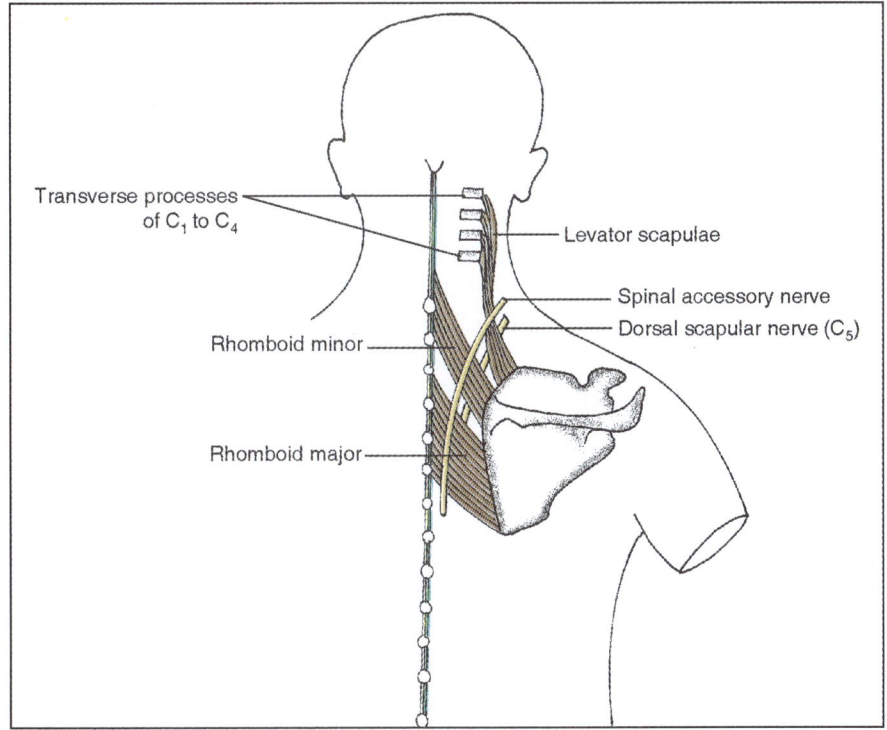

Fig. 8.3 Levator scapulae and rhomboids

Levator scapulae

Origin	Posterior tubercles of the transverse processes of upper 4 cervical vertebrae.
Insertion	Medial border of scapula above the root of spine of scapula.
Nerve	Cervical plexus ($C_{3, 4}$) and dorsal scapular nerve (C_5).
Actions	With upper fibres of trapezius it elevates the scapula. With rhomboids it causes medial rotation of scapula.

Rhomboid minor

Origin.	7th Cervical and 1st thoracic spines with supraspinous ligament and adjacent ligamentum nuchae.
Insertion.	Medial border of scapula opposite the root of spine.
Nerve.	Dorsal scapular nerve (C_5).
Action.	Retraction and medial rotation of scapula.

Rhomboid major

Origin.	2nd to 5th Thoracic spines with supraspinous ligaments.
Insertion.	Medial border of scapula below the root of spine.
Nerve.	Dorsal scapular nerve (C_5).
Action.	Retraction and medial rotation of scapula.

MUSCLE ATTACHING SCAPULA TO RIBS

Serratus anterior

Origin	8 Digitations from upper eight ribs.
Insertion	Costal surface of the medial border of scapula.
	Levels of insertion to the scapula are as follows,
	Upper two digitations – The superior angle.
	3rd and 4th digitations – The medial border. } of scapula.
	Lower four digitations – The inferior angle
Nerve	Long thoracic nerve ($C_{5, 6, 7}$).
Actions	Protraction.
	Lower four digitations act with upper and lower fibres of trapezius and cause lateral rotation of scapula.
Applied	Paralysis of muscle makes the medial border of scapula prominent (winging of scapula).The medial border of scapula can be made visibly more prominent in such cases by asking the patient to push against the wall.

MUSCLES ATTACHING THE SCAPULA TO HUMERUS

Six muscles are considered here, i.e., deltoid, subscapularis, teres major, supraspinatus,, inraspinatus and teres minor.

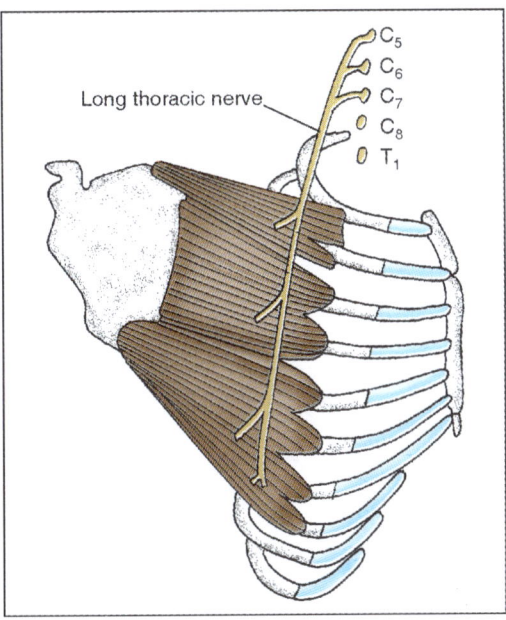

Fig. 8.4 Serratus anterior

DISSECTION STEPS: SHOULDER REGION

Remove fascia from the surface of deltoid and define its attachments and note its fibres. Separate the deltoid from the spine of the scapula and turn it down. Remove fascia over the infraspinatus. Clean and define the inferior border of ifraspinatus muscle and identify the teres major and minor muscles. Define the boundaries of the quadrangular space and note its contents. Expose and define the long head of triceps. Divide the remaining fibres of the deltoid, turn it downwards and define subscapularis. Clean and define the boundaries of the upper triangular space. Clean and define the boundaries of the lower triangular space.

Deltoid

Origin	*Anterior fibres* (parallel) – Anterior margin of lateral 1/3 of the clavicle.
	Posterior fibres (parallel) – Inferior margin of crest of spine of scapula.
	Middle fibres (multipennate) – Lateral margin of acromion process and intermuscular septa.
Insertion	Deltoid tuberosity of humerus.
Actions	Brings about following movements at the shoulder joint.
	Anterior fibres – Fexion.
	Posterior fibres – Extension.
	Acromial fibres – Abduction.
Applied	Paralysis of deltoid results into loss of abduction at shoulder.

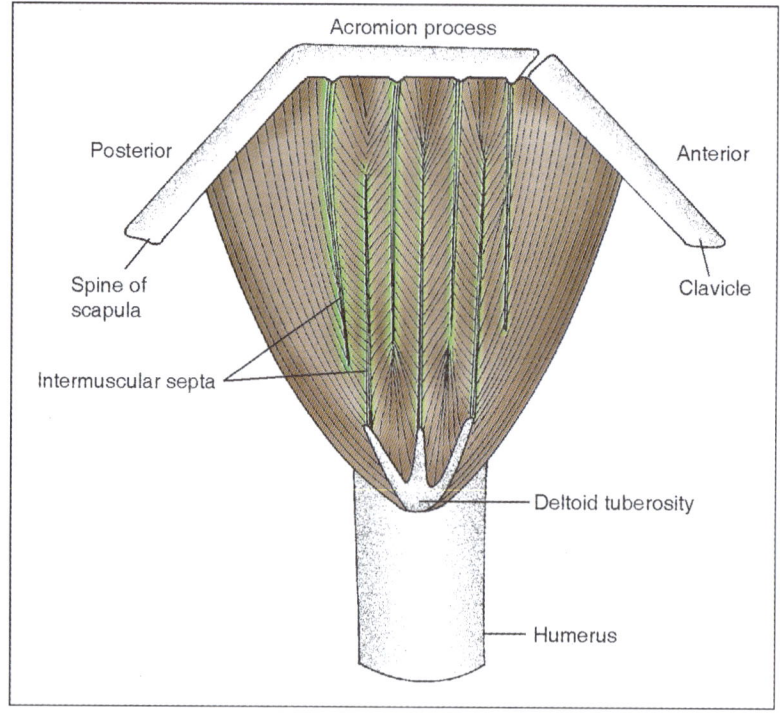

Fig. 8.5 Attachments of deltoid (lateral view)

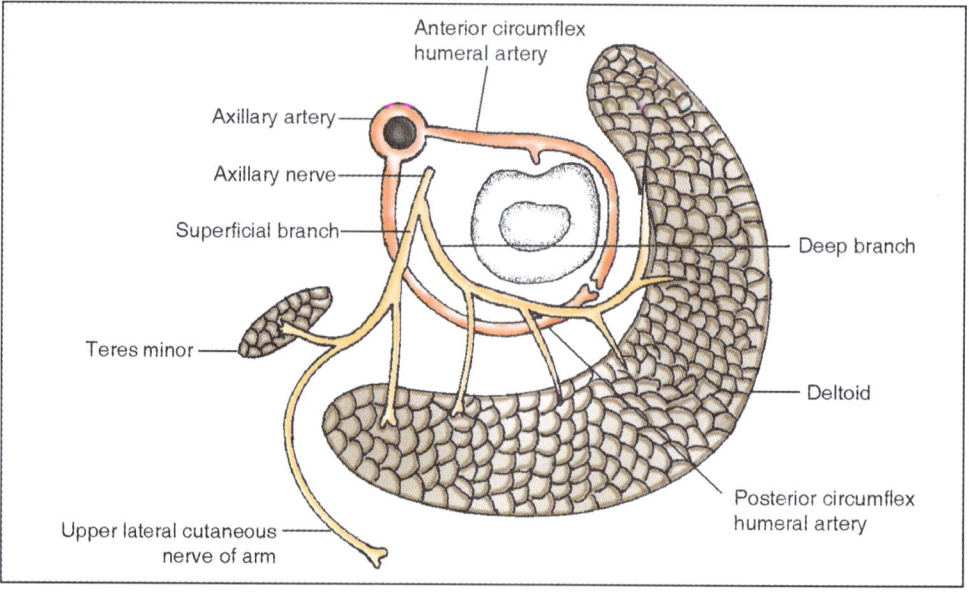

Fig. 8.6 Deep relations of deltoid

Subscapularis

Origin	Costal surface of scapula (medial 2/3) and intermuscular septa.
Insertion	Lesser tuberosity of humerus.
Nerve	Upper and lower subscapular nerves ($C_{5, 6}$).
Actions	It stabilizes shoulder and helps in the medial rotation of arm.
Subscapular bursa	It is located deep to the lateral part of the muscle and invariably communicates with the cavity of shoulder joint.

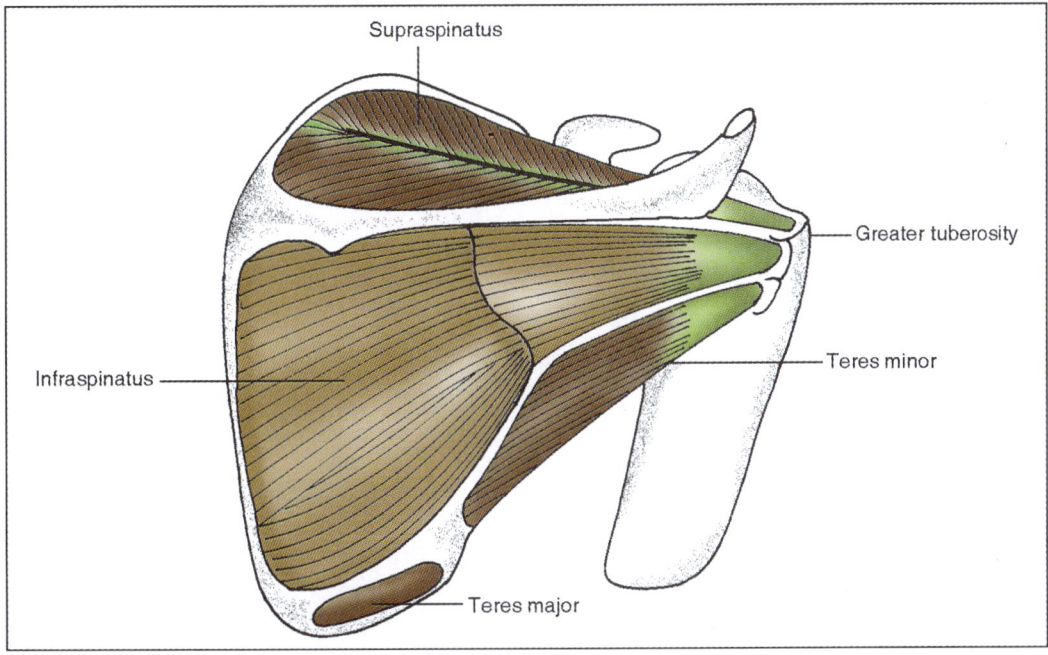

Fig. 8.7 Scapular muscles getting attached to the greater tuberosity of humerus

Teres major

Origin.	Lateral margin of scapula (dorsal aspect of lower 1/3)
Insertion.	Medial lip of intertubercular sulcus.
Nerve.	Lower subscapular nerve ($C_{5, 6}$).

Actions

1. To steady the shoulder during movements of the limb.
2. Medial rotation of arm.
3. Adduction.
4. With teres minor, holds down the head of humerus to neutralize its upward pull by deltoid during abduction.

Supraspinatus

Origin. Medial 2/3 of supraspinous fossa of scapula.

Insertion. Upper facet of the greater tuberosity of humerus.

Nerve. Suprascapular nerve (C_5, $_6$).

Actions 1. To stabilize the shoulder joint.

2. To initiate the abduction.

Bursae 1. Deep to its lateral part.

2. Above the muscle (subdeltoid or subacromial bursa).

Applied anatomy. Rupture of the supraspinatus tendon is common.

Infraspinatus

Origin. Medial 2/3 of infraspinous fossa of scapula.

Insertion. Middle facet of greater tuerosity of humerus.

Nerve. Suprascapular nerve ($C_{5,\ 6}$).

Actions 1. To stabilize shoulder joint.

2. Lateral rotation of arm.

Bursa. It is located deep to its lateral part.

Teres minor

Orign. Upper 2/3 of lateral border of scapula.

Insertion. Lower facet on the greater tuberosity of humerus.

Nerve. Axillary nerve ($C_{5,\ 6}$).

Actions 1. To stabilize shoulder.

2. Adduction and lateral rotation of arm.

3. To hold down the head of humerus to neutralize its upward pull by deltoid during abduction.

ROTATOR CUFF

Tendons of four muscles namely, subscapularis, supraspinatus, infraspinatus and teres minor fuse with the lateral part of capsule of the shoulder joint to form rotator cuff. The cuff plays most important role in the stability of the shoulder joint. The rotator cuff is deficient inferiorly making the shoulder joint more prone to inferior dislocation.

MOVEMNETS OF SCAPULA

Three sets of movements occur in scapula i.e., elevation/depression, protraction/retraction and medial/lateral rotations.

Elevation. It is produced by trapezius (upper fibres) and levator scapulae.

Depression. It is caused by pectoralis minor, pectoralis major (lower fibres) and gravity.

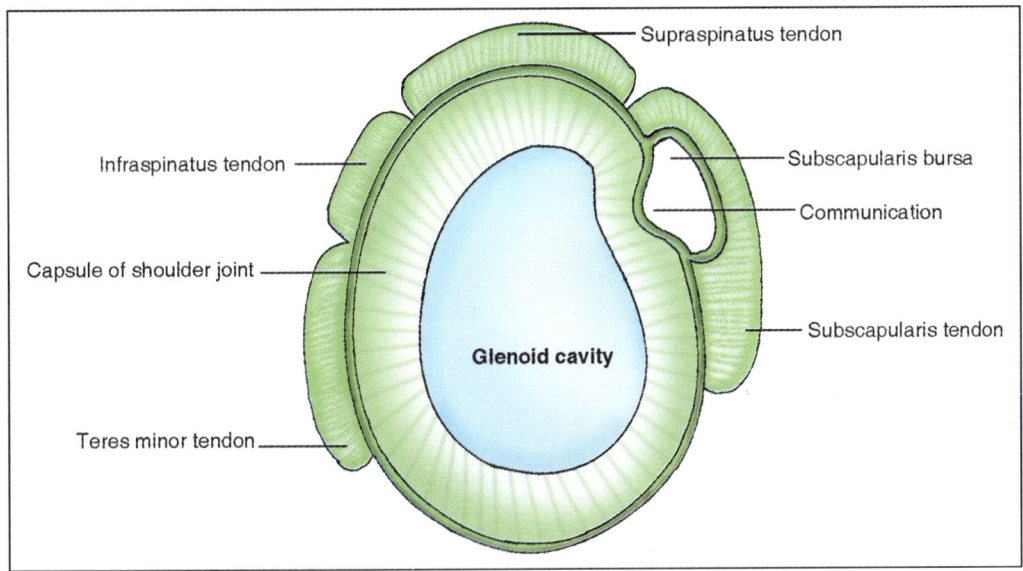

Fig. 8.8 Rotator cuff

Protraction and retraction. These are forward and backward movements of scapula respectively around a vertical axis passing through conoid ligament. Main protractor is serratus anterior. Rhomboids along with middle fibres of trapezius bring about retraction.

Rotation. Scapula rotates around a horizontal axis passing through the center of spine and sternoclavicular joint. During medial rotation the inferior angle of scapula moves medially and it is brought about by the levator scapulae, rhomboids and gravity. During lateral rotation, the inferior angle of scapula moves laterally and the glenoid cavity faces further upwards. It is brought about by the upper and lower fibres of trapezius and lower four digitations of serratus anterior. Lateral rotation is required for abduction of arm above head.

SCAPULAR ANASTOMOSES

Three arteries participate in the formation of anastomoses around scapula.

1. *Suprascapular artery*. It is a branch of thyrocervical trunk which itself arises from Ist part of subclavian artery. This artery crosses the suprascapular notch above the suprascapular ligament (suprascapular nerve passes below the ligament) and then the spinoglenoid notch to supply the dorsum of scapula.

2. *Dorsal scapular artery*. It is a direct branch of 3rd part of subclavian artery. It descends along the medial border of scapula with dorsal scapular nerve deep to levator scapulae and rhomboids and supplies both costal and dorsal aspects of scapula.

3. *Subscapular artery*. It arises from the 3rd part of axillary artery and descends along the lateral border of scapula. It terminates into circumflex scapular artery (which passes through upper triangular space) and thoracodorsal artery. Nerve to teres major passes through the angle between these terminal branches.

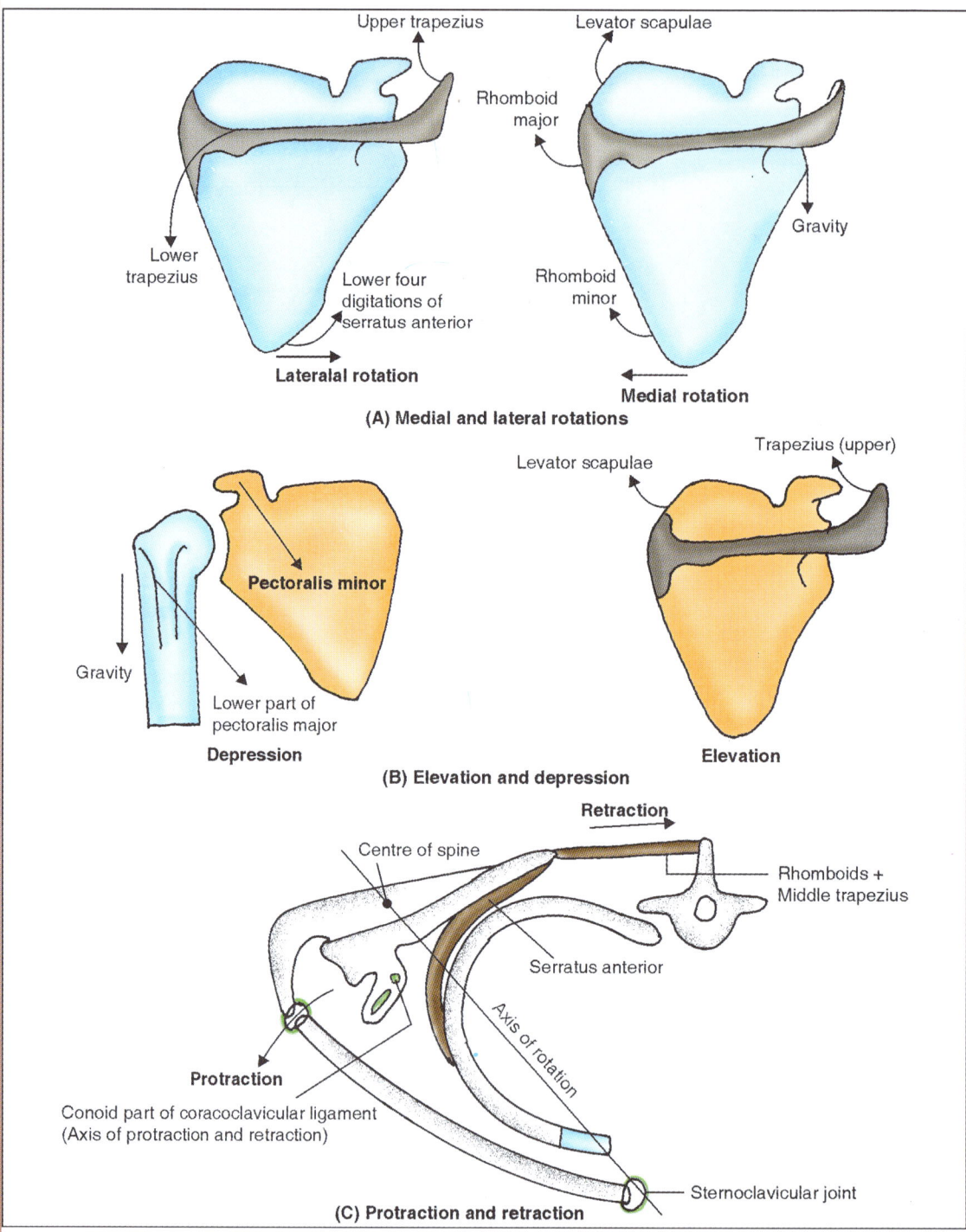

Fig. 8.9 Movements of scapula (A) Medial and lateral rotations (B) Elevation and depression. (C) Protraction and retraction

Applied anatomy

- Collaterals develop to overcome the arterial supply of limb in case of obstruction to main arteries (between distal subclavian and proximal axillary arteries).

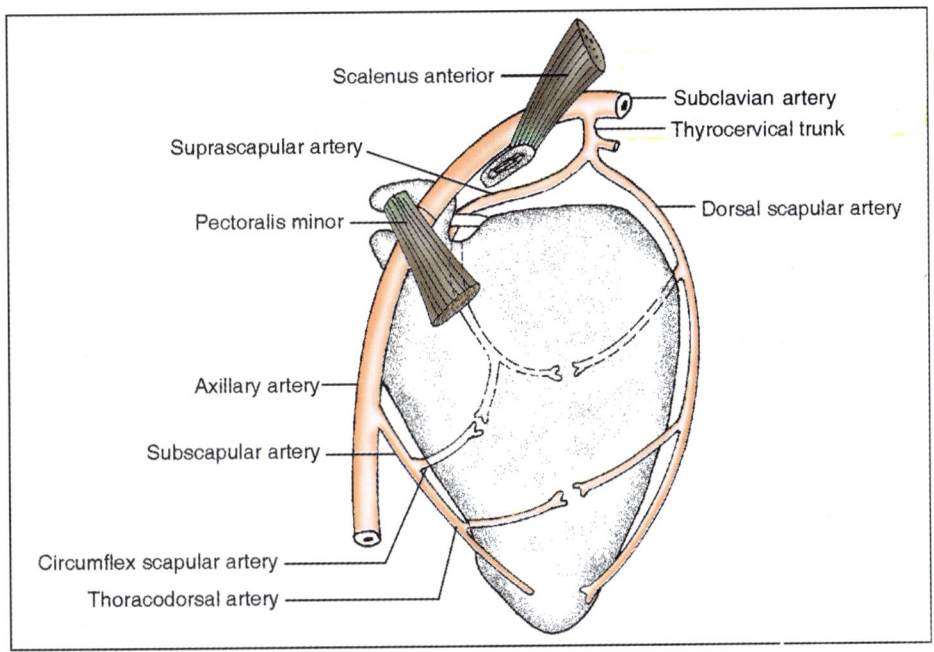

Fig. 8.10 Scapular anastomoses

SUPRASCAPULAR NERVE

It arises by two roots (C_5, $_6$) and crosses two notches (suprascapular and spinoglenoid) and supplies two muscles (supraspinatus and infraspinatus). It always crosses the suprascapular notch below the suprascapular ligament (artery passes above the ligament) to enter the dorsum of scapula.

AXILLARY NERVE

Root value C_5, $_6$

Course and relations. It arises from the posterior cord of the brachial plexus in the axilla and passes through the quadrangular space in close relation to the surgical neck of humerus. In the quadrangular space it lies immediately below the capsule of shoulder joint.

Branches
1. An articular branch from the trunk of the nerve supplies the shoulder joint.
2. Two terminal branches (anterior and posterior).
   (a) Anterior (deep) branch passes deep to deltoid and supplies it.
   (b) Posterior (superficial) branch passes superficial to deltoid and supplies teres minor and deltoid. Posterior branch continues as upper lateral cutaneous nerve of arm.

Applied anatomy

- Axillary nerve may be damaged during downward dislocation of humeral head or fracture at the surgical neck of humerus. Due to paralysis of deltoid there is loss of abduction at the shouder joint.

INTERMUSCULAR SPACES

Quadrangular space

Boundaries

Medial. Long head of triceps.

Lateral. Surgical neck of humerus.

Inferior. Teres major.

Superior. Subscapularis, teres minor, capsule of shoulder joint.

Contents

Axillary nerve.

Posterior circumflex humeral vessels.

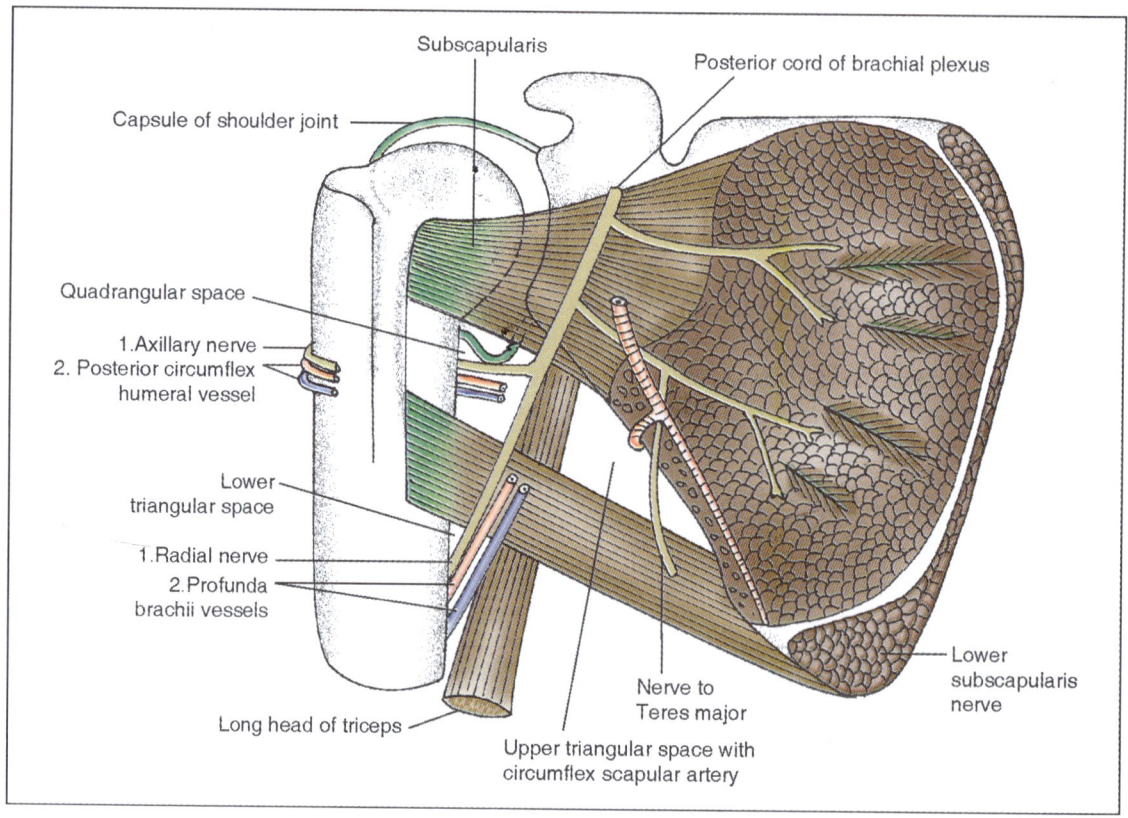

Fig. 8.11 Intermuscular spaces

Upper triangular space

Boundaries

Lateral – Long head of triceps.

Medial – Lateral border of scapula.

Inferior – Teres major.

Contents

Circumflex scapular artery.

Lower triangular space

Boundaries

Medial – Long head of triceps.

Superior – Teres major.

Lateral – Humerus.

Contents

1. Radial nerve
2. Profunda brachii vessels

9

Cutaneous Veins, Lymphatics and Nerves of Upper Limb

SUPERFICIAL VEINS

Dorsal venous net. It is a venous plexus over the dorsum of hand. It receives dorsal digital veins from dorsal aspects of digits. Intercapitular veins lie between distal ends of medial 4 metacarpals and connect palmar digital veins with the dorsal digital veins.

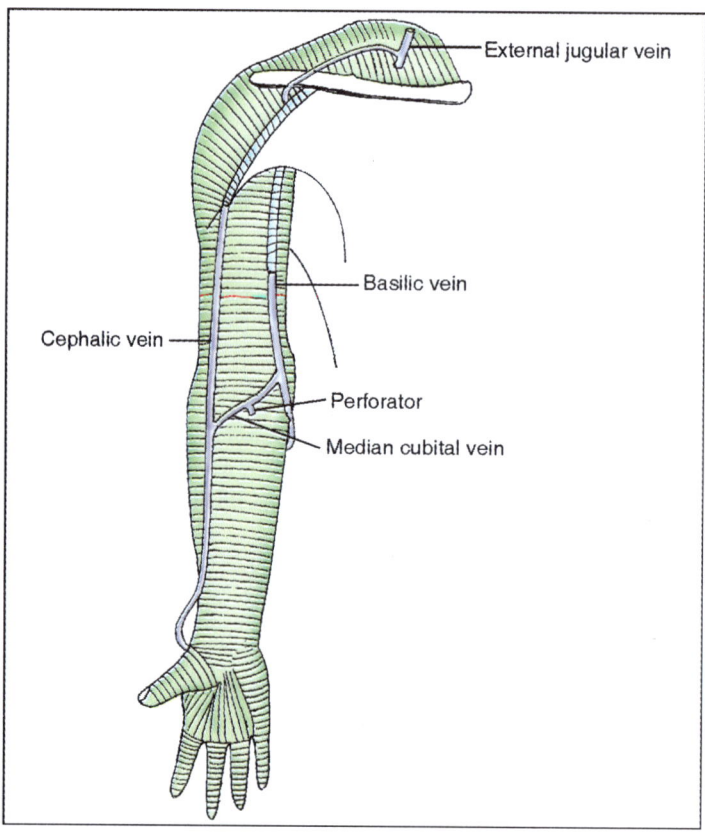

Fig. 9.1 Superficial veins of the upper limb

Blood is carried proximally from dorsal net by two prominent veins namely cephalic vein from its lateral aspect and basilic vein from its medial aspect.

Cephalic vein

It runs across the anatomical snuff box to ascend along the anterolateral aspect of upper limb. It pierces the deep fascia at the lower end of deltopectoral groove. It then ascends in this groove to reach infraclavicular fossa where it pierces the clavipectoral fascia to join the axillary vein.

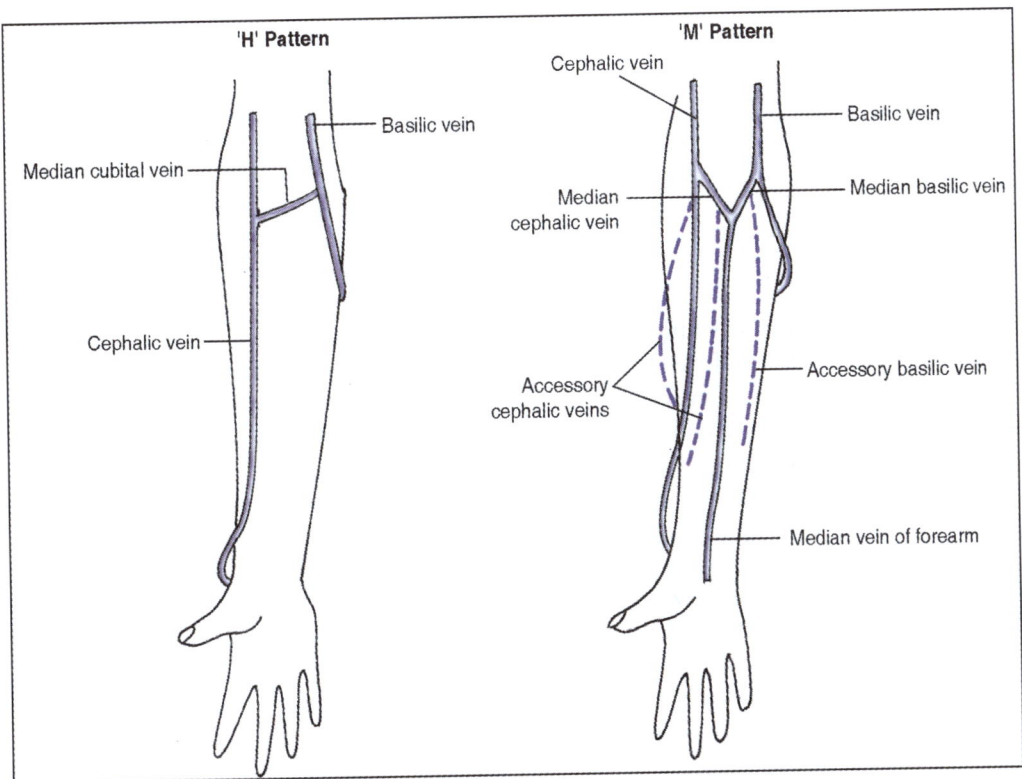

Fig. 9.2 Two common patterns of connecting veins

Basilic vein

It runs in the posteromedial aspect of forearm. Close to elbow, it winds round the medial aspect of forearm and then ascends along anteromedial aspect of arm. It pierces deep fascia in the middle of arm. It continues as the axillary vein beyond the lower border of the teres major.

Connecting veins

1. *Between superficial veins*
   (a) **'H'** pattern – Connecting vein between cephalic and basilic veins at the elbow is called the median cubital vein.

(b) **'M'** pattern – Median vein of forearm ascends on the front of forearm to reach the elbow where it splits into median cephalic and median basilic veins to join cephalic and basilic veins respectively.

2. *Between superficial and deep veins.* These are called perforators.

3. *Between cephalic vein and external jugular vein.* This vein if present crosses the clavicle and may be trapped between fractured ends of clavicle leading to profuse bleeding.

Accessory veins

Veins parallel to cephalic vein (accessory cephalic vein) or basilic vein (accessory basilic vein) can be noticed.

Applied anatomy

- Superficial veins are of great clinical significance for their use in intravenous injections and catheterization.

LYMPHATIC DRAINAGE

Superficial lymphatics

Lymphatics form a rich palmar lymphatic plexus and ascend mainly to lateral axillary group of lymph nodes except few which pass to dorsum of hand. Lymphatics from back of hand, forearm and arm wind round the corresponding sides to reach the front. Of these, majority drain into lateral axillary lymph nodes. Few of them accompany either cephalic or basilic veins. Former drain into deltopectoral and infraclavicular lymph nodes while latter drain into cubital lymph nodes. Efferents of infraclavicular lymph nodes end into apical while those of cubital into lateral axillary lymph nodes. Superficial lymphatics from pectoral region drain into anterior group and those from scapular region drain into posterior group of axillary lymph nodes.

Deep lymphatics

Deep lymphatics from hand, forearm and arm drain into lateral group of axillary lymph nodes.

Applied anatomy

- Lymphatics form the commonest route for the spread of infection and malignancy.
- Inflammation of lymphatics is called lymphangitis.
- Inflammation of lymph nodes is called lymphadenitis.

CUTANEOUS NERVES

Root of limb

1. Lateral supracalvicular nerve ($C_{3, 4}$).
2. Upper lateral cutaneous nerve of arm ($C_{5, 6}$).
3. Intercostobrachial nerve (T_2).

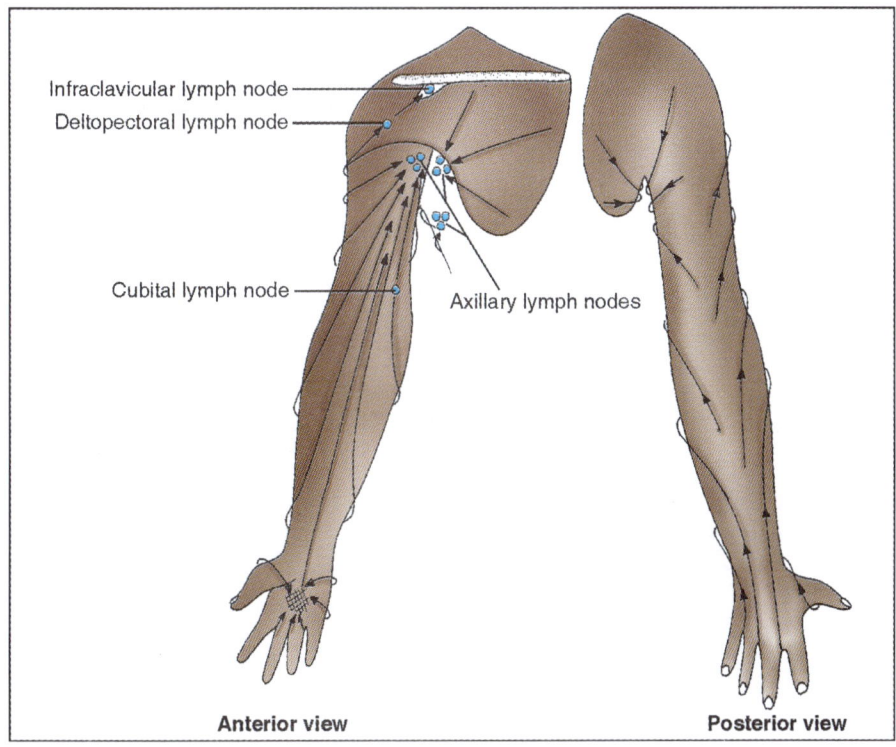

Infraclavicular lymph node

Deltopectoral lymph node

Cubital lymph node

Axillary lymph nodes

Anterior view

Posterior view

Fig. 9.3 Superficial lymphatics of upper limb

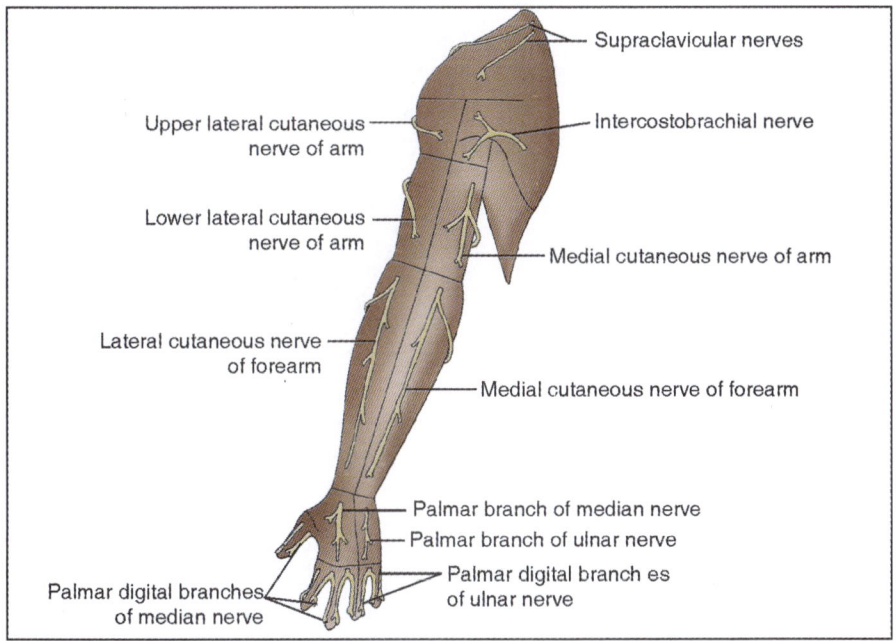

Supraclavicular nerves

Upper lateral cutaneous nerve of arm

Intercostobrachial nerve

Lower lateral cutaneous nerve of arm

Medial cutaneous nerve of arm

Lateral cutaneous nerve of forearm

Medial cutaneous nerve of forearm

Palmar branch of median nerve

Palmar branch of ulnar nerve

Palmar digital branch es of ulnar nerve

Palmar digital branches of median nerve

Fig. 9.4 Cutaneous nerves of the upper limb (anterior view)

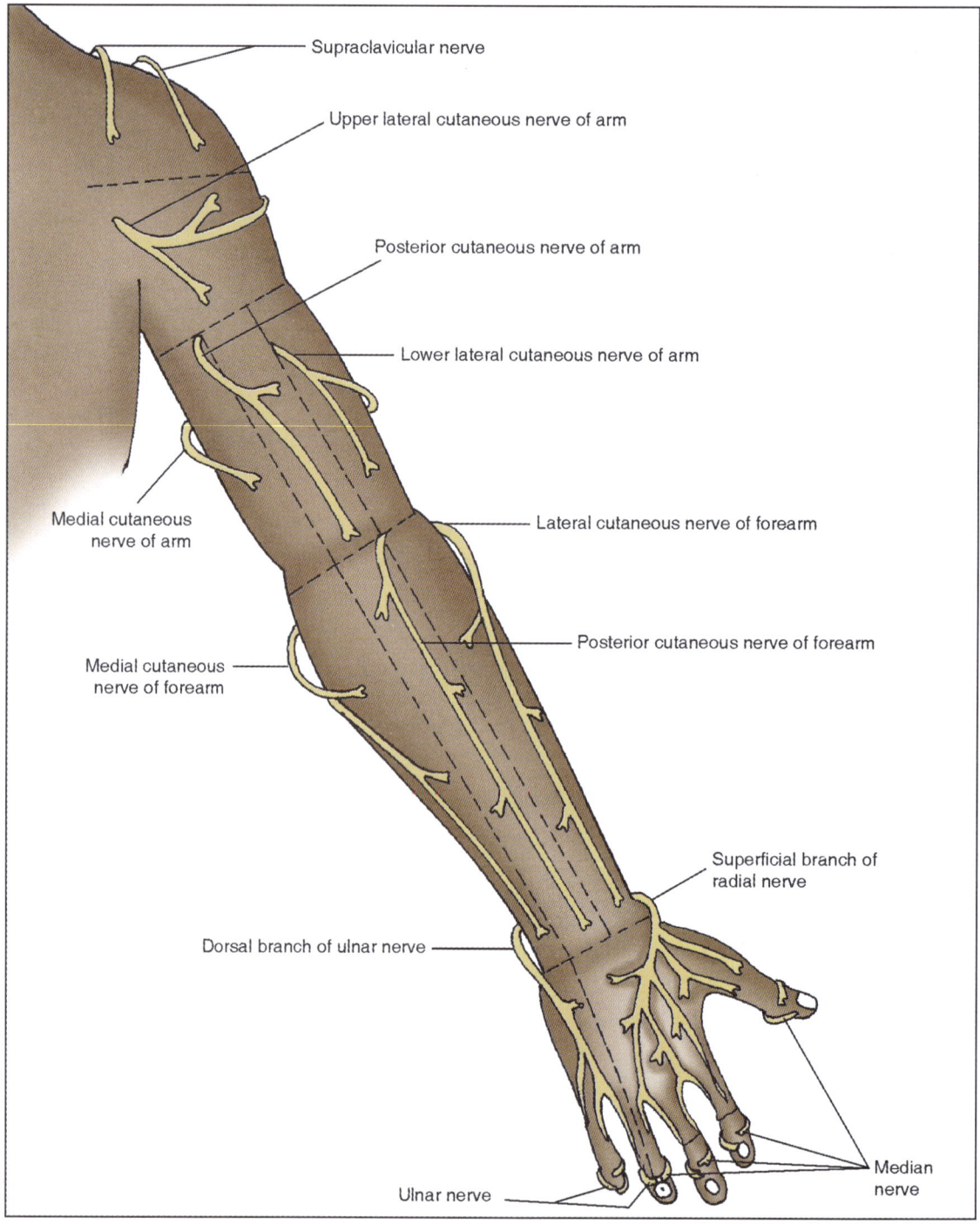

Supraclavicular nerve

Upper lateral cutaneous nerve of arm

Posterior cutaneous nerve of arm

Lower lateral cutaneous nerve of arm

Medial cutaneous
nerve of arm

Lateral cutaneous nerve of forearm

Posterior cutaneous nerve of forearm

Medial cutaneous
nerve of forearm

Superficial branch of
radial nerve

Dorsal branch of ulnar nerve

Median
nerve

Ulnar nerve

Fig. 9.5 Cutaneous nerves of the upper limb (posterior view)

Rest of the limb

Region	Location	Nerves	Root values
Arm	Lateral	Lower lateral cutaneous nerve of arm	$C_{5,\,6}$
	Medial	Medial cutaneous nerve of arm	$T_{1,\,2}$
	Posterior	Posterior cutaneous nerve of arm	C_5
Forearm	Lateral	Lateral cutaneous nerve of forearm	$C_{5,\,6}$
	Medial	Medial cutaneous nerve of forearm	C_8, T_1
	Posterior	Posterior cutaneous nerve of forearm	$C_{6,\,7,\,8}$
Hand			
Palm	Medial $\frac{1}{3}$	Palmar branch of ulnar nerve	$C_{7,\,8}$
	Lateral $\frac{2}{3}$	Palmar branch of median nerve	$C_{6,\,7,\,8}$
Dorsum	Medial $\frac{1}{3}$	Dorsal branch of ulnar nerve	$C_{7,\,8}$
	Lateral $\frac{2}{3}$	Superficial branch of radial nerve	$C_{6,\,7,\,8}$
Digits	Medial $1\frac{1}{2}$	Palmar and dorsal digital branches of ulnar nerve,	$C_{7,\,8}$
	Lateral $3\frac{1}{2}$	Palmar aspect—palmar digital branches of median nerve	$C_{6,\,7,\,8}$
		Dorsal aspect—dorsal digital branches of superficial	
		branch of radial nerve	$C_{6,\,7,\,8}$

DERMATOMES

Area of the skin supplied by single spinal nerve is called a dermatome. Dermatomes are distributed in an orderly numerical sequence because of outgrowth of limb from the side of the trunk and migration of dermatomes on it.

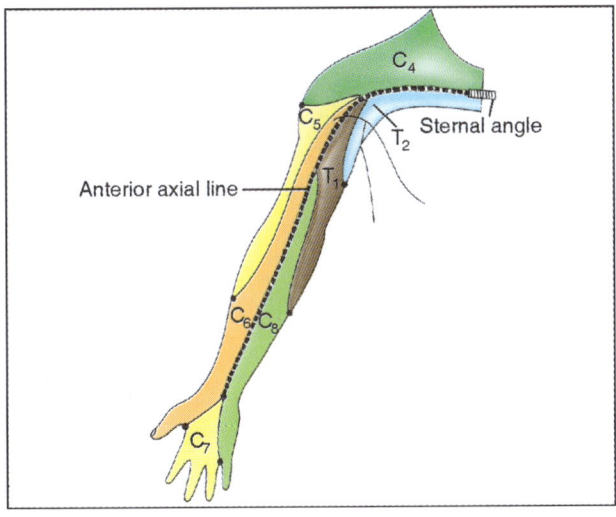

Fig. 9.6 Dermatomes of the upper limb (anterior view)

Axial lines are junctions between dermatomes supplied by discontinuous spinal segments. Anterior axial line extends from the sternal angle of Louis to the wrist. Posterior axial line starts at the vertebra prominence (7th cervical vertebra) on the back and ends at the middle of the arm. There is no overlapping between areas supplied by discontinuous segments, (testing anaesthesia across the axial lines is more fruitful) while those supplied by continuous segments do overlap and therefore missing the area of anaesthesia in case of single spinal segment lesion.

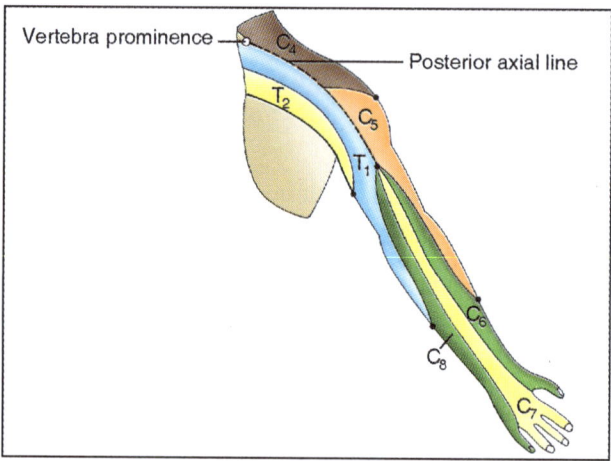

Fig. 9.7 Dermatomes of the upper limb (posterior view)

10

Joints of Clavicle

STERNOCLAVICULAR JOINT

Type. Modified saddle type of synovial joint.

Articular surfaces

(a) Medial end of the clavicle is concavo-convex and is called sternal articular facet (here articular cartilage is fibrocartilage).

(b) Manubrium and Ist costal cartilage provide articular facet for clavicle. Here articular cartilage is hyaline.

Ligaments

Capsule	–	Attached to margins of articular surfaces.
Sternoclavicular ligament	–	Anterior and posterior.
Interclavicular ligament	–	It connects medial ends of two clavicles and occupies the suprasternal notch.
Costoclavicular (rhomboid) ligament	–	It connects 1st rib's anterior end with the rhomboid fossa of clavicle. It is bilaminar.
Articular disc	–	It is fibrocartilage in nature. It divides the joint cavity into medial and lateral compartments.

Arteries

Internal thoracic artery.

Suprascapular artery.

Nerve. Medial supraclavicular nerve.

Movements. The medial end of clavicle moves as follows,

In the lateral compartment – upward and downward.

In the medial compartment – forward and backward and rotation of 40°.

Applied anatomy. Forward dislocation is common.

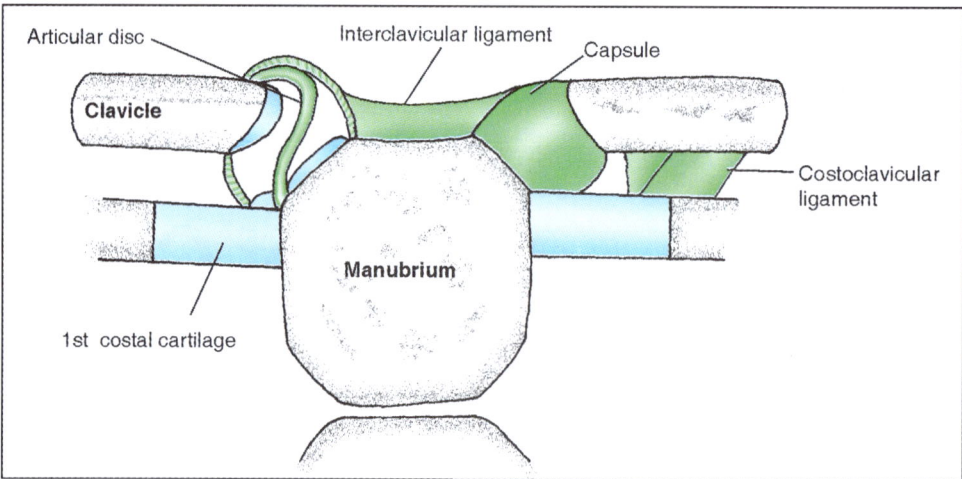

Fig. 10.1 Sternoclavicular joint

ACROMIOCLAVICULAR JOINT

It is a plane synovial joint between lateral end of clavicle and acromion process of scapula. Both the articular surfaces are covered with fibrocartilage. Like sternoclavicular joint, the interior of the joint presents an articular disc but unlike that of sternoclavicular joint, it is incomplete. Conoid and trapezoid parts of coracoclavicular ligament strengthen the joint. It receives arterial supply from supraclavicular and thoracoacromial arteries and is innervated by the lateral supraclavicular nerve.

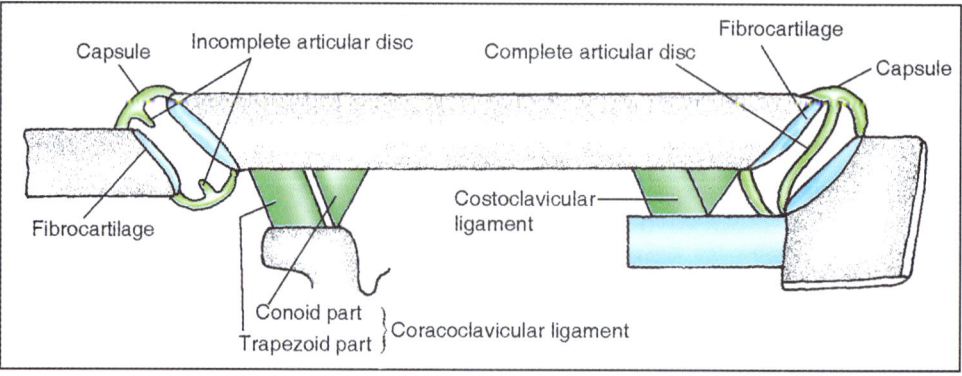

Fig. 10.2 Acromioclavicular joint versus sternoclavicular joint

Applied anatomy

- The acromioclavicular joint is made optimally accessible by asking the patient to adduct the arm and keep the hand on the opposite shoulder.
- Subluxation of the joint makes the lateral end of clavicle more prominent.
- In cases of osteoarthritis of this joint, patient feels pain when arm is abducted above right angle.

11

Shoulder Joint

DISSECTION STEPS: SHOULDER JOINT

Cut across the subscapularis at the neck of the scapula and reflect it down. Expose and clean the coracoclavicular ligament and identify the articular capsule of the shoulder joint. Give vertical incision through the posterior part of the capsule of the joint. Rotate the arm medially. Disarticulate the head of the humerus through the cut in the capsule and identify the intracapsular tendon of long head of biceps brachii and labrum glenoidale. Workout the relations of the shoulder joint.

Type. Ball and socket type of synovial joint.

Articular surfaces. Head of humerus (ball) articulates with the glenoid cavity of scapula (socket). Concavity of the latter is accentuated by the presence of labrum glenoidale along its margin. Articular cartilage over the head as well as glenoid cavity are hyaline in nature. Thickness of cartilage reduces from centre to periphery over the head but just opposite to it in the glenoid cavity.

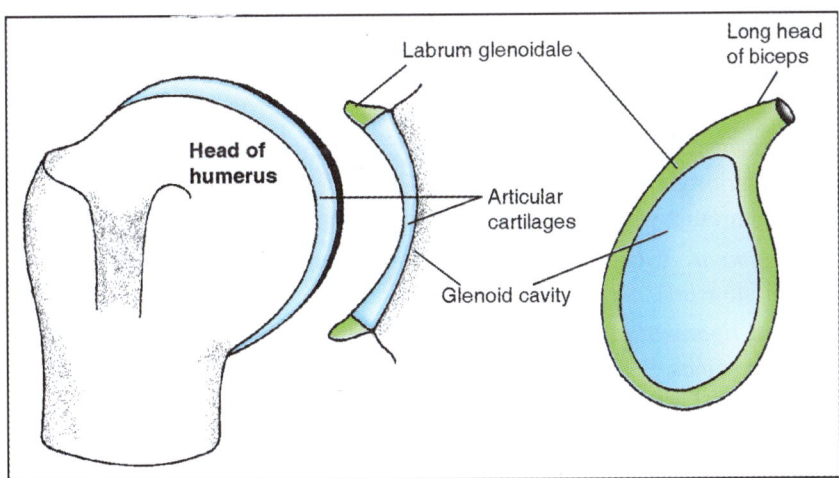

Fig. 11.1 Articular surfaces of shoulder joint

Capsule

It is attached to both scapular glenoid cavity and humeral head along the articular margins with some exceptions e.g., at the upper end of the glenoid cavity it encloses the supraglenoid tubercle (long head of biceps is intracapsular) and on the humerus it extends for about 1 cm on its medial aspect. At the upper end of the intertubercular sulcus it is deficient for the passage of long head of biceps.

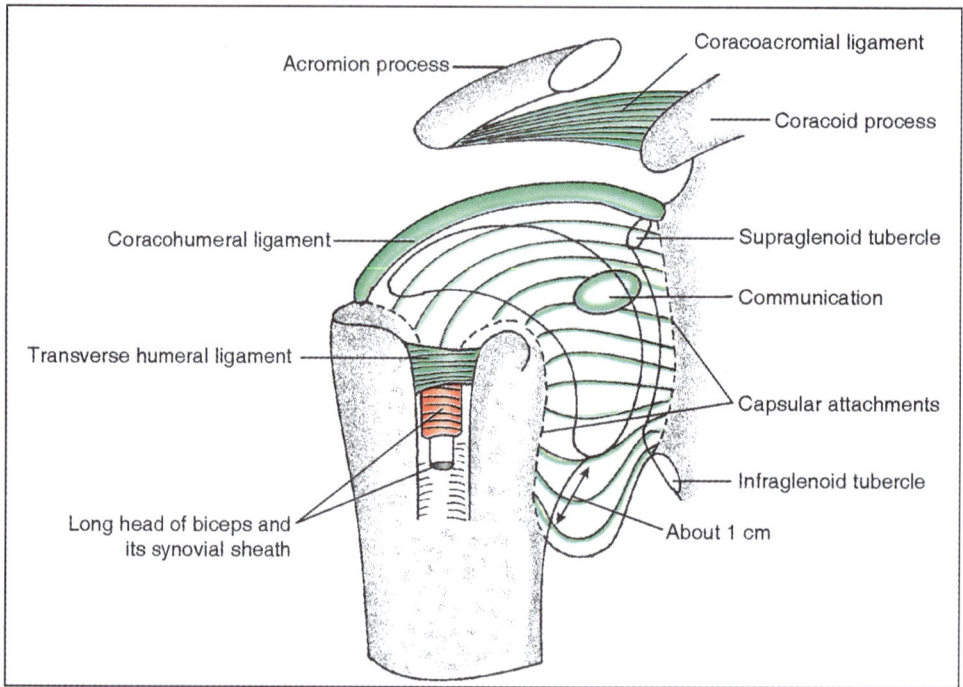

Fig. 11.2 Shoulder joint (capsular attachments and ligaments)

LIGAMENTS

Glenohumeral ligaments: There are three thickenings in the anterior wall of capsule namely superior, middle and inferior glenohumeral ligaments. Between the superior and middle components there is an opening through which subscapular bursa communicates with the cavity of shoulder joint.

Coracohumeral ligament: It connects the root of coracoid precess with the upper part of greater tuberosity of humeurs.

Transverse humeral ligament: It is transversely running fibrous band bridging the upper end of intertubercular sulcus. Passage deep to this ligament is meant for the emergence of long head of biceps.

Coracoacromial ligament: It is triangular ligament whose base is attached to lateral margin of coracoid process and apex to the tip of acromion process.

Labrum glenoidale: It is a fibrocartilaginous ring attached to the margin of glenoid cavity and further deepening it.

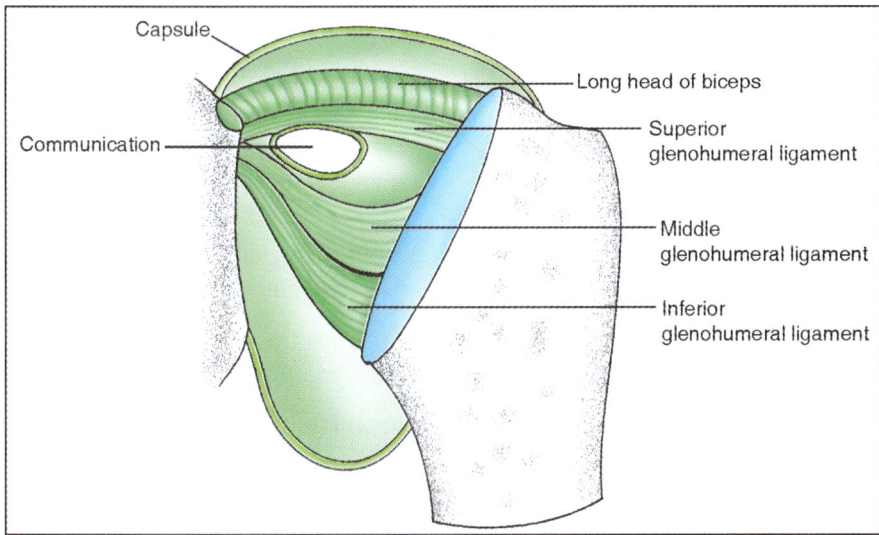

Fig. 11.3 Glenohumeral ligaments (anterior capsule visualized from posterior aspect)

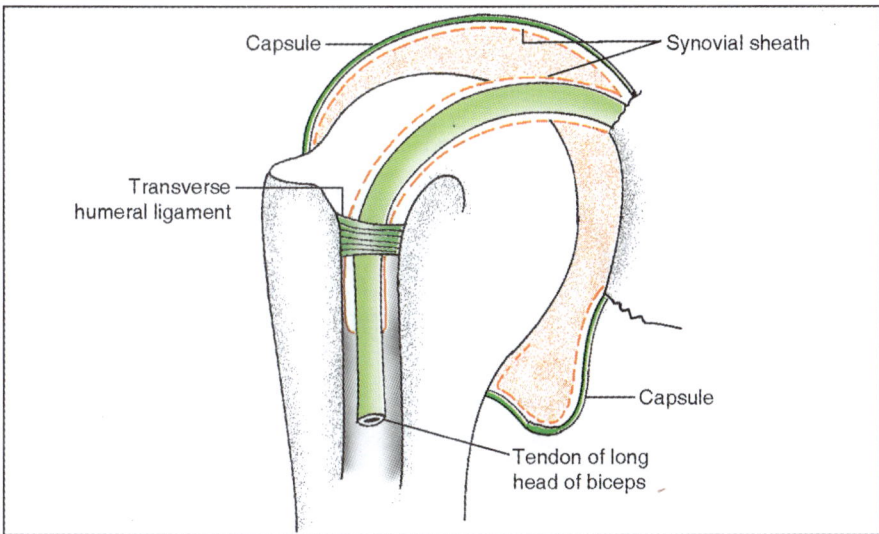

Fig. 11.4 Synovial membrane (sheath) of the shoulder joint

Synovial membrane

It lines the capsule and covers the intracapsular parts of non-articular bones. It herniates through openings and forms tubular sheath around the long head of biceps.

Bursae

1. Subscapularis bursa is located between the lateral part of subscapularis and capsule of shoulder joint. It communicates invariably with the joint.

2. Supraspinatus in its lateral part is sandwiched between subacromial bursa (superiorly) and suparspinatus bursa (inferiorly).
3. Bursa can also be observed in relation to coracoid process and several muscles adjacent to the joint e.g. infraspinatus, coracobrachialis, long head of triceps, latissimus dorsi, and teres major.

Relations

Long head of biceps is intracapsular from its attachment to supraglenoid tubercle to the upper end of bicipital groove. It appears outside the capsule under transverse humeral ligament and then runs in the bicipital groove.

External relations

Superior. Coracoacromial arch (coracoid process + acromion process + coracoacromial ligament), subacromial bursa, deltoid and supraspinatus.

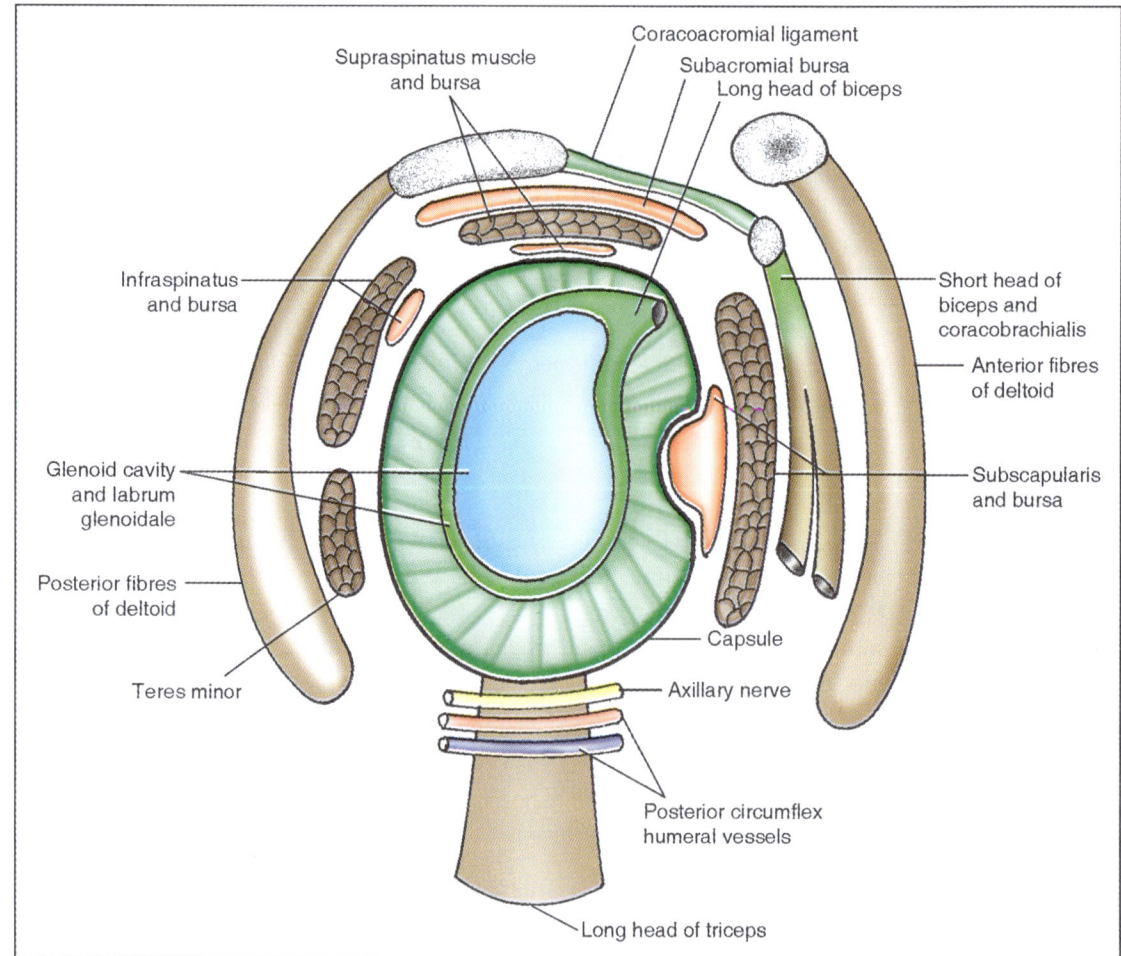

Fig. 11.5 Relations of the shoulder joint

Inferior. Long head of triceps, axillary nerve and posterior circumflex humeral vessels.

Anterior. Subscapularis, short head of biceps, coracobrachialis and deltoid.

Posterior. Infraspinatus, teres minor and deltoid.

Blood supply

Circumflex humeral (anterior and posterior), suprascapular and subscapular vessels.

Nerves

Axillary, suprascapular, musculocutaneous and lateral pectoral nerves.

Movements

According to conventional concept the abduction and adduction movements take place in coronal plane while flexion and extension occur in sagittal plane. But truly speaking abduction and adduction take place in scapular plane and flexion and extension occur in a plane perpendicular to scapular plane. In other words during abduction, arm moves forwards and laterally and during flexion the arm moves forwards and medially.

Total range of abduction is 180°, of which 2/3rd (120°) occurs at glenohumeral joint while the remaing (60°) is due to lateral rotation of scapula. It is interesting to note that for every 15° (1/3rd) abduction , 10° is glenohumeral and 5° is scapular.

According to recent studies, first 30° of abduction is glenohumeral, while remaining 120° is 50% (60°) glenohumeral and 50% (60°) scapular (involving sternoclavicular and acromioclavicular joints). Last 30° of abduction is due to contralateral flexion of vertebral column.

Total range of flexion is about 120°. **Extension** is the movement opposite to flexion. In terms of biomechanics, abduction and adduction are sliding movements while flexion and extension are spin movements occurring between humeral head and glenoid cavity.

Rotation (medial and lateral) of arm takes place along the vertical axis passing through humerus. Its range is 90°. Rotation is said to be medial when front of arm goes medially.

Stability

1. *Muscular factor*. It plays most important role in the stability of joint. Rotator cuff strengthens the joint anteriorly, superiorly and posteriorly. Long head of biceps supports the head from above, and long head of triceps supports the head from below in 90° abducted arm.
2. *Ligaments*. Coracoacromial ligament prevents upward displacement of head.
3. *Bony surfaces*. These play little role in its stability due to the shallowness of glenoid cavity and relatively large head of humerus.
4. *Atmospheric pressure*. It keeps the two articular surfaces against each other. In an attempt to separate them creates a negative pressure inside the joint.

Applied anatomy

- Shoulder triangle is formed by the union of three bony points, tip of coracoid, tip of acromion and prominence of greater tuberosity. The points are important in clinical diagnosis of lesion in the neighbourhood of shoulder joint.
- Examination of shoulder joint is usually done from behind due to easy garsp of elbow and scapula if necessary.
- When testing the rotation at shoulder, forearam should be 90° flexed to avoid pronation or supination of forearm.
- Valuable information can be gained by watching a patient abducting his arm slowly
  - If patient is able to take the arm above his head, there could not be any severe problem associated with shoulder. Patient is asked to bring the palms of two hands together above the head.
  - If the mid part of the range (60°-120°) is accompanied by pain and the remainder of the movement being painless (painful arm syndrome), supraspinatus tendinitis, subacromial bursitis or fracture of greater tuberosity are the causes.
  - If the abduction is limited to 40°-50°, a partial or complete tear of supraspinatus is likely.
  - If the arm can be raised only very slightly and patient supports the injured limb with his other hand, the fracture or dislocation is certain.
  - If the shoulder is painful throughout the movement, arthritis is probable.
- Supraspinatus tendon forms roof of shoulder joint and floor of subacromial bursa and therefore, when tendon ruptures an open communication results between the two cavities.
- Excessive fluid in the subacromial bursa presents as fluctuant swelling around the shoulder. In this case head of the humerus can be easily palpated, a finding which differentiates it from effusion in the shoulder joint.
- Dislocation of shoulder joint follows a fall on outstretched hand. The common dislocation is anterior.
- Dislocation of shoulder may be associated with injury to nerve (axillary) or compression of axillary vessels.

Arm

DISSECTION STEPS: FRONT OF ARM

Cut vertically through the deep fascia on the anterior surface of the arm upto elbow and cut transversely through it at this level. Reflect the flap and and uncover the biceps brachii. Lift the biceps brachii and identify the brachialis, musculocutaneous nerve between biceps and brachialis, brachial artery and the median nerve. Trace the musculocutaneous nerve. Remove the fascia from the brachialis and identify the musculocutaneous nerve (passing through coracobrachialis), brachioradialis, radial nerve and the extensor carpi radialis logus.

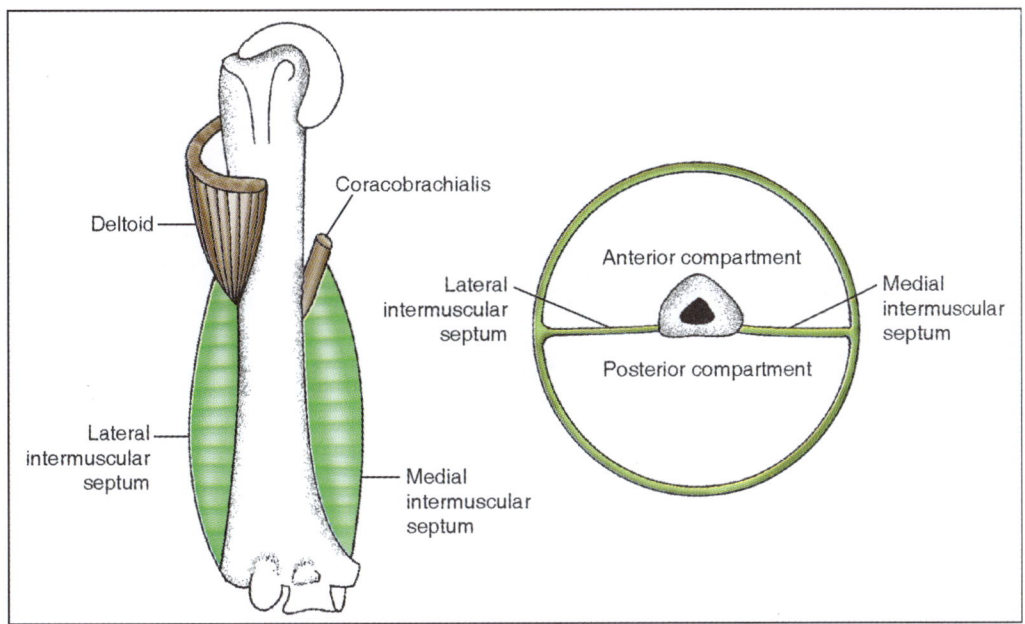

Fig. 12.1 Compartments of arm

COMPARTMENTS

The flexor and extensor compartments of arm lie on front and behind the humerus and intermuscular septa (medial and lateral) respectively.

Flexor compartment

Brachialis

Origin. Lower half of front of humerus and medial intermuscular septum.

Insertion. Front of coronoid process of ulna.

Nerve. Musculocutaneous nerve and radial nerve (proprioceptive).

Actions. Flexion at elbow.

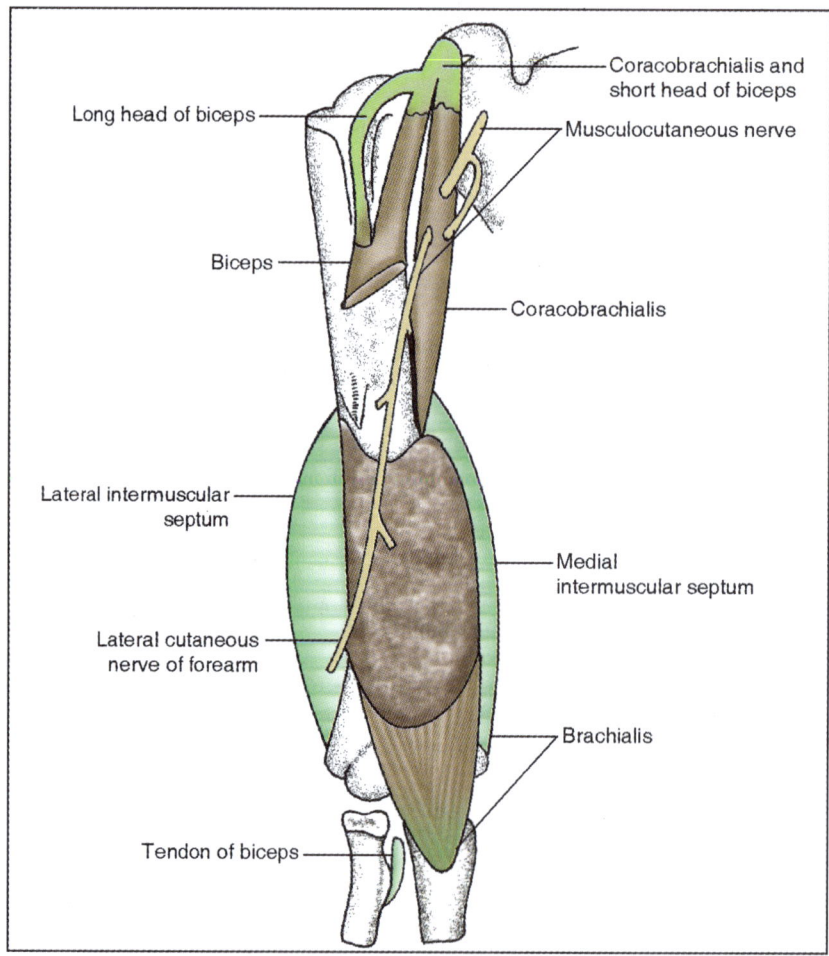

Fig. 12.2 Brachialis and coracobrachialis

Coracobrachialis

Origin. Tip of coracoid process (along with short head of biceps brachii).

Insertion. Middle of the medial margin of humerus.

Nerve. Musculocutaneous nerve.

Actions. Adduction and flexion at shoulder joint.

Biceps brachii

Origin

Short head. Tip of coracoid process.

Long heaed. Supraglenoid tubercle of scapula.

Insertion

Tendon. Directly to the posterior aspect of radial tuberosity.

Bicipital aponeurosis. Indirectly to the posterior border of ulna through deep fascia.

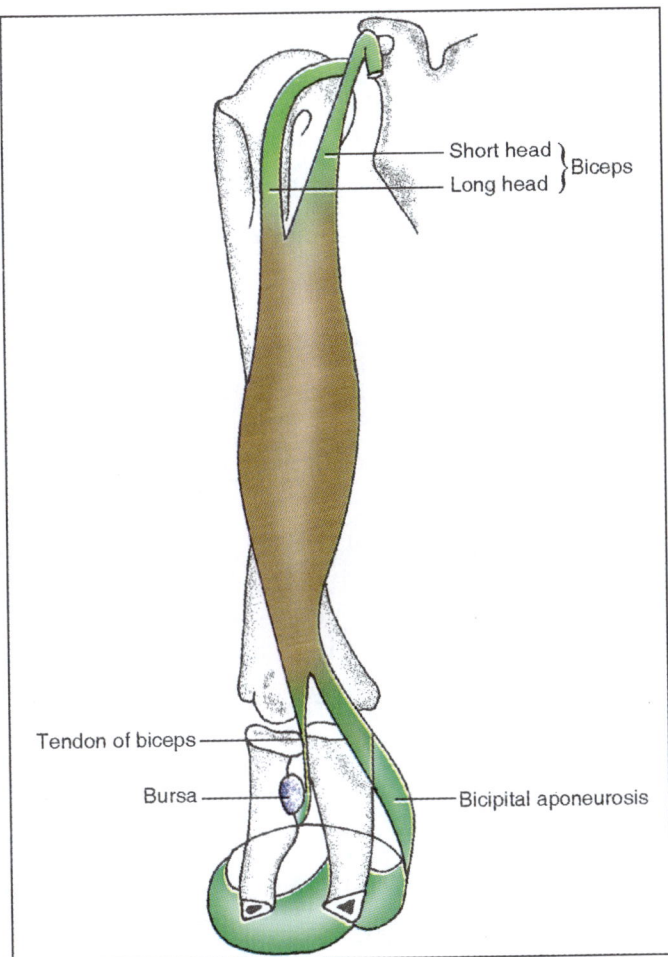

Fig. 12.3 Biceps brachii

Nerve. Musculocutaneous nerve.

Actions

1. Flexion at elbow and shoulder.
2. Supination of flexed forearm.

Brachial artery

Commencement. It is continuation of axillary artery at the lower border of teres major.

Termination. It divides into two terminal branches at the level of neck of radius.

Course and relations. Brachial artery is medial to humerus in the upper part of arm but comes to lie in front in its lower part. It passes deep to bicipital aponeurosis and is sandwiched between the median nerve (medial) and tendon of biceps brachii (lateral) at the elbow. (The relation is **NAT** from medial to lateral, i.e. median **N**erve, brachial **A**rtery and biceps **T**endon).

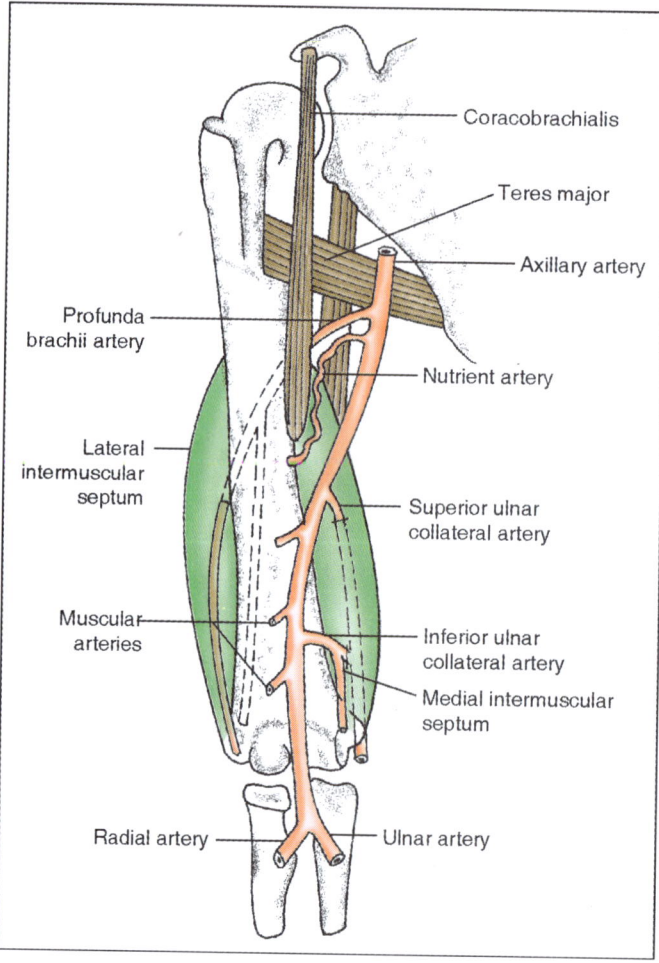

Fig. 12.4 Brachial artery

Branches

1. *Profunda brachii*. It accompanies the radial nerve to enter the posterior compartment of arm through lower triangular space.
2. *Nutrient artery:* It follows coracobrachialis to enter the nutrient foramen in the humerus just below its insertion.
3. *Superior ulnar collateral artery*. It pierces the medial intermuscular septum along with the ulnar nerve to reach the back of the medial epicondyle of humerus.
4. *Inferior ulnar collateral artery*. It originates about 5 cm above the elbow and descends in front of the medial epicondyle of humerus.
5. *Muscular branches*.
6. *Terminal branches*. Radial artery and ulnar artery.

Musculocutaneous and other nerves

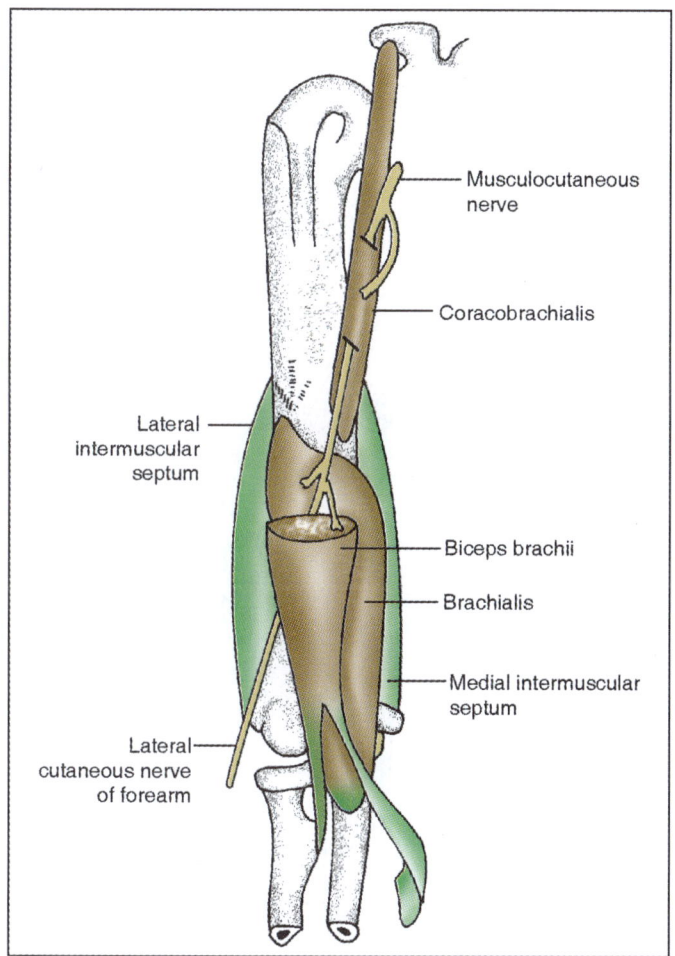

Fig. 12.5 Musculocutaneous nerve

1. **Musculocutaneous nerve**. It pierces coracobrachialis to reach between brachialis and biceps. It supplies all the three muscles of the flexor compartment of arm. The nerve continues as the lateral cutaneous nerve of forearm.

2. **Median nerve**. It descends along the lateral aspect of upper part of the brachial artery, crosses it in the middle of arm and then descends along its medial side upto elbow.

3. **Ulnar nerve**. It descends on the medial aspect of upper part of the brachial artery but disappears by piercing the medial intermuscular septum.

4. **Radial nerve**. It descends in the groove between brachialis (medially) and brachioradialis and extensor carpi radialis longus (laterally). After supplying all these three muscles it terminates into superficial and deep branches at the level of lateral epicondyle of humerus.

Extensor compartment

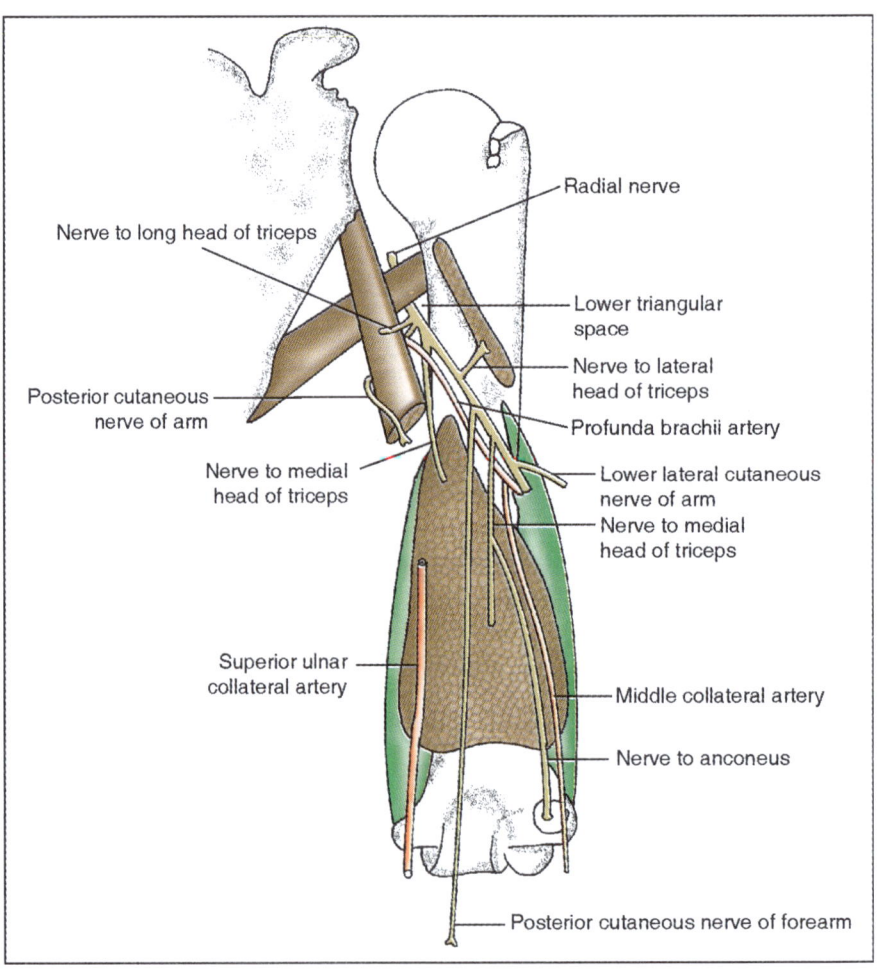

Fig. 12.6 Extensor compartment of arm

DISSECTION STEPS: BACK OF THE ARM

Remove the deep fascia from the back of the arm. Expose and define the three heads of triceps. Find the radial nerve in the axilla posterior to the axillary artery. Trace the radial nerve in the radial groove and separate the triceps lateral head along the line of the nerve in the groove. Divide and reflect the parts of the lateral head of triceps to expose the radial nerve. Follow the ulnar nerve in the posterior compartment behind the medial intermuscular septum and trace it to the back of the medial epicondyle of humerus.

Triceps

Origin

Long head. From the infraglenoid tubercle of scapula.

Lateral head. Back of humerus above the radial groove.

Medial head. Back of humerus below the radial groove and both intermuscular septa.

Insertion. Superior surface of olecranon process of ulna. Some deep fibres (articularis cubiti) get attached directly to the capsule of the elbow joint.

Nerve. Radial nerve.

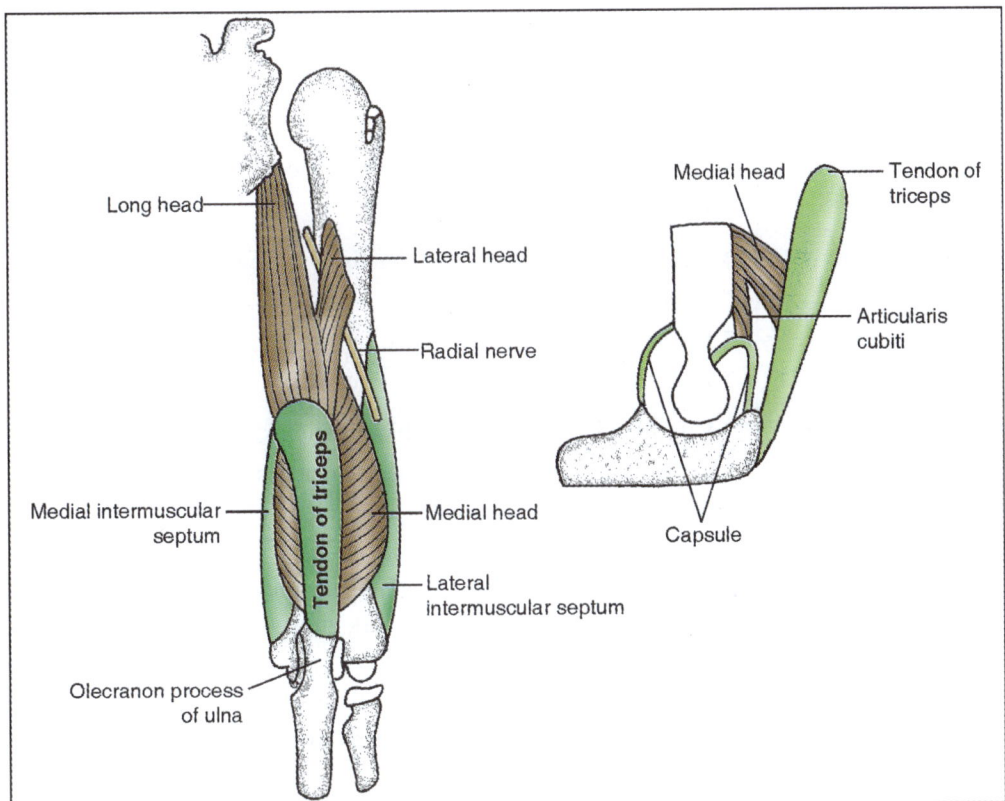

Fig 12.7 Triceps

Actions.

1. Extension at elbow joint.
2. Protection of the capsule of elbow joint (by articularis cubiti).

Profunda brachii artery

After arising from the brachial artery, it passes through the lower triangular space and radial groove with the radial nerve. It provides a number of **muscular branches** and terminates into following two terminal branches.

1. **Middle collateral artery**. It follows the course of nerve to anconeus to reach the back of lateral epicondyle of humerus.
2. **Radial collateral artery**. It accompanies the radial nerve, pierces the lateral intermuscular septum and descends in the arm's flexor compartment to reach the front of lateral epicondyle of humerus.

Radial nerve $(C_{5,6,7,8}.T_1)$

Course. It passes through lower triangular space to reach the radial groove where it runs under the cover of lateral head of triceps. The nerve then pierces the lateral intermuscular septum to descend in the flexor compartment of arm.

Branches

Part of the radial nerve	Branches
Proximal to radial groove	* Nerve to medial and long heads of triceps. * Posterior cutaneous nerve of arm
In the radial groove	* Nerve to medial and lateral heads of triceps. * Nerve to anconeus. * Lower lateral cutaneous nerve of arm. * Posterior cutaneous nerve of forearm.
Distal to radial groove	* Muscular. To brachialis, brachioradialis, extensor carpi-radialis longus. * Terminal—Superficial and deep branches. * Articualr—To elbow joint.

Applied anatomy

- Radial nerve may be involved in fracture of humeral shaft, gunshot wound of axilla and arm or due to pressure by crutch (crutch palsy).
- For complete radial nerve palsy, it must be interrupted in the axilla.
- If the lesion is situated at the middle third of humerus (a common site of fracture), the brachioradialis is spared.
- The charateristic deformity of radial nerve palsy is called "wrist drop".
- Radial nerve at the wrist is commonly thickened in lepromatous leprosy.

Cubital Fossa

It is a triangular depressed area in front of the upper forearm. It has an upper base, lower apex and medial and lateral margins.

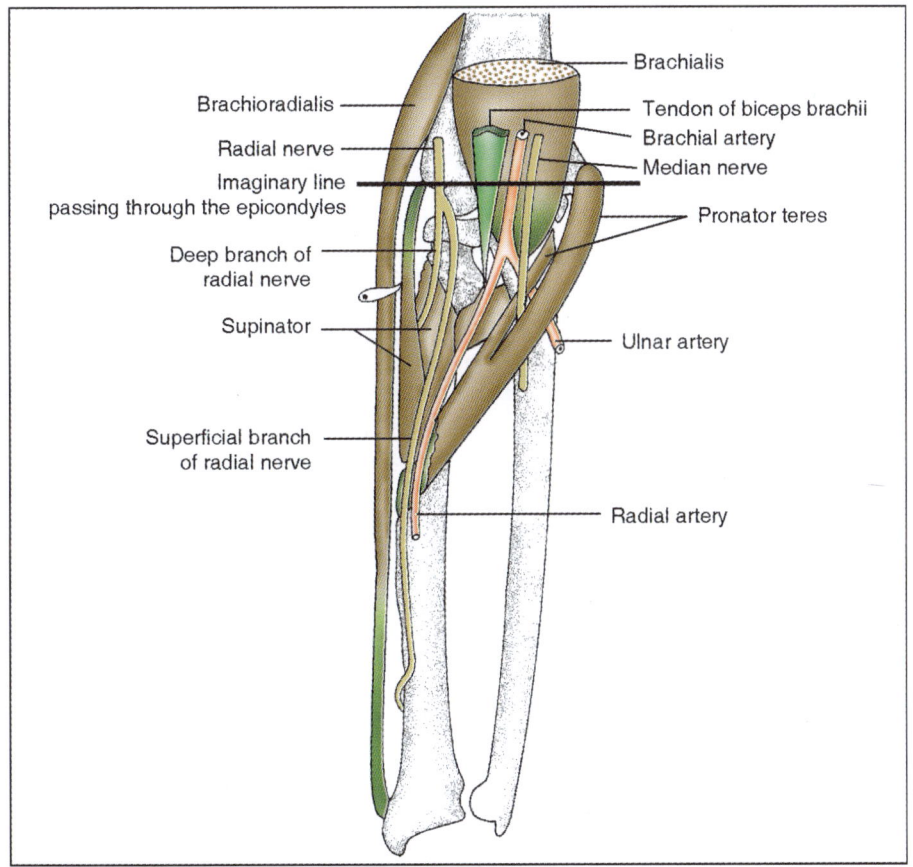

Fig. 13.1 Cubital fossa

DISSECTION STEPS: CUBITAL FOSSA

Clean and define the boundaries of the cubital fossa. Clean and define the structures in the roof. Clean and define the contents of the fossa. Clean the muscular floor (brachialis and supinator) of the fossa.

Boundaries

Medial. Pronator teres.
Lateral. Brachioradialis.

Base

Imaginary line joining two epicondyles of humerus.

Apex

Where medial and lateral margins meet.

Roof

Deep fascia.

Floor

Brachialis and supinator.

Contents

From medial to lateral these are median nerve, brachial artery and its two terminal branches (radial and ulnar arteries), tendon of biceps, radial nerve and its two terminal branches (superficial and deep branches).

14

Arterial Anastomoses Around Elbow

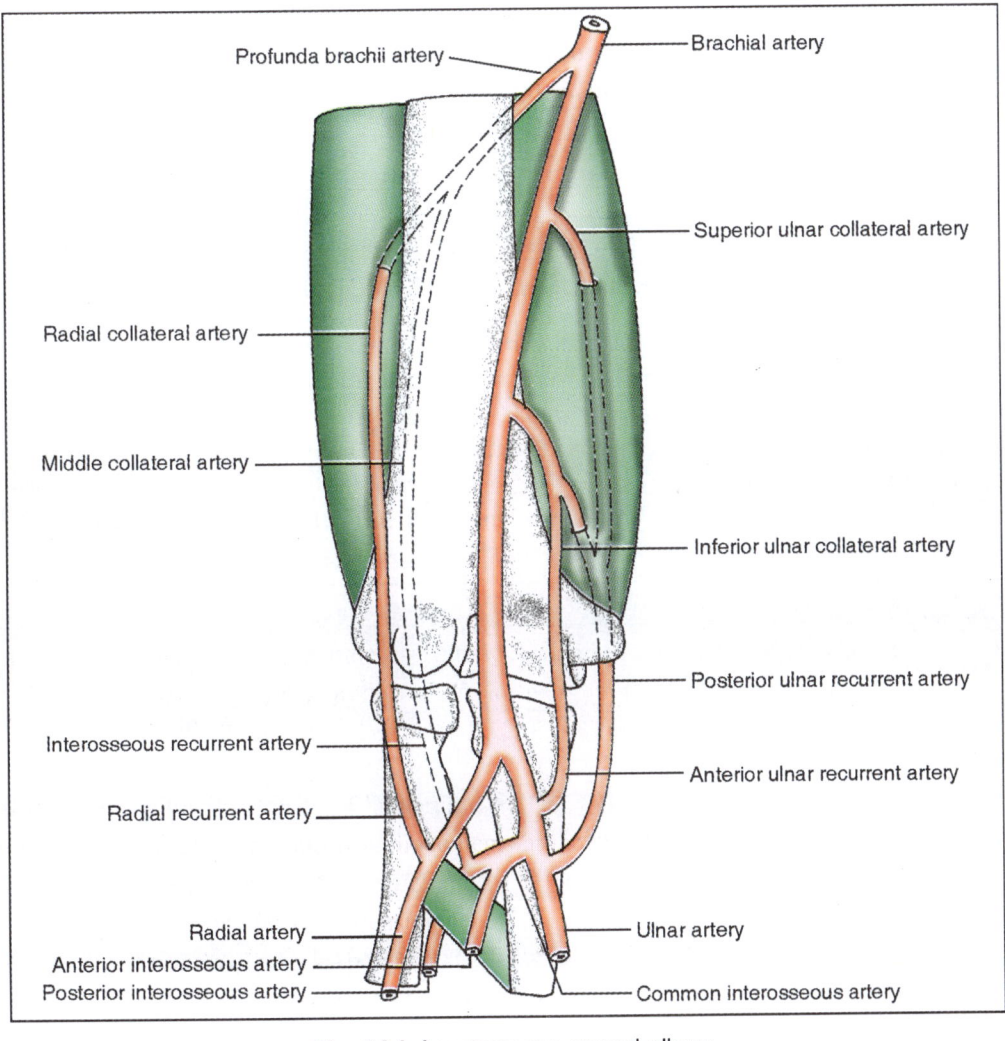

Fig. 14.1 Anastomoses around elbow

Four decending arteries anastomose with four ascending arteries in relation to humeral epicondyles. Anastomosis occurs:

1. **Behind the medial epicondyle**

   Between descending superior ulnar collateral artery (*from brachial artery*) and ascending posterior ulnar recurrent artery (*from ulnar artery*).

2. **In front of medial epicondyle**

   Between descending inferior ulnar collateral artery (*from brachial artery*) and ascending anterior ulnar recurrent artery (*from ulnar artery*).

3. **In front of lateral epicondyle**

   Between descending radial collateral artery (*from profunda brachii artery*) and ascending radial recurrent artery (*from radial artery*).

4. **Behind the lateral epicondyle**

   Between descending middle collateral artery (*from profunda brachii artery*) and ascending interosseous recurrent artery (*from posterior interosseous artery*).

15

Flexor Compartment of Forearm and Palm

FOREARM

Compartments. Two compartments, flexor and extensor are roughly located in front and behind the two bones (radius and ulna) and interosseous membrane respectively. Medial limit of the two compartments is the posterior border of ulna while laterally they are demarcated by the superficial branch of the radial nerve.

DISSECTION STEPS
FRONT OF FOREARM (FLEXOR COMPARTMENT)

Give a vertical midline incisions at the elbow (incision 5, Fig. 3.13) extending upto the wrist and extend it transversely across the wrist. Divide the deep fascia of the forearm to expose the superficial muscles. Clean and define the ulnar nerve and vessels between the flexor carpi ulnaris and flexor digitorum superficialis. Pull the brachioradialis laterally to expose the extensor carpi radialis longus. Between the brachioradialis and extensor carpi radialis longus identify the radial artery. Cut the tendons of the flexor carpil radialis and palmaris longus about 5 cm proximal to the wrist. Expose and define the radial artery, and flexor digitorum superficialis. Push aside the flexor digitorum superficialis and identify the deep flexors and the median nerve. Clean and define the flexor retinaculum.

SUPERFICIAL MUSCLES OF FLEXOR COMPARTMENT

Pronator teres

Origin

Humeral head (superficial fibres)	–	Common flexor origin from the front of humeral medial epicondyle and medial supracondylar ridge.
Ulnar head (deep fibres)	–	Coronoid process of ulna (medial aspect).

Insertion. Middle of the lateral aspect of radius.

Nerve. Median nerve.

Actions. Flexion and pronation of forearm.

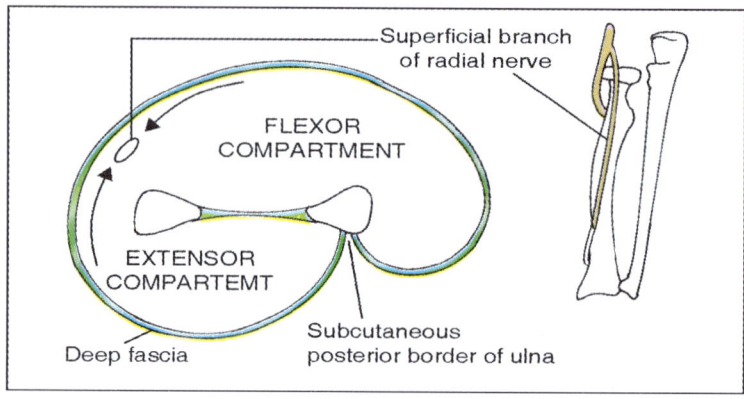

Fig. 15.1 Compartments of the forearm

Flexor carpi radialis

Origin. Common flexor origin (front of the humeral medial epicondyle).

Insertion. Palmar aspects of the bases of 2nd and 3rd metacarpals.

Nerve. Median nerve.

Actions. With flexor carpi ulnaris causes flexion of hand.

With extensor carpi radialis helps in abduction of hand.

Palmaris longus

Origin. Common flexor origin.

Insertion. Flexor retinaculum, continues into palm as palmar aponeurosis.

Nerve. Median nerve.

Actions. Flexion of hand.

Tenses palmar aponeurosis.

Flexor carpi ulnaris

Origin

Humeral fibres – Common flexor origin.

Ulnar fibres – Posterior border of ulna.

Insertion. Pisiform bone.

Nerve. Ulnar nerve.

Actions. With flexor carpi radialis causes flexion of hand.

With extensor carpi ulnaris causes adduction of hand.

Flexor digitorum superficialis

Origin. Medial epicondyle of humerus, medial collateral ligament of elbow, sublime tubercle of coronoid process, tendinous arch (from sublime tubercle to the upper end of anterior oblique line of radius) and anterior oblique line of radius.

Insertion. Provides 4 tendons which get inserted into the bases of middle phalanges of medial 4 digits of hand. Before insertion each tendon provides passage for the flexor digitorum profundus tendon.

Nerve: Median nerve.

Actions. Flexion of middle and proximal phalanges and hand.

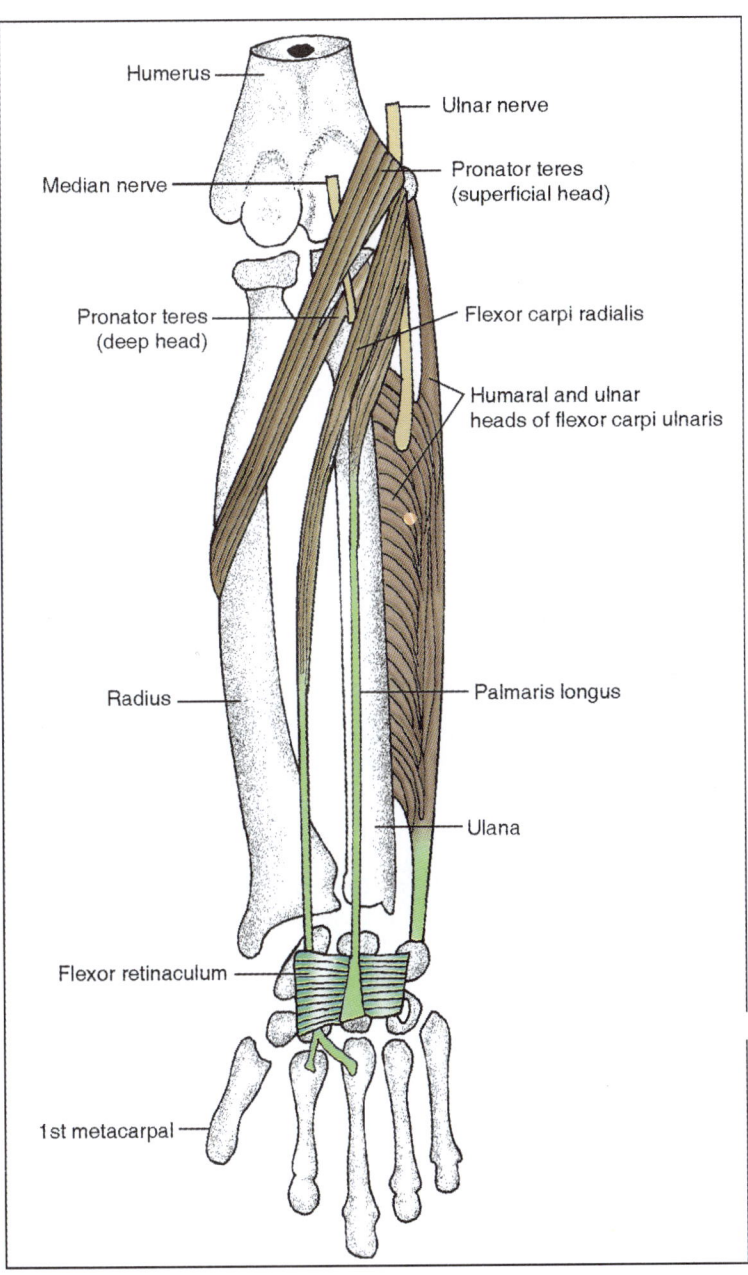

Fig. 15.2 Superficial group of muscles of the flexor compartment of forearm

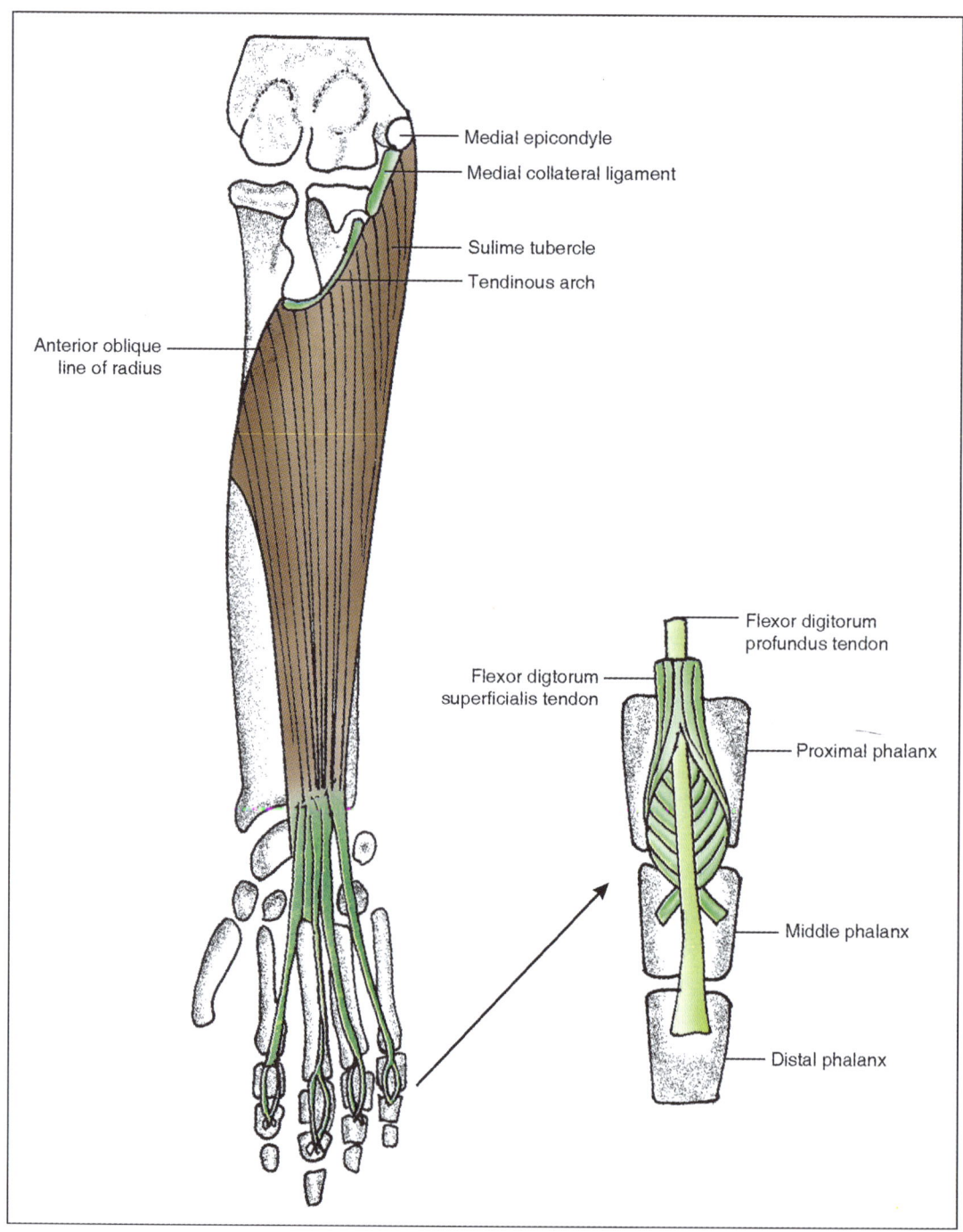

Fig. 15.3 Flexor digitorum superficialis

> ## DISSECTON STEPS: FRONT OF FOREARM AND PALM
>
> Proximal to the flexor retinaculum trace the radial artery lateral to the tendon of flexor carpi radialis. Identify the ulnar nerve and vessels between the flexor carpi ulnaris and flexor digitorum superficialis and trace them to the palm passing superficial to the flexor retinaculum. Clean and trace the structures deep to the flexor retinaculum. Continue incision 5 (Fig. 3.13) over the palm and reflect the skin flaps. Clean the superficial and deep fascia and identify the palmar aponeurosis. Separate the palmar aponeurosis from the thenar and hypothenar muscles. Cut the aponeurosis near flexor retinaculum, turn it distally and identify the superficial palmar ach. Clean and define the thenar and hypothenar muscles. Cut the palmaris brevis. Dissect out the tendons of flexor digitorum superficialis and flexor digitrum profundus upto their insertions and identify the deep branch of ulnar nerve, lumbricals arising from the tendons of flexor digitorum porfundus, synovial sheaths and the deep palmar arch.

DEEP MUSCLES OF FLEXOR COMPARTMENT

Flexor pollicis longus

Origin. Anterior surface of upper 3/4th of radius and adjacent interosseous membrane.

Insertion. Base of terminal phalanx of thumb.

Nerve. Anterior interosseous nerve (a branch of median nerve).

Actions. Flexion of terminal phalanx of thumb.

Flexor digitorum profundus

Origin. Anterior and medial surfaces of the upper 3/4th of ulna and adjacent interosseous membrane; posterior border of ulna.

Insertion. Provides 4 tendons each of which passes through the passage in the corresponding tendon of flexor digitorum superficialis. Tendons get inserted to the bases of distal phalanges of medial 4 digits of hand.

Nerve. *Medial half* – Ulnar nerve.

Lateral half – Anterior interosseous branch of the median nerve.

Actions.

1. Primarily flexion of distal phalanges.
2. Flexion of wrist and other joints of the hand.
3. It is a chief gripping muscle.

Pronator quadratus

Origin. Lower ¼th of front of ulna.

Insertion. Front and medial aspect of lower ¼th of radius.

Nerve. Anterior interosseous nerve.

Actions. Pronation of the forearm.

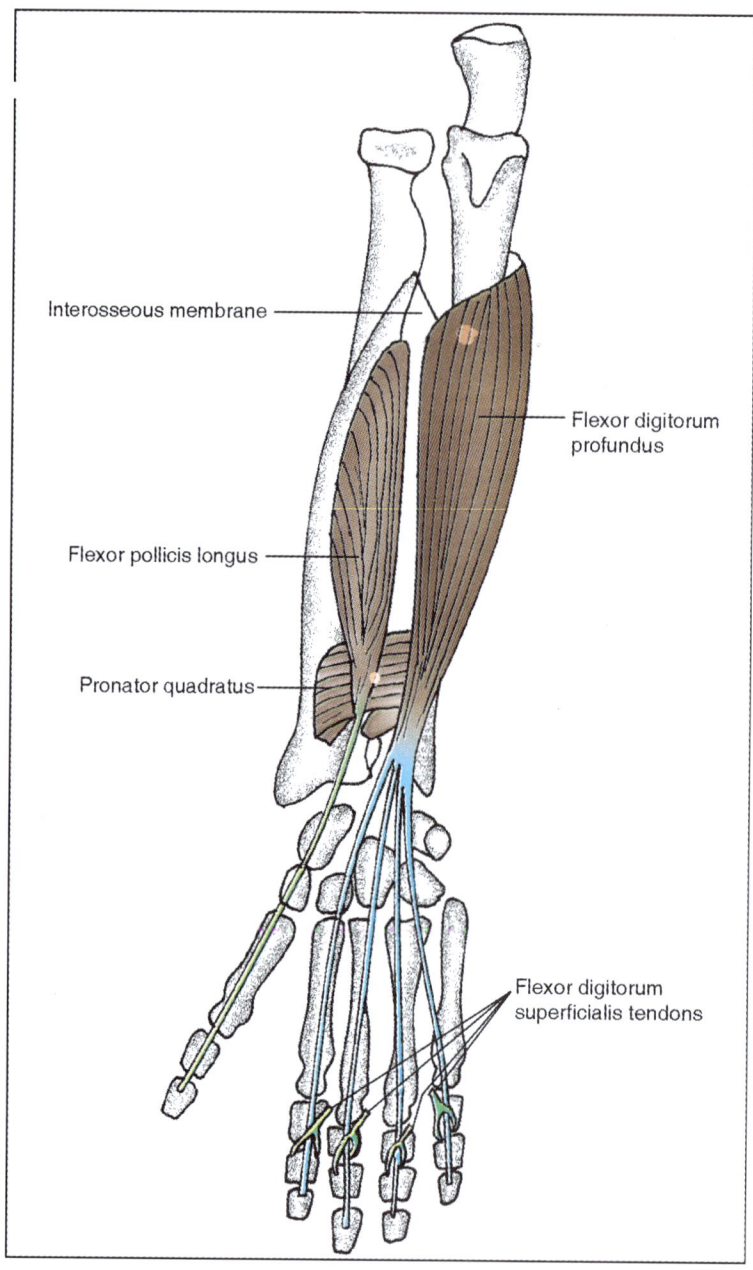

Interosseous membrane

Flexor digitorum profundus

Flexor pollicis longus

Pronator quadratus

Flexor digitorum superficialis tendons

Fig. 15.4 Deep muscles of the flexor compartment of forearm

SYNOVIAL SHEATHS OF THE FLEXOR TENDONS

At the wrist all eight tendons of long flexors (four each for flexor digitorum superficialis and profundus, l ng superficial and deep respectively) pass through the carpal tunnel. Here the tendons are surrounded by *common synovial sheath* (also called the *ulnar bursa*). The sheath extends from distal part of the forearm to the middle of the palm. Tendon of flexor pollicis longus possesses its own synovial sheath (*radial bursa*).

Over the digits the tendons of long flexors are surrounded by *a common digital synovial sheath*, each one of which extends from the level of metacarpophalangeal joint to base of distal pahalanx. However, the digital sheath of the little finger is continuous proximally with the ulnar bursa.

Applied anatomy

1. Infection of little finger and thumb are more dangerous because they can spread into the palm and even upto 2.5 cm above the wrist. In about 50% cases the two bursae (*ulnar and radial*) communicate with each other behind the flexor retinaculum.
2. Infection of the thumb may spread to the radial bursa and then to the ulnar bursa. It can be drained by an incision along the medial margin of the thenar eminence. This incision should be restricted proximally to avoid injury to the branch of the median nerve to the thenar muscles.
3. Infected digital synovial sheath is drained by opening the sheath at its both ends. This may be achieved by making transverse incision, one on the distal palmar crease and other on the crease of distal interphalangeal joint.
4. Infection of ulnar bursa is usually secondary to the infection of the little finger, and this in turn may spread to space of Parona resulting into an hour-glass swelling (two swellings, one each in palm and forearm joined by narrow region behind the flexor retinaculum in the middle).
5. Ulnar bursa is approached by an incision along the lateral margin of the hypothenar eminence.

PALMAR ASPECT OF HAND

DEEP FASCIA

Location	Name
Over carpus	Flexor retinaculum
Over metacarpus	Thick palmar aponeurosis in the middle but thinner fascia over thenar and hypothenar eminences
Over phalanges	Fibrous flexor sheath

Applied anatomy

*   Volkmann's ischaemic contracture (fibrosis and contracture of flexor muscles) is due to vascular injuries which result into muscle infarction (death of muscle fibres) followed by fibrosis.
*   If there is division of flexor digitorum superficialis tendons only, there is no loss of flexion. But division of both long flexor tendons results into loss of flexion of finger and muscle repair is required.
*   In Dupuytren's contracture, palmar aponeurosis is thickened and contracted. Typically the condition affects the ring finger (which is permanently flexed) but later the little finger also becomes implicated.

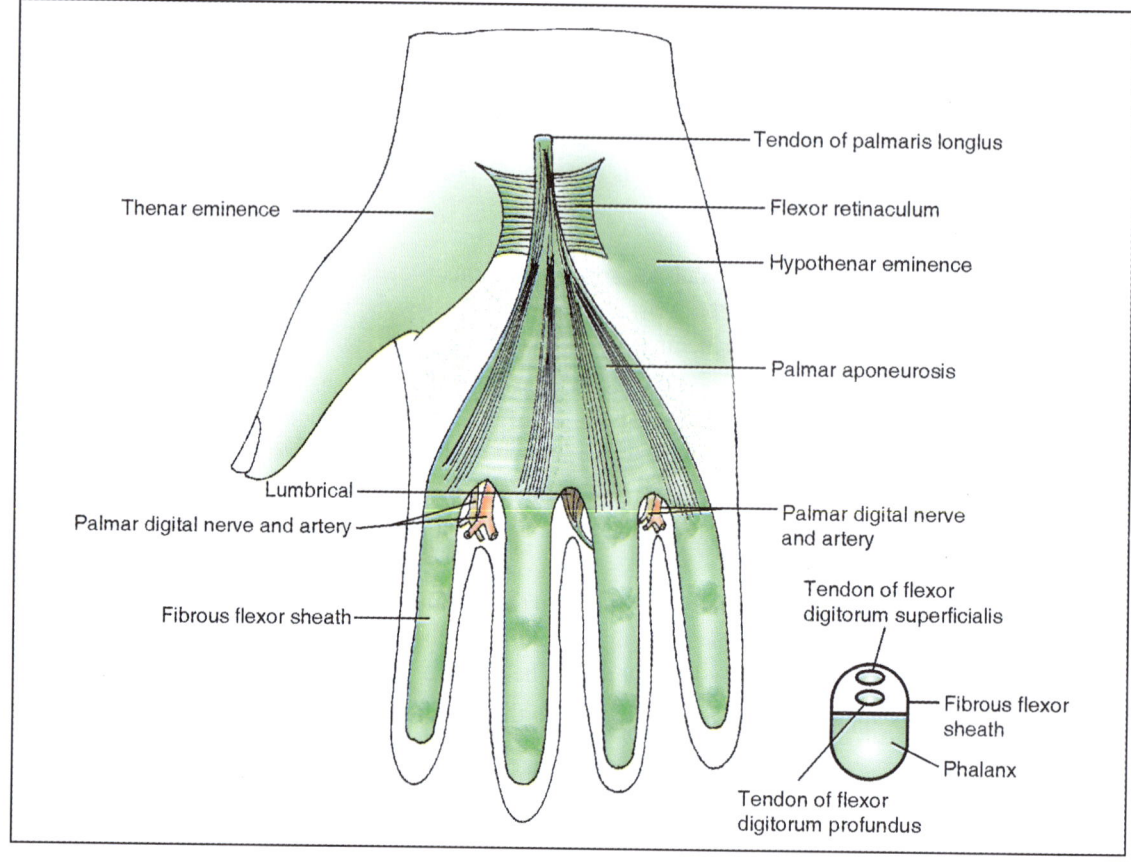

Labels in figure:
- Tendon of palmaris longlus
- Flexor retinaculum
- Hypothenar eminence
- Palmar aponeurosis
- Thenar eminence
- Palmar digital nerve and artery
- Tendon of flexor digitorum superficialis
- Lumbrical
- Palmar digital nerve and artery
- Fibrous flexor sheath
- Fibrous flexor sheath
- Phalanx
- Tendon of flexor digitorum profundus

Fig. 15.5 Deep fascia of the palm

FLEXOR RETINACULUM

It is the deep fascia over the front of carpus. It is quadrangular in shape with its angles attached to four bony prominences, i.e. pisiform, hook of hamate, tubercle of scaphoid and crest of terapezium.

Relations

Anterior: Thenar and hypothenar muscles, palmaris longus tendon, ulnar nerve and artery, palmar cutaneous branches of the median and ulnar nerves and superficial palmar branch of the radial artery.
Posterior (carpal tunnel): Tendons of flexor digitorum superficialis and flexor digitorum profundus (4 each) with their common synovial sheath, median nerve. Between the two laryers of flexor retinaculum lies the tendon of flexor carpi radialis.

LATERAL MUSCLES OF PALM

It includes muscles of thenar eminence (*Abductor pollicis brevis, flexor pollicis brevis* and *opponens pollicis*) and *adductor pollicis.*

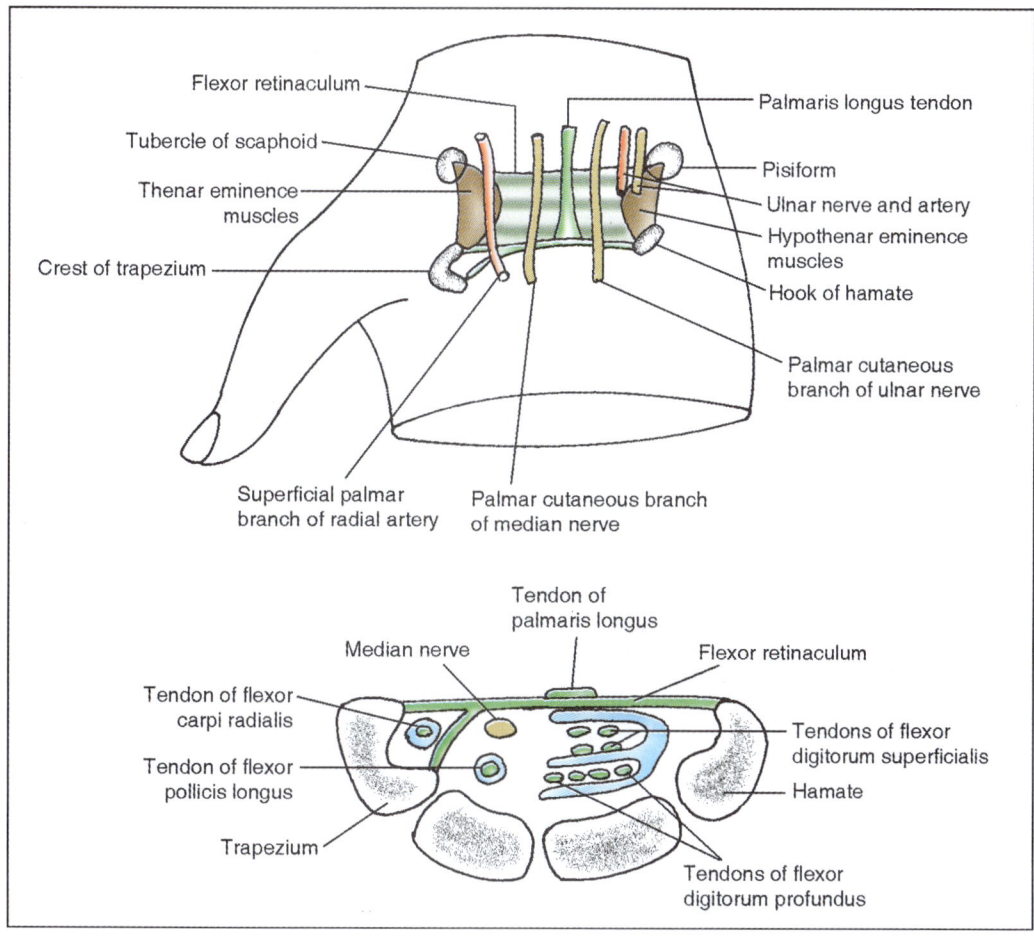

Fig. 15.6 Flexor retinaculum

Muscles of thenar eminence originate from the lateral part of flexor retinaculum, tubercle of scaphoid and crest of trapezium. Ist two (abductor and flexor) are inserted to the anteromedial aspect of the base of proximal phalanx of thumb. Opponens pollicis is inserted to the shaft of 1st metacarpal. All the above are supplied by the median nerve (flexor pollicis brevis can get additional twig from the deep branch of ulnar nerve). Their actions are attributed to their names i.e., *flexor pollicis brevis* causes *flexion, abductor pollicis brevis* causes *abduction* and *opponens* helps in *opposition* (medial rotation) of thumb.

ADDUCTOR POLLICIS

Origin

Transverse head. Shaft of 3rd metacarpal.

Oblique head. Bases of 2nd and 3rd metacarpals and capitate.

Insertion. Posteromedial aspect of base of proximal phalanx of thumb.

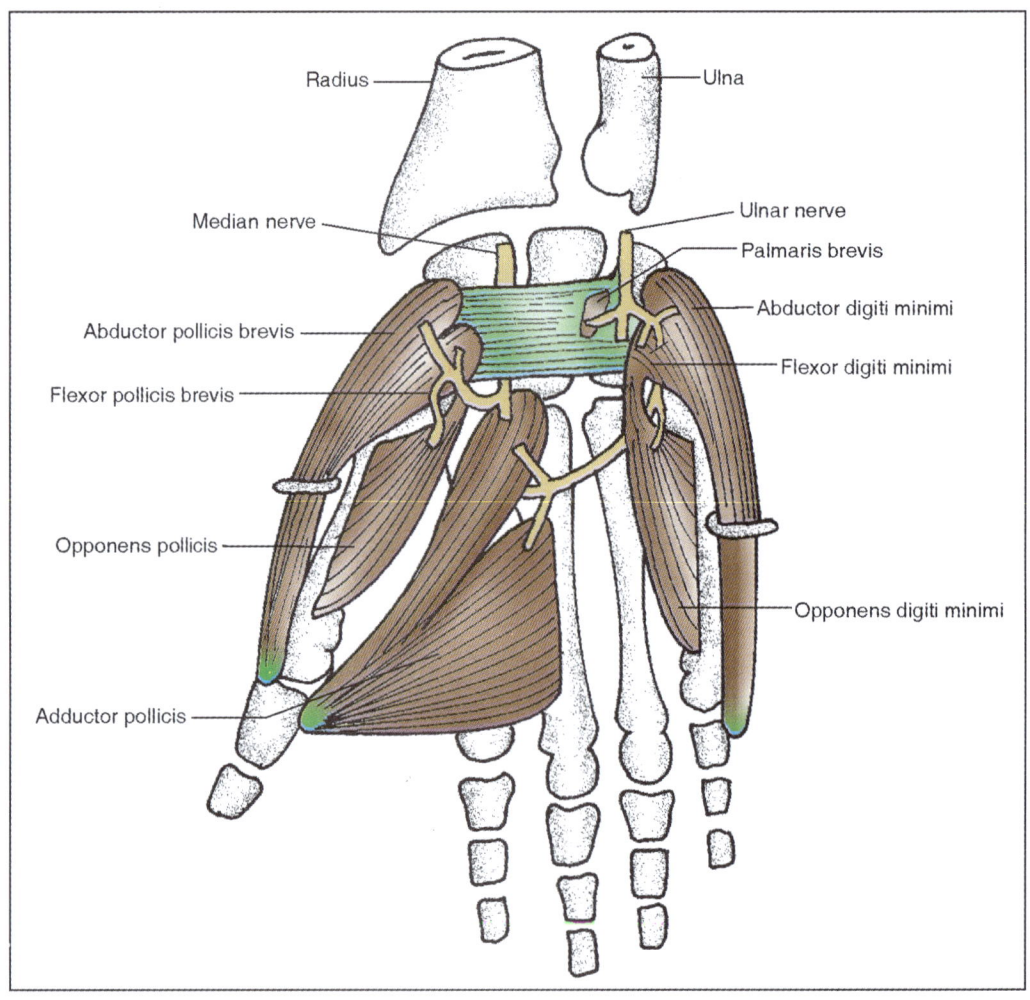

Fig. 15.7 Lateral and medial muscles of palm

Nerve. Deep branch of ulnar nerve.

Actions. Adduction of thumb.

MEDIAL MUSCLES OF PALM

It includes *abductor digiti minimi, flexor digiti minimi* and *opponens digiti minimi*. All originating from the medial part of flexor retinaculum, pisiform and hook of hamate. First two (abductor and flexor) get inserted to the anteromedial aspect of base of proximal phalanx of little finger. Opponens digiti minimi gets inserted to the shaft of 5th metacarpal. All are supplied by the deep bra..ch of ulnar nerve. Their actions are attributed to their names i.e., *abductor digiti minimi* causes *abdution* and *flexor digiti minimi* causes *flexion* of little finger. *Opponens digiti minimi rotates* the 5th metacarpal externally (cupping palm). Lying in the superficial fascia is palmaris brevis muscle cannecting the skin of the medial margin of palm with flexor retinaculum. It is supplied by the only muscular branch of superficial branch of ulnar nerve.

Applied anatomy

- Wasting of muscles due to nerve injury is a striking sign. Wasting of thenar eminence is observed in cases of median nerve injury (e.g. carpal tunnel syndrome) and that of hypothenar eminence is noticed in cases of ulnar nerve lesion (e.g., elbow tunnel syndrome).
- *Froment's sign*. It demonstrates the paralysis of adductor pollicis. The patient is asked to grasp a f 'ded news paper firmly between thumb and index finger. On paralysed side, thumb is flexed at the interphalangeal joint due to contraction of flexor pollicis longus.

ULNAR ARTERY IN THE FOREARM AND HAND

Course. It arises from brachial artery at the level of neck of radius in the cubital fossa. Passes medially deep to the pronator teres and descends under the tendinous arch for flexor digitorum superficialis to join ulnar nerve. Ulnar artery crosses the superficial aspect of flexor retinaculum lateral to the pisiform and terminates by dividing into *superficial and deep branches*.

Branches

1. *Common interosseous artery*. It divides into following two branches.
   (*a*) *Posterior interosseous artery*. It passes back above the upper border of the interosseous membrane to enter the posterior compartment.
   (*b*) *Antererior interosseous artery*. It descends in front of the interosseous membrane and gives following branches,
      (i) Muscular
      (ii) Nutrient artery to both radius and ulna.
      (iii) Branch to palmar carpal arch.
      (iv) Continues into posterior compartment through a foramen in the lower part of interosseous membrane.
2. *Anterior ulnar recurrent artery*. Ascends to reach the front of medial epicondyle.
3. *Posterior ulnar recurrent artery*. Ascends along ulnar nerve to reach the back of medial epicondyle.
4. *Palmar carpal branch to palmar carpal arc*.
5. *Dorsal carpal branch to dorsal carpal arch*.
6. *Muscular branches*.
7. *Terminal branches:*
   (*a*) Deep branch. It completes deep palmar arch with the radial artery.
   (*b*) Superficial branch. It continues as superficial palmar arch. Superficial palmar arch provides a proper palmar digital artery to the medial side of little finger and three common palmar digital arteries to medial three interdigital clefts where they split into proper palmar digital arteries.

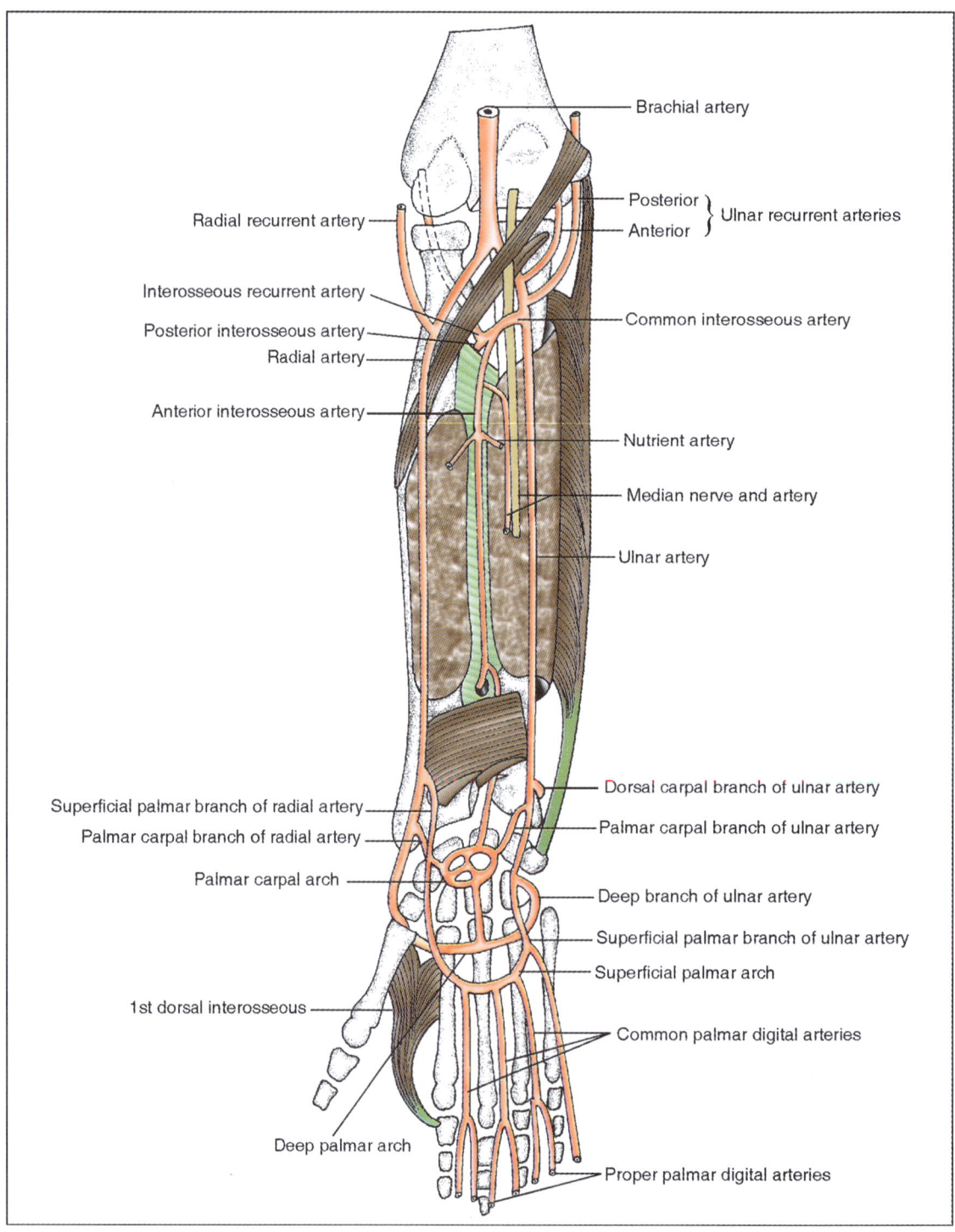

Brachial artery

Radial recurrent artery

Posterior } Ulnar recurrent arteries
Anterior }

Interosseous recurrent artery

Posterior interosseous artery

Radial artery

Common interosseous artery

Anterior interosseous artery

Nutrient artery

Median nerve and artery

Ulnar artery

Superficial palmar branch of radial artery

Palmar carpal branch of radial artery

Palmar carpal arch

Dorsal carpal branch of ulnar artery

Palmar carpal branch of ulnar artery

Deep branch of ulnar artery

Superficial palmar branch of ulnar artery

Superficial palmar arch

1st dorsal interosseous

Common palmar digital arteries

Deep palmar arch

Proper palmar digital arteries

Fig. 15.8 Arteries of flexor compartment of forearm and hand

RADIAL ARTERY IN THE FOREARM AND HAND

Course. It arises from the brachial artery at the level of neck of radius. It passes laterally and descends superficial to the insertion of pronator teres under the cover of brachioradialis to reach the front of the lower end of radius where it can be easily palpated lateral to the tendon of flexor carpi radialis. It crosses the anatomical snuff box to reach the dorsum of hand. It enters the palmar aspect of hand by passing through the 1st intermetacarpal space between two heads of 1st dorsal interosseous muscle. It terminates by continuing as deep palmar arch.

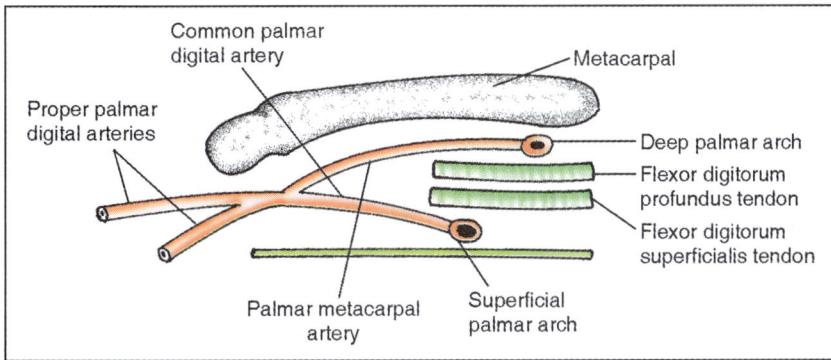

Fig. 15.9 Orientation of palmar arches

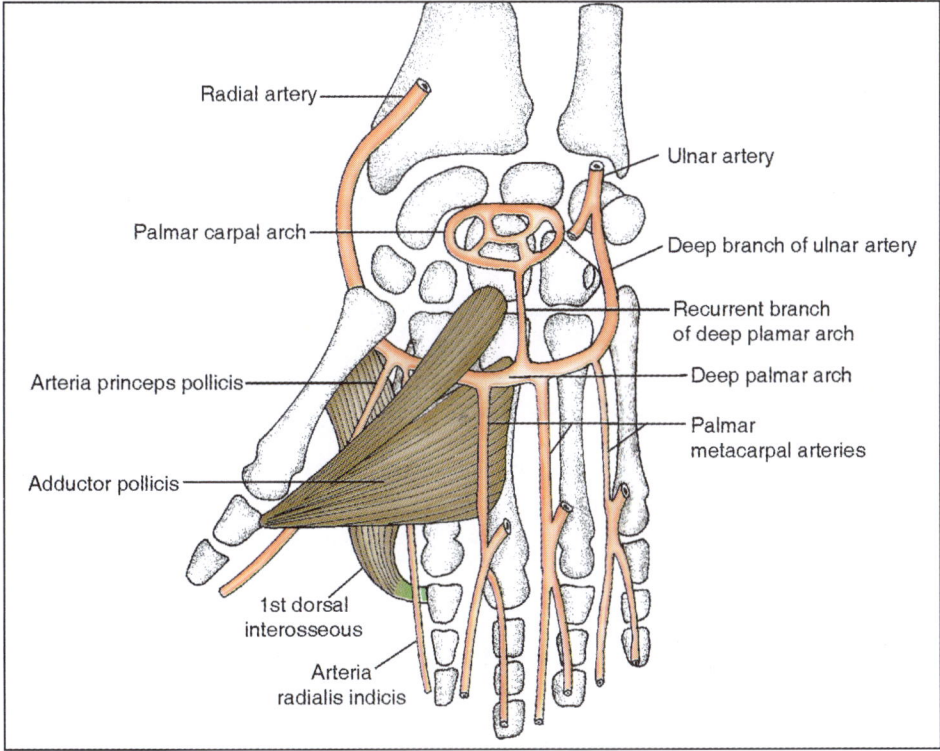

Fig. 15.10 Deep palmar arch

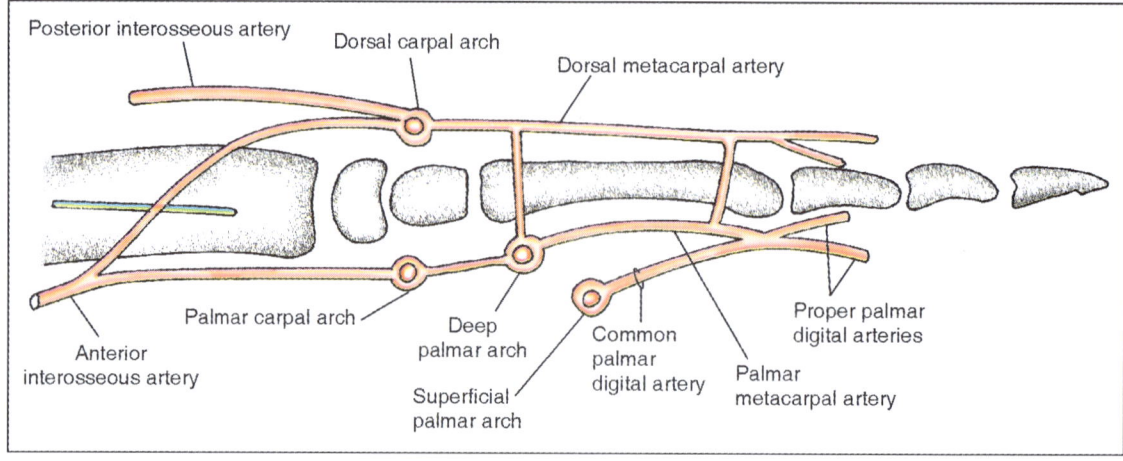

Posterior interosseous artery
Dorsal carpal arch
Dorsal metacarpal artery
Palmar carpal arch
Anterior interosseous artery
Deep palmar arch
Common palmar digital artery
Proper palmar digital arteries
Palmar metacarpal artery
Superficial palmar arch

Fig. 15.11 Main arteries in relation to hand

Branches

1. *Radial recurrent artery.* Ascends to reach the front of lateral epicondyle.
2. *Muscular branches.*
3. *Superficial palmar branch.* It enters the palm superficial to the flexor retinaculum, turns medially to complete the superficial palmar arch with superficial branch of ulnar artery deep to palmar aponeurosis.
4. *Palmar carpal branch.* It joins palmar carpal arch.
5. *Dorsal carpal branch.* It arises in the anatomical snuff box and joins the dorsal carpal arch.
6. *Arteria princeps pollicis.* It goes to the thumb.
7. *Arteria radialis indicis.* It passes to the radial side of index finger.
8. *Deep palmar arch.* It runs medially against the bases of middle three metacarpals along deep branch of ulnar nerve. It gives a recurrent branch to the palmar carpal arch and 3 palmar metacarpal arteries each of which joins the corresponding common palmar digital artery from superficial palmar arch.

ULNAR NERVE IN THE FOREARM AND HAND

Course. Ulnar nerve enters the forearm by passing between the two heads of flexor carpi ulnaris. It then descends under the cover of same muscle medial to the ulnar artery to reach the lateral aspect of pisiform superficial to flexor retinaculum. Here it terminates into its two terminal branches.

Branches in the forearm

1. *Articular.* To the elbow joint.
2. *Muscular.* To flexor carpi ulnaris and medial half of flexor digitorum profundus.
3. *Cutaneous.* Palmar and dorsal cutaneous branches which supply the medial 1/3rd of corresponding aspects of hand respectively.

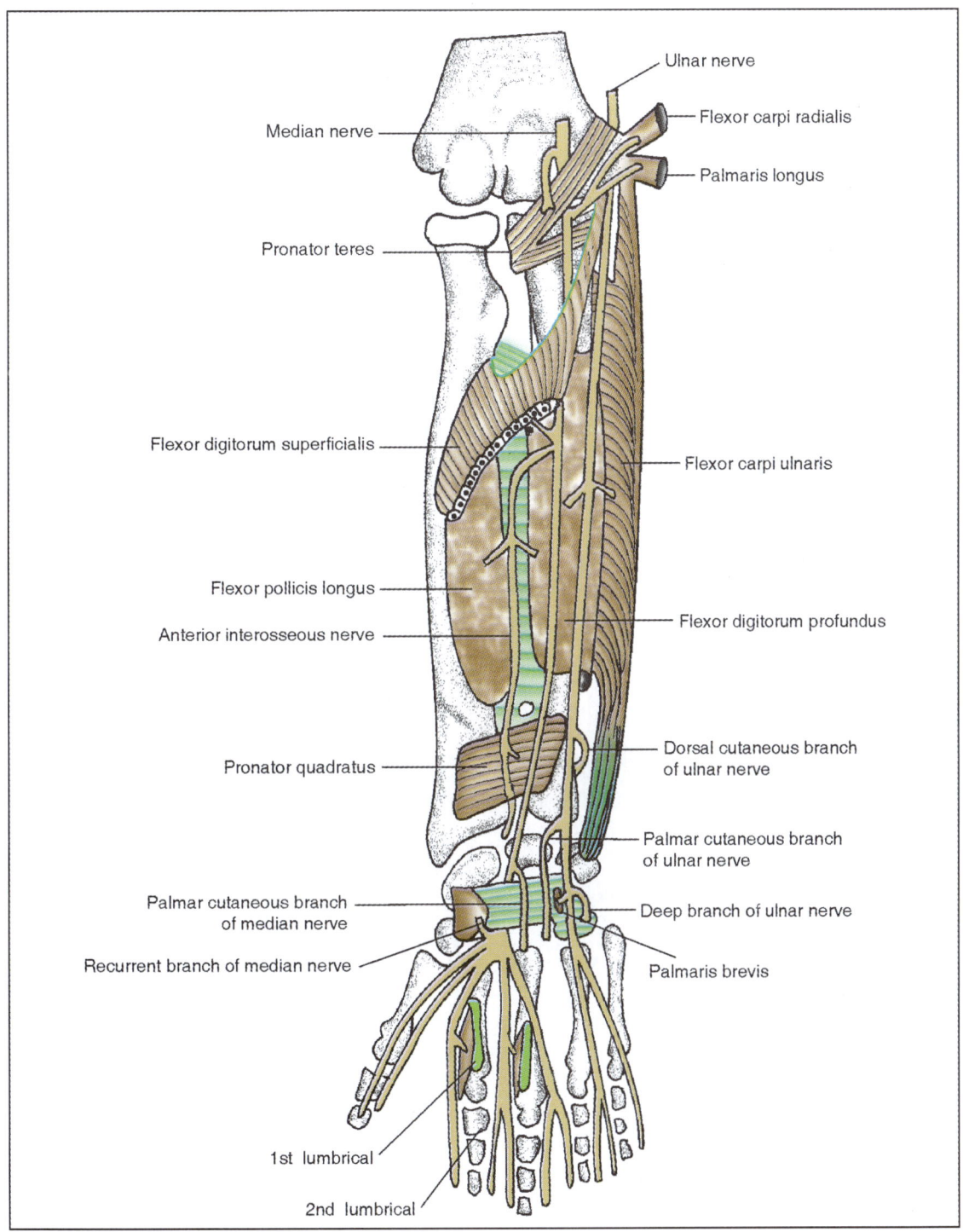

Median nerve

Pronator teres

Flexor digitorum superficialis

Flexor pollicis longus

Anterior interosseous nerve

Pronator quadratus

Palmar cutaneous branch
of median nerve

Recurrent branch of median nerve

1st lumbrical

2nd lumbrical

Ulnar nerve

Flexor carpi radialis

Palmaris longus

Flexor carpi ulnaris

Flexor digitorum profundus

Dorsal cutaneous branch
of ulnar nerve

Palmar cutaneous branch
of ulnar nerve

Deep branch of ulnar nerve

Palmaris brevis

Fig. 15.12 Nerves of flexor compartment of forearm and hand

Branches in the hand

Ulnar nerve terminates by dividing into superficial and deep branches which cross the flexor retinaculum.

   I. Superficial branch. It gives rise to following branches,

       1. *Muscular branch* to palmaris brevis.

       2. *Cutaneous branches*. To medial 1½ digits (by common and proper palmar digital nerves).

   II. Deep branch. Passes between abductor digiti minimi and flexor digiti minimi, crosses the ulnar aspect of hook of hamate and then runs laterally under opponens digiti minimi and long flexor tendons over the bases of middle 3 metacarpals in the concavity of the deep palmar arch. It supplies all the medial (hypothenar eminence) and intermediate (lumbricals and interossei) muscles of palm (*except lateral two lumbricals*), adductor pollicis and some times flexor pollicis brevis.

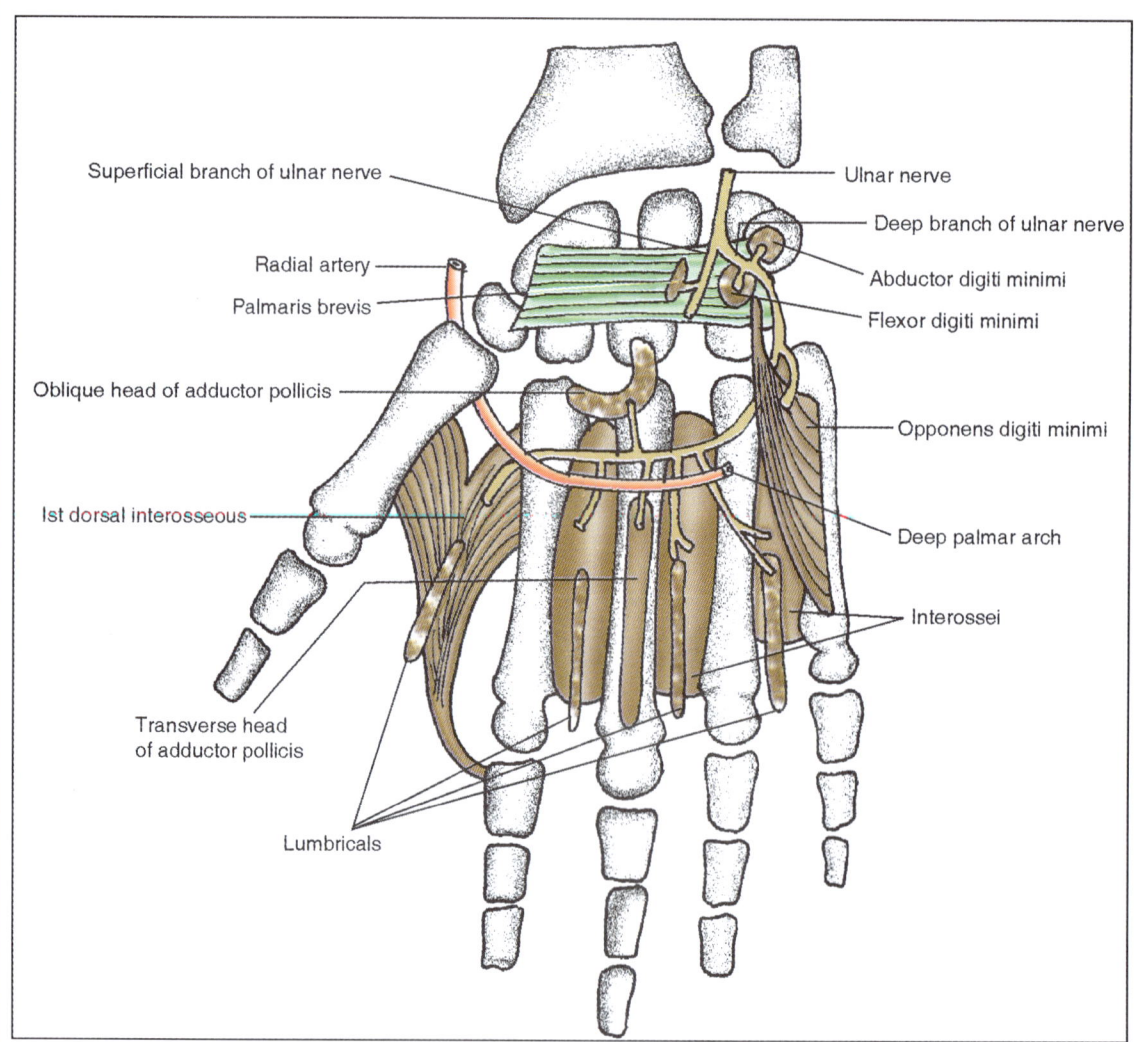

Fig. 15.13 Deep branch of the ulnar nerve

Applied anatomy

- *Levels of ulnar nerve lesion.* Ulnar nerve may be involved at higher level near the elbow and lower level at the wrist. In the former case, flexor carpi ulnaris and medial half of flexor digitorum profundus are also involved in addition to small muscles of the hand. Involvement at the wrist spares above mentioned 1½ muscles of forearm.

- *Ulnar claw-hand.* It is the deformity of the hand in cases of ulnar nerve lesions. The little and ring fingers are hyperextended at the metacarpophalangeal joints and are flexed at the interphalangeal joints. It is different from true claw-hand which also involves the middle and index fingers and is observed in the lesions of both the median and the ulnar nerves.

- *Ulnar nerve paradox.* It is said that higher the lesion (more ulnar nerve fibres are involved) the lesser the deformity produced. It is because of paralysis of ulnar half of flexor digtorum profundus leading to less flexion of medial two fingers.

- Lesion of ulnar nerve leads to paralysis and wasting of interossei, which leads to marked hollowing between metacarpals on the dorsum of hand.

- In leprosy (Hansen's disease) the thickened ulnar nerve can be easily felt behind the medial epicondyle of humerus.

MEDIAN NERVE IN THE FOREARM AND HAND

Course. Median nerve leaves the cubital fossa by passing between the two heads of pronator teres and under the tendinous arch for flexor digitorum superficialis. It runs deep to the latter muscle and follows the course of tendon of the palmaris longus to enter the hand under the flexor retinaculum.

Branches in the forearm

1. *Muscular.* To all superficial muscles except flexor carpi ulnaris.
2. *Articular.* To the elbow and proximal radioulnar joints.
3. *Anterior interosseous nerve.* It descends in front of interosseous membrane along with the anterior interosseous artery. It supplies all deep muscles (except medial half of flexor digitorum profundus) and also gives articular branches to the wrist, distal radio-ulnar and carpal joints.
4. *Palmar cutaneous branch.* It crosses the flexor retinaculum superficially and supplies lateral 2/3 rd of palm.
5. *Communicating branch* to the ulnar nerve.

Branches in the hand

1. *Recurrent branch.* It is the most lateral branch for muscles of thenar eminence.
2. *Proper palmar digital nerves (three).* Two for the thumb and one for the lateral aspect of the index finger. The latter also supplies the 1st lumbrical.
3. *Common palmar digital nerves (two).* Towards 2nd and 3rd interdigital clefts (*the one going to the 2nd cleft also supplies 2nd lumbrical*) where they split into proper palmar digital nerves to supply the adjacent sides of 2nd, 3rd and 4th fingers.

Applied anatomy

- Inability of the patient to pick up pin with thumb and index finger is a constant feature in cases of median nerve lesion. This is partly due to associated sensory loss.

- If the lesion is located in or above the cubital fossa, there is loss of power to flex the interphalangeal joints of index finger. This can be demonstrated by Ochsner's clasping test. When the patient is asked to clasp his hands firmly, he is unable to flex the index finger on the affected side.

- Lesion at the wrist spares flexor muscles of forearm but the thenar muscles are paralysed. '*Pen-touching test*' is performed to confirm the paralysis of adductor pollicis. Patient's dorsum of hand is resting on the table and then he is unable to raise (abduct) the thumb to touch the pen held just above it.

- *Ape-like thumb*. This is a sign of prolonged median nerve lesion in or above the cubital fossa. The thumb is in the same plane as the rest of the palm. It is due to unopposed action of extensor pollicis longus and adductor pollicis.

- Chronic lesion of median nerve at wrist leads to wasting of thenar eminence.

- *Carpal tunnel syndrome*. It denotes a compression neuropathy of the median nerve as it passes beneath the flexor retinaculum. Interestingly, there is hyperaesthesia over the distribution of the median nerve. Sensation in the palm is normal as the palmar cutaneous branch emerges from the median nerve proximal to the flexor retinaculum. Higher lesions of median nerve can be differentiated because such conditions are associated with anaesthesia of palm.

- Median nerve can be palpated at the bottom of a groove between flexor carpi radialis and palmaris longus tendons. A thickened median nerve just above the flexor retinaculum may be indicative of *leprosy*.

Extensor Compartment of Forearm and Dorsum of Hand

DISSECTION STEPS
BACK OF THE FOREARM (EXTENSOR COMPARTMENT)

Remoeve the skin and fascia from the back of the forearm leaving the extensor retinaculum intact and define its attachments. Separate the extensor muscles from each other at the wrist. Separate the brachioradialis, extensor carpi radialis longus and extensor carpi radialis brevis from extensor digitorum. Expose and clean the supinator muscle. Expose the posterior interosseous nerve emerging from supinator. Work out dorsal digital expansion.

Externsor retinaculum

Attachments

Lateral. Anterolateral border of lower part of radius.

Medial. Triquetral and pisiform bones.

Relations

Superficial branch of the radial nerve and dorsal branch of ulnar nerve cross it superficially. Septa from the deep surface extend to radius and ulna forming six compartments which are as follows from lateral to medial.

Compartment	Structures
1	Tendons of abductor pollicis longus and extensor pollicis brevis.
2	Tendons of extensor carpi radialis longus and extensor carpi radialis brevis.
3	Tendon of extensor pollicis longus.
4	Tendons of extesor digitorum and extensor indicis, posterior interosseous nerve and anterior interosseous artery.
5	Tendon of extensor digiti minimi.
6	Tendon of extensor carpi ulnaris.

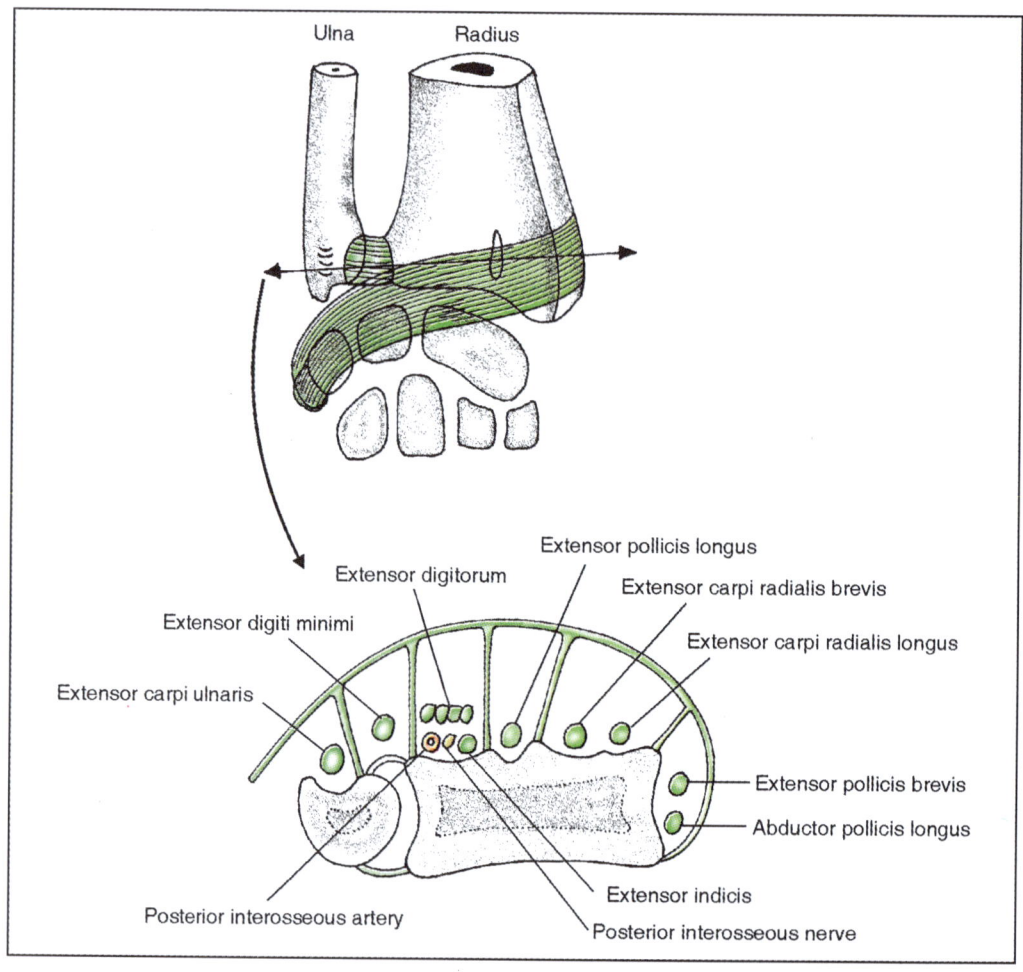

Fig. 16.1 Extensor retinaculum

Extensor expansion

It is triangular thickening of deep fascia on the dorsal aspect of medial four digits.

Base. It covers the dorsum and sides of head of metacarpal and gets attached to the deep transverse metacarpal ligaments.

Aex. It gets attached to the dorsal aspect of base of distal phalanx.

Contribution to joints. The expansion contributes to the dorsal aspects of the capsules of metacarpophalangeal and interphalangeal joints.

Muscles joining the base. Long extensor tendon joins the middle of the base and splits into three slips. Central slip gets attached to the base of middle phalanx. Marginal (collateral) slips unite and extend to the base of distal phalanx. Basal angles are joined by the lumbricals and interossei muscles.

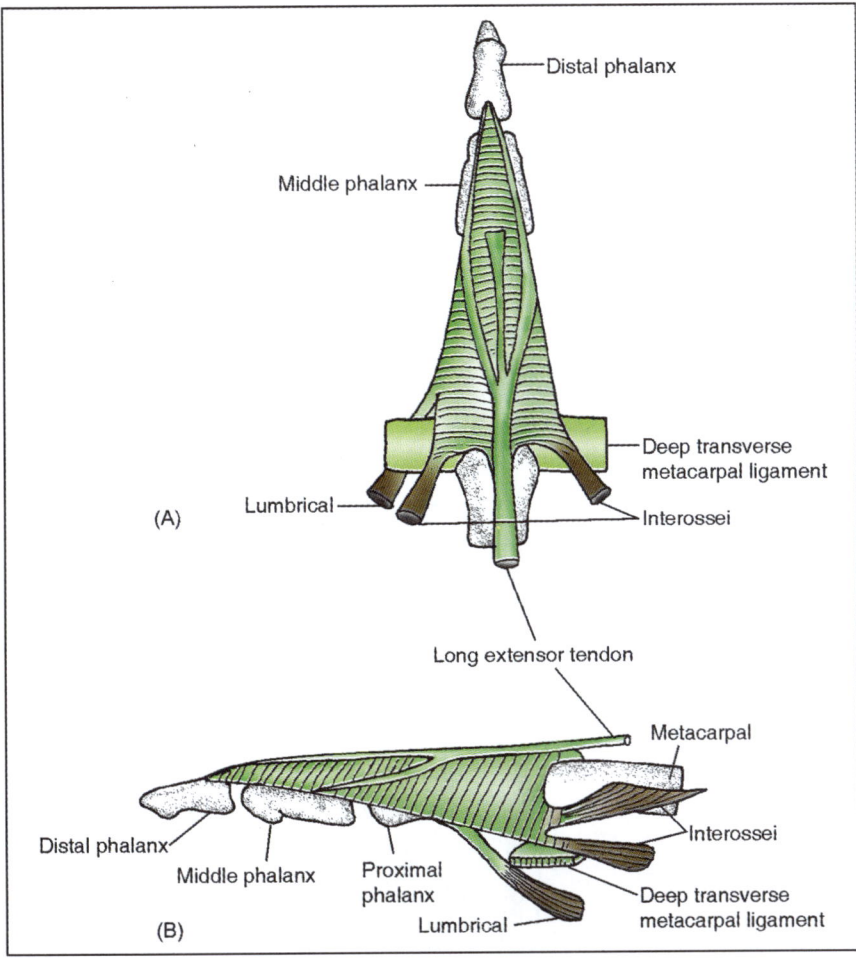

Fig. 16.2 Extensor expansion: (A) Dorsal view; (B) Side view

SUPERFICIAL MUSCLES OF EXTENSOR COMPARTMENT

Brachioradialis

Origin. Upper 2/3 rd of lateral supracondylar ridge of humerus.

Insertion. Just above the radial styloid process.

Nerve. Radial nerve.

Actions. Flexion of elbow. Brings fully supinated and pronated forearm to midprone position.

Applied anatomy. flexion of elbow is weakened if this muscle is paralysed. When the patient is asked to flex his elbow joint against resistance, the brachioradialis no longer springs up to bridge the angle between arm and forearm as it does normally.

Extensor carpi radialis longus

Origin. Lower 1/3 rd of lateral supracondylar ridge of humerus.

Insertion. Dorsal aspect of the base of 2nd metacarpal.

Nerve. Radial nerve.

Actions. With the extensor carpi ulnaris, causes extension at the wrist.

With the flexor carpi radialis causes abduction at the wrist.

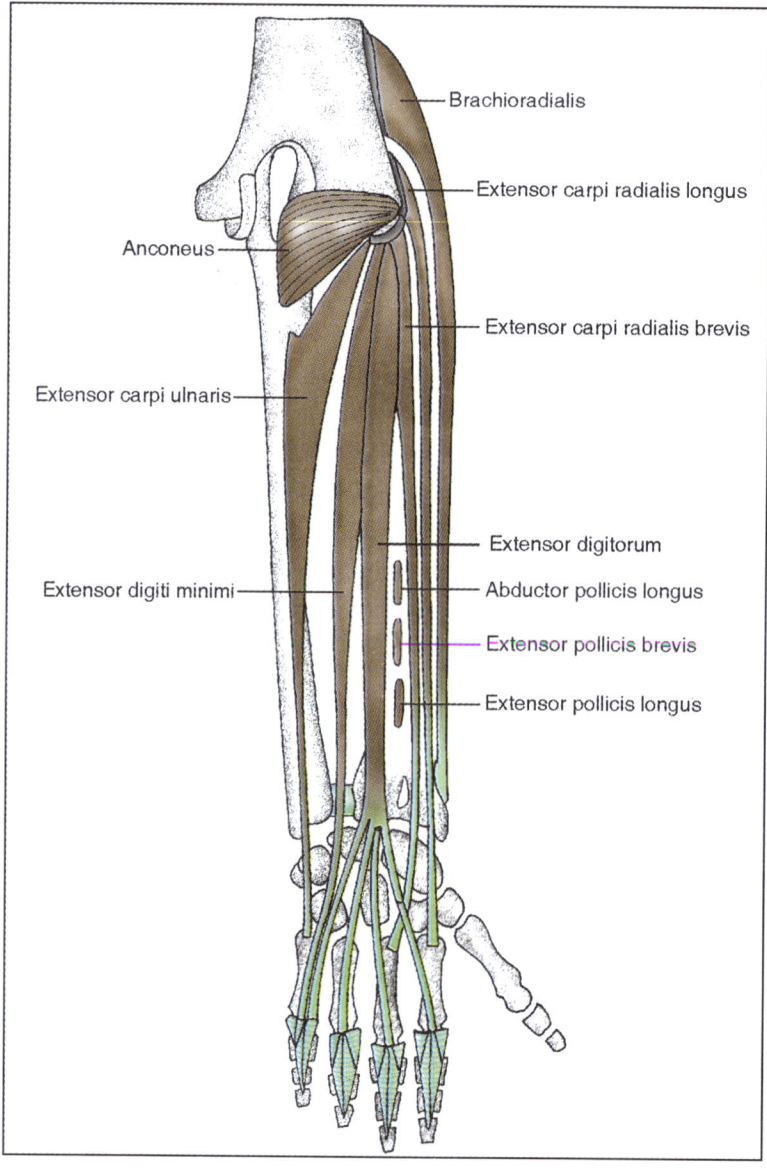

Fig. 16.3 Superficial muscles of the extensor compartment of forearm

Extensor carpi radialis brevis

Origin. Front of lateral epicondyle of humerus (common extensor origin).

Insertion. Dorsal aspect of the base of 3rd metacarpal.

Nerve. Deep branch of radial nerve.

Actions. With extensor carpi ulnaris, causes extension at wrist.

With flexor carpi radialis, causes abduction at wrist.

Extensor digitorum

Origin. Common extensor origin.

Insertion. It gives rise to 4 tendons for medial 4 digits. Each tendon gets attached to corresponding middle and distal phalanges through extensor expansion.

Nerve. Posterior interosseous nerve.

Action. Extension of medial four digits and wrist.

Applied anatomy. If paralysed, the patient is unable to prevent the examiner from flexing the extended fingers easily.

Extensor digiti minimi

Origin. Common extensor origin.

Insertion. Through extensor expansion to middle and distal phalanges of little finger.

Nerve. Posterior interosseous nerve.

Actions. Extension of little finger and wrist.

Extensor carpi ulnaris

Origin

Humeral head. Common extensor origin.

Ulnar head. Posterior border of ulna (There is a common aponeurotic origin for the flexor digitorum profundus, flexor carpi ulnaris and extensor carpi ulnaris).

Insertion. Dorsal aspect of the base of 5th metacarpal.

Nerve. Posterior interosseous nerve.

Actions. With extensor carpi radialis longus and brevis causes extension at wrist.

With flexor carpi ulnaris causes adduction at wrist.

Anconeus

Origin. Posterior surface of lateral epicondyle of humerus.

Insertion. Lateral aspect of olecranon process.

Nerve. Nerve to medial head of triceps from the radial nerve.

Actions. Abduction of ulna during pronation of forearm.

Weak extensor at the elbow.

DEEP MUSCLES OF EXTENSOR COMPARTMENT

Abductor pollicis longus

Origin. Upper part of posterior surfaces of radius and ulna and interosseous membrane.

Insertion. Base of the 1st metacarpal.

Nerve. Posterior interosseous nerve.

Actions. Abduction of thumb (at carpometacarpal joint).

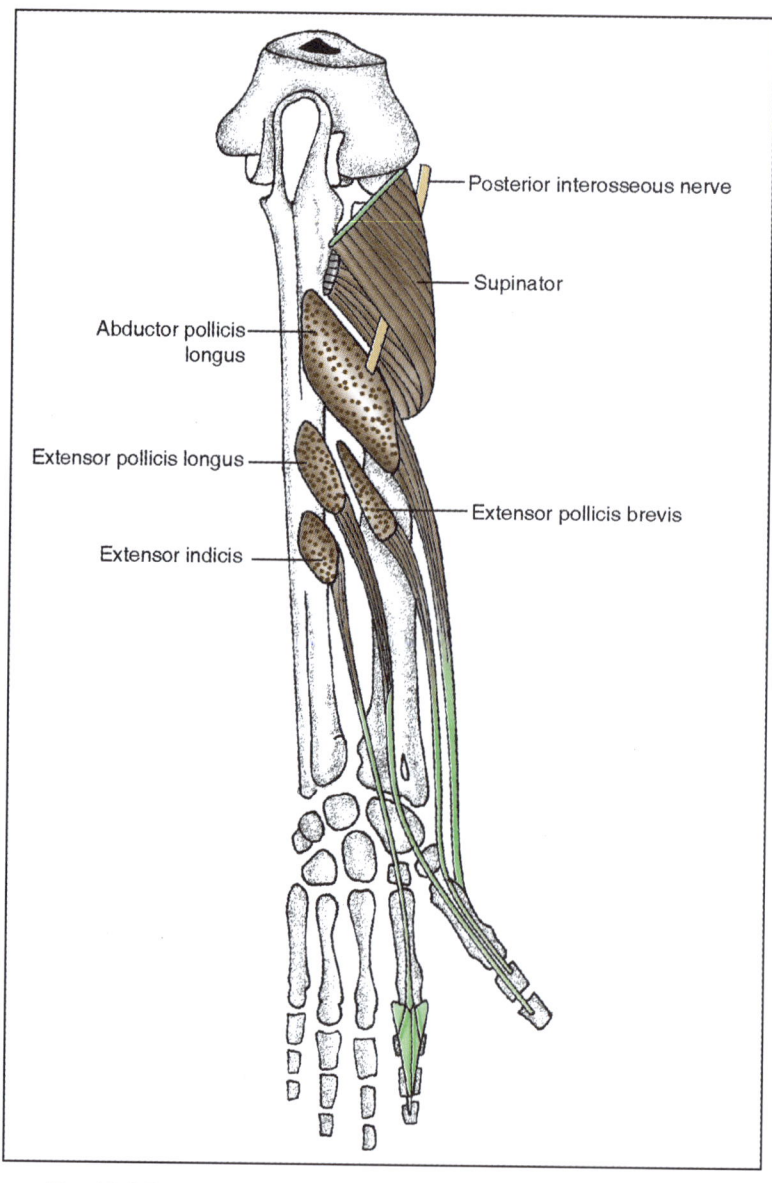

Fig. 16.4 Deep muscles of the extensor compartment of forearm

Applied anatomy. de Quervain's disease (stenosing synovitis) is a painful condition affecting the common tendon sheath of abductor pollicis longus and extensor pollicis brevis which become chronically inflamed and stenosed at radial styloid process. Passive flexion of thumb across palm induces pain.

Extensor pollicis brevis

Origin. Posterior surface of radius and adjacent interosseous membrane just below the origin of abductor pollicis longus.
Insertion. Base of the proximal phalanx of thumb.
Nerve. Posterior interosseous nerve.
Actions. Extension of proximal phalanx of thumb.
Applied. Involved in de Quervain's disease (see abductor pollicis longus).

Extensor pollicis longus

Origin. Posterior surface of ulna and adjacent interosseous membrane, jut below the origin of abductor pollicis longus and extensor pollicis brevis.
Insertion. Base of the distal phalanx of thumb.
Nerve. Posterior interosseous nerve
Applied anatomy. In case of rupture of extensor pollicis longus, patient feels pain at the base of thumb. Thumb falls simply against palm. Terminal joint is flexed and cannot be extended. It is usually due to rheumatoid arthritis.

Extensor indicis

Origin. Posterior surface of ulna and adjacent interosseous membrane just below the origin of extensor pollicis longus.
Insertion. Middle and distal phalanges of index finger, through extensor expansion.
Nerv. Posterior interosseous nerve.
Actions. Extension of index finger and wrist.

Supinator

Origin
> *Superficial head*. Lateral epicondyle of humerus, radial collateral ligament of elbow and annular ligament of radius.
> *Deep head*. Supinator crest and fossa of ulna.

Insertion. Lateral surface of radius between two oblique lines.
Nerve. Deep branch of radial nerve.
Actions. Supination of extended forearm.

SYNOVIAL SHEATHS OF EXTENSOR TENDONS

Like flexor tendons the tendons of extensor aspect while passing under the extensor retinaculum are also surrounded by *synovial sheaths*. Normally there are six sheaths corresponding to the number of compartments. Hower, each tendon of 1st and 2nd compartments may have individual sheaths. Proximally the sheath extends just proximal to extensor retinaculum. Distally, its termination is variable. The sheaths of tendons that gain insertion into the bases of the metacarpal bones extends upto the insersion. And that of the extensor pollicis brvis to the base of the 1st metacarpal bone. The sheaths for the tendons of long extensors including extensor pollicis longus extend to the level of the middle of metacarpus.

NERVES OF EXTENSOR COMPARTMENT

Deep branch of radial nerve

Course. As one of the terminal branch of radial nerve at the level of lateral epicondyle of humerus, it pierces the supinator. The nerve runs a course between two heads of supinator and appears on the back as posterior interosseous nerve.

Branches: To extensor carpi radialis brevis and supinator.

Posterior interosseous nerve

Course: nerve passes deep to the superficial group of extensor muscles. It first crosses abductor pollicis longus and extensor pollicis brevis superficially and then runs deep to extensor pollicis longus and extensor indicis to enter the 4th compartment deep to the extensor retinaculum.

Branches

Muscular. To all muscles of extensor compartment of forearm except anconeus, brachioradialis, extensor carpi radialis longus, extensor carpi radialis brevis and supinator.

Articular. To dorsal aspect of wrist and carpal joints.

Applied anatomy

- *Higher lesions of radial nerve (in axilla).* It causes paralysis of triceps. To test triceps, patient is asked to keep the arm on the table, flex the forearm at 90° and extend it against resistance. Paralysis of the brachioradialis weakens the flexion at elbow and the prominence made by this muscle in the angle between arm and forearm during flexion of forearm in midprone position is lost. The characteristic deformity noticed is wrist drop.

- *A lesion at the middle 3rd of humerus* (a frequent site of fracture) spares both triceps and brachioradialis, but wrist drop deformity is obvious similar to higher lesion.

- *Further lower lesion* involves posterior interosseous nerve and usually spares both the extensor carpi radialis longus and brevis and therefore typical *'wrist-drop'* deformity is not present.

- *Anaesthesia* in the territory of superficial branch of radial nerve is a constant feature in cases of its direct involvement or lesion of radial nerve.

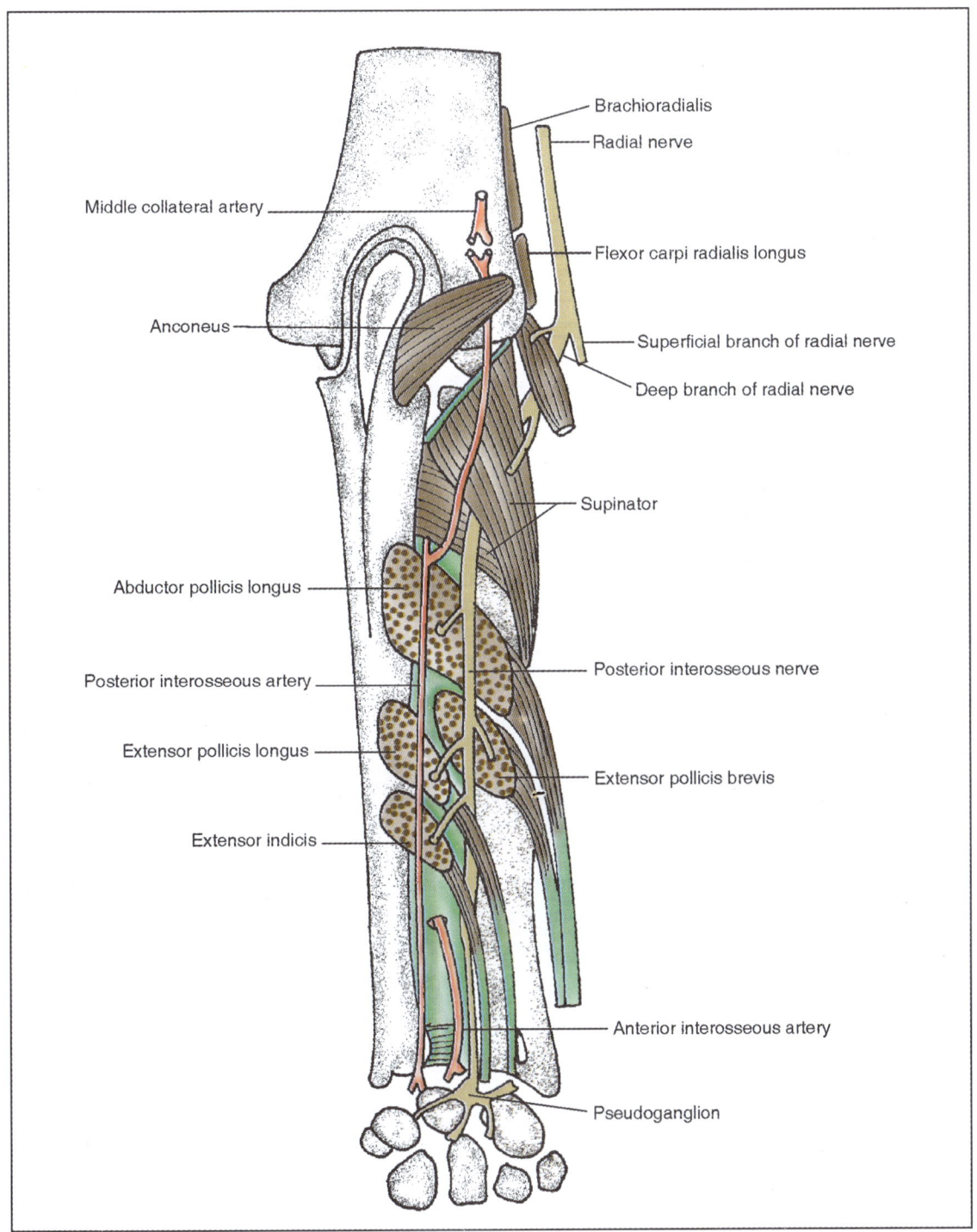

Fig. 16.5 Nerves and vessels of the extensor compartment of forearm

ARTERIES OF EXTENSOR COMPARTMENT

Posterior interosseous artery

Course. The artery appears below the lower border of supinator and descends between superficial and deep group of muscles.

Branches

1. *Muscular.*
2. *Interosseous recurrent artery.*
3. *Extends to dorsal carpal arch (rete).*

Anterior interosseous artery

It appears through a foramen in the lower part of interosseous membrane and descends through 4th compartment under extensor retinaculum to join the dorsal carpal arch.

17

Carpal Rete/Arch

Palmar and dorsal carpal arches are network of arteries in relation to the dorsal and palmar aspects of carpal bones. These supply adjacent carpal bones and joints. Dorsal carpal arch boosts the supply of dorsum of hand and digits.

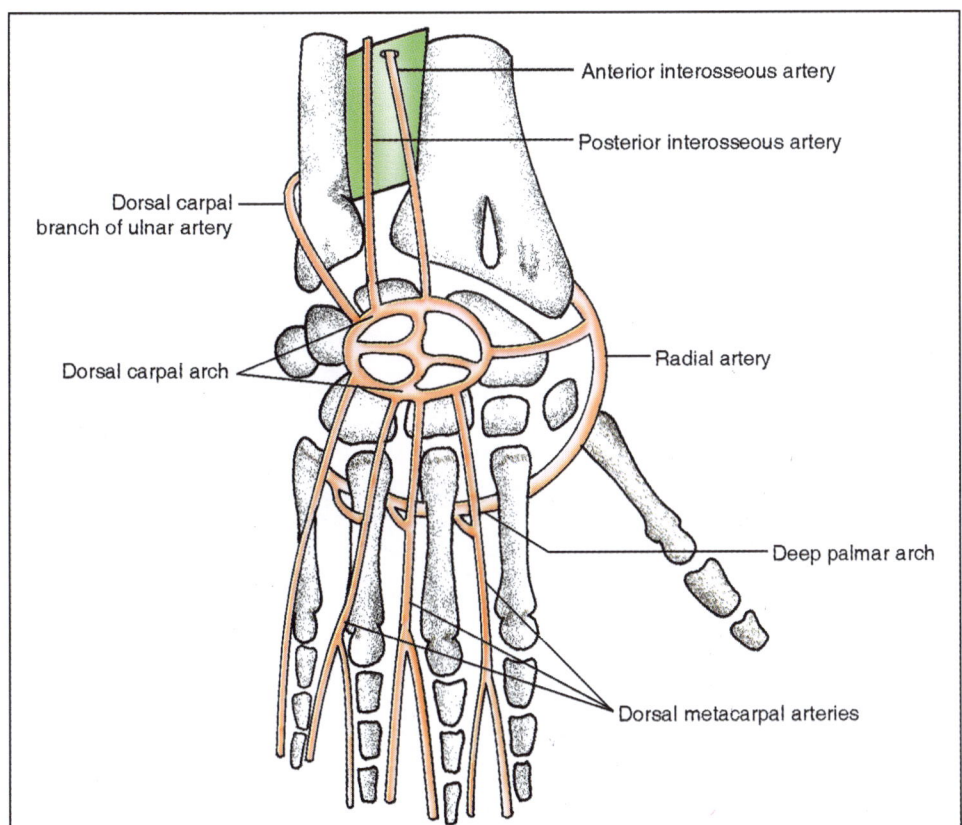

Fig. 17.1 Dorsal carpal arch

PALMAR CARPAL ARCH

Formation. It is formed by the following arteries,

1. Palmar carpal branch of radial artery.
2. Palmar carpal branch of ulnar artery.
3. Recurrent branch from deep palmar arch.
4. Descending branch from anterior interosseous artery.

DORSAL CARPAL ARCH

Formation. Following arteries contribute to this arch,

1. Anterior interosseous artery.
2. Posterior interosseous artery.
3. Dorsal carpal branch of radial artery.
4. Dorsal carpal branch of ulnar artery.

Branches

1. *Dorsal digital artery.* To the ulnar side of little finger.
2. *Dorsal metacarpal arteries (three).* To 2nd, 3rd and 4th interdigital clefts where these split into dorsal digital arteries to the adjacent sides of medial 4 digits. Dorsal metacarpal arteries are connected to deep palmar arch and palmar metacarpal arteries through perforators.

18

Intermediate Group of Muscles of Palm

It includes four lumbricals, three palmar interossei and four dorsal interossei. These muscles are numbered from lateral to medial side.

LUMBRICALS

Origin. Lumbricals arise from tendons of flexor digitorum profundus. Lateral two lumbricals are unipennate in nature and medial two are bipennate. The former originate from the radial sides of corresponding tendons. 3rd lumbrical arise from adjacent sides of 2nd and 3rd tendons while 4th lumbrical from the corresponding sides of 3rd and 4th profundus tendons.

Insertion. Each lumbrical gets attached to the radial side of corresponding extensor expansion.

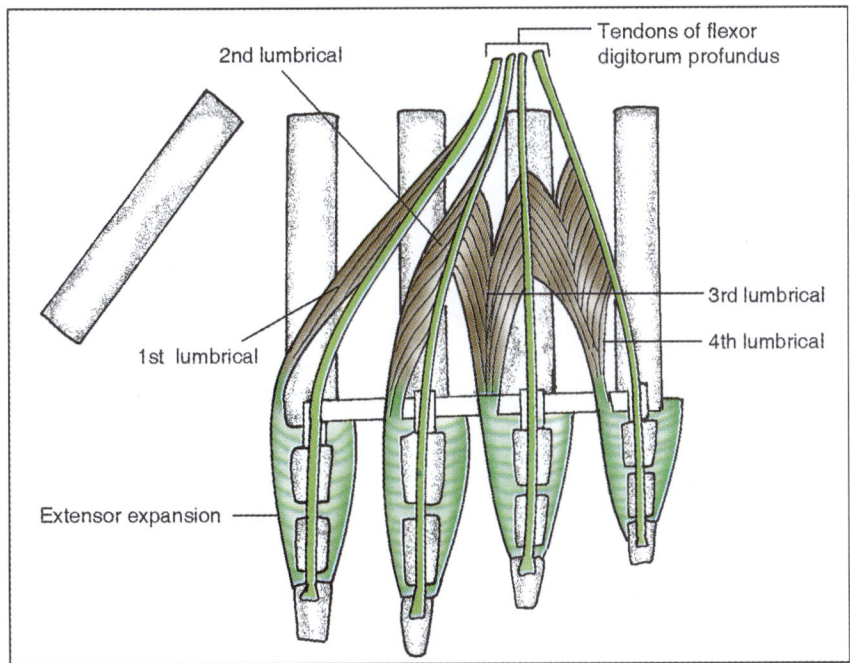

Fig. 18.1 Lumbricals

Nerve. Lateral two lumbricals are supplied by the median nerve and medial two lumbricals by the deep branch of the ulnar nerve.

Actions. Flexion at the metacarpophalangeal joints and extension at the interphalangeal joits of medial four digits.

PALMAR INTEROSSEI

Origin. Three palmar interossei arise from central finger sides of 2nd, 4th and 5th metacarpals.

Insertion. Three palmar interossei are inserted into central finger sides of proximal phalanges and extensor expansions of 2nd, 4th and 5th digits respectively.

Nerve. Deep branch of ulnar nerve.

Actions. Flexion at metacarpophalangeal joints, extension at the interphalangeal joints and adduction (movement towards middle finger) of 2nd, 4th and 5th digits respectively.

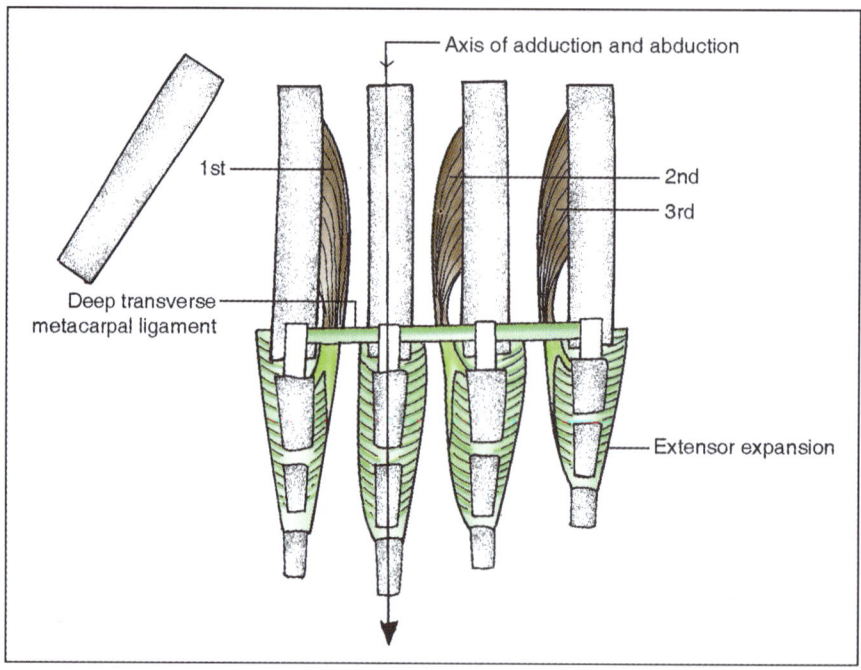

Fig. 18.2 Palmar interossei

DORSAL INTEROSSEI

Origin. Four dorsal interossei occupy the corresponding intermetatarsal spaces and arise from adjacent metacarpals.

Insertions

Lateral two.   To the radial sides of bases of proximal phalanges and extensor expansions of 2nd and 3rd digits.

Medial two. To the ulnar sides of bases of proximal phalanges and extensor expansions of 3rd and 4th digits.

Nerve. Deep branch of ulnar nerve.

Actions. Flexion at the metacarpophalangeal joints of middle three digits. 1st dorsal interosseous abducts (moves away from the central finger) the 2nd digit; 2nd and 3rd dorsal interossei abduct the central finger itself while last dorsal interosseous abducts the 4th digit.

Applied anatomy. All the interossei and medial two lumbricals are paralysed when ulnar nerve is injured. Lateral two lumbricals are paralysed due to median nerve lesion. *'Claw-hand'* deformity is a constant feature. In paralysed cases wasting of interossei is noticed in the form of depression in the intermetacarpal spaces appreciated from dorsal aspect.

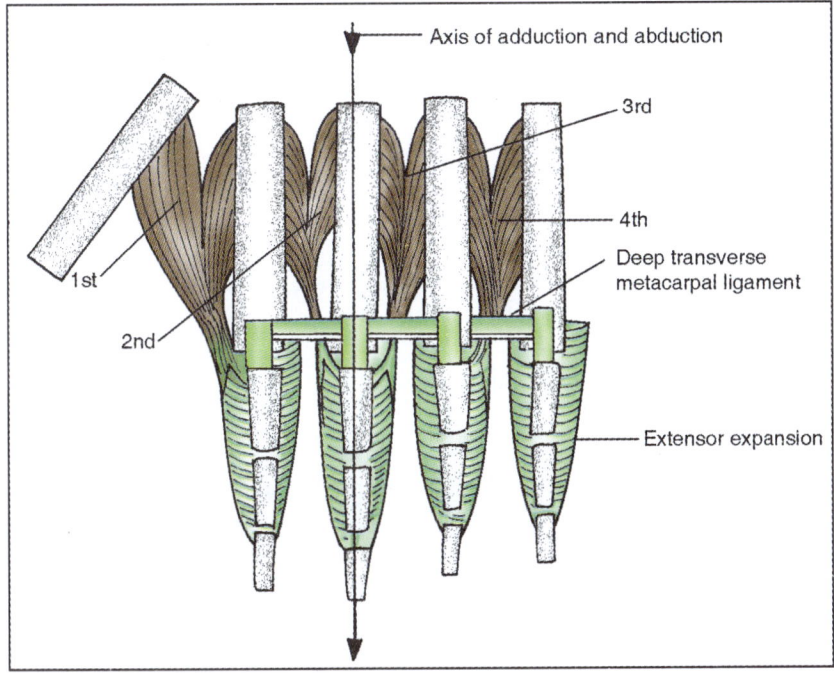

Fig. 18.3 Dorsal interossei

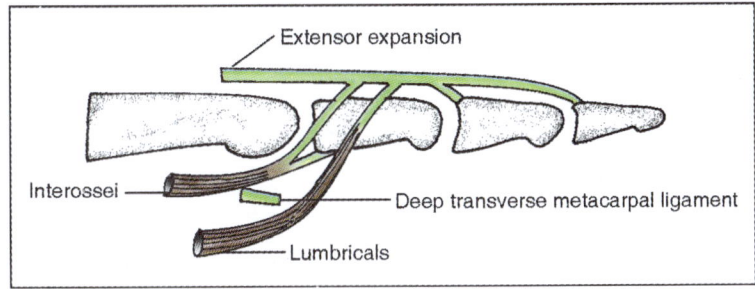

Fig. 18.4 Relations of lumbricals and interossei with joints of phalanges

19

Fascial Compartments

CLASSIFICATION

1. Forearm space of Parona.
2. Palmar spaces of hand,
    (a) Mid-palmar space.
    (b) Thenar space.
3. Dorsal spaces of hand,
    (a) Dorsal subcutaneous space.
    (b) Dorsal subaponeurotic space.
4. Pulp space.
5. Fascial compartment of thenar muscles.
6. Fascial compartment of hypothenar muscles.

FOREARM SPACE OF PARONA

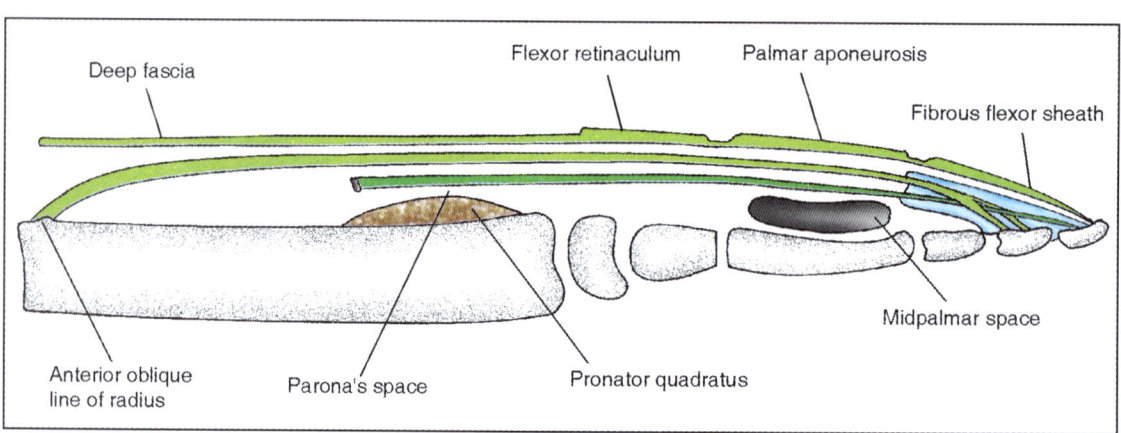

Fig. 19.1 Parona's space

Boundaries

Anterior. Long flexor tendons.

Posterior. Pronator quadratus.

Superior. Anterior oblique line of radius.

Inferior. Continues with carpal tunnel.

MIDPALMAR SPACE

Boundaries

Anterior

1. Common synovial sheath for flexor digitorum superficialis and profundus tendons.
2. Superficialis and profundus tendons for medial 3 digits with associated lumbricals.
3. Palmar aponeurosis.

Posterior

1. Fascia over the transverse head of adductor pollicis and interossei in 3rd and 4th intermentacarpal spaces
2. 3rd and 4th metacarpals

Lateral. Intermediate palmar septum.

Medial. Hypothenar muscles.

Distal. Distal palmar crease.

Proximal. Inferior margin of flexor retinaculum.

Lumbrical sheath. This is the tubular covering of lumbrical muscles. 2nd, 3rd and 4th lumbrical sheaths are considered as diverticula from the midpalmar space.

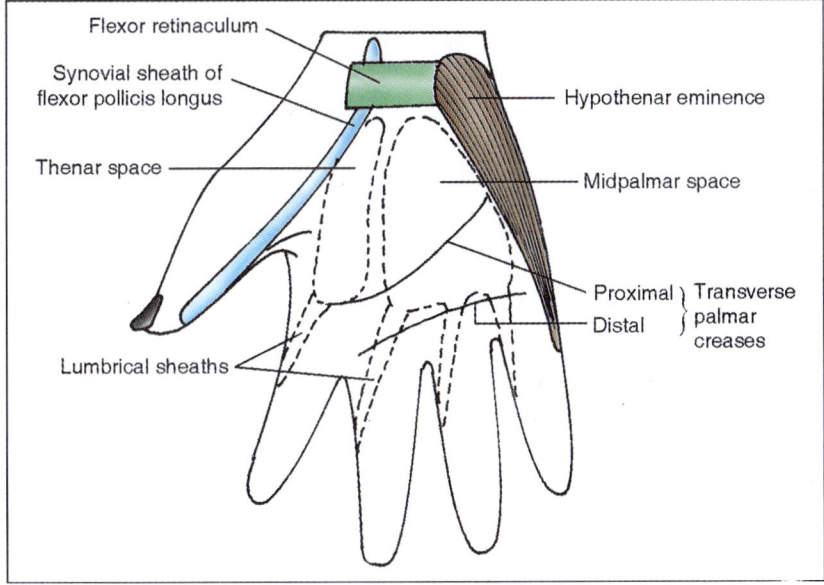

Fig. 19.2 Outline of the fascial compartments of palm

THENAR SPACE

Boundaries

Anterior. Thenar muscles, palmar aponeurosis, common synovial sheath, long flexor tendons for index finger and 1st lumbrical.

Posterior. Transverse head of adductor pollicis.

Lateral. Tendon of flexor pollicis longus with synovial sheath.

Medial. Intermediate palmar septum.

Distal. Proximal transverse palmar crease.

Proximal. Distal margin of flexor retinaculum.

Ist lumbrical sheath. It is considered to be a diverticulum from the thenar sapace.

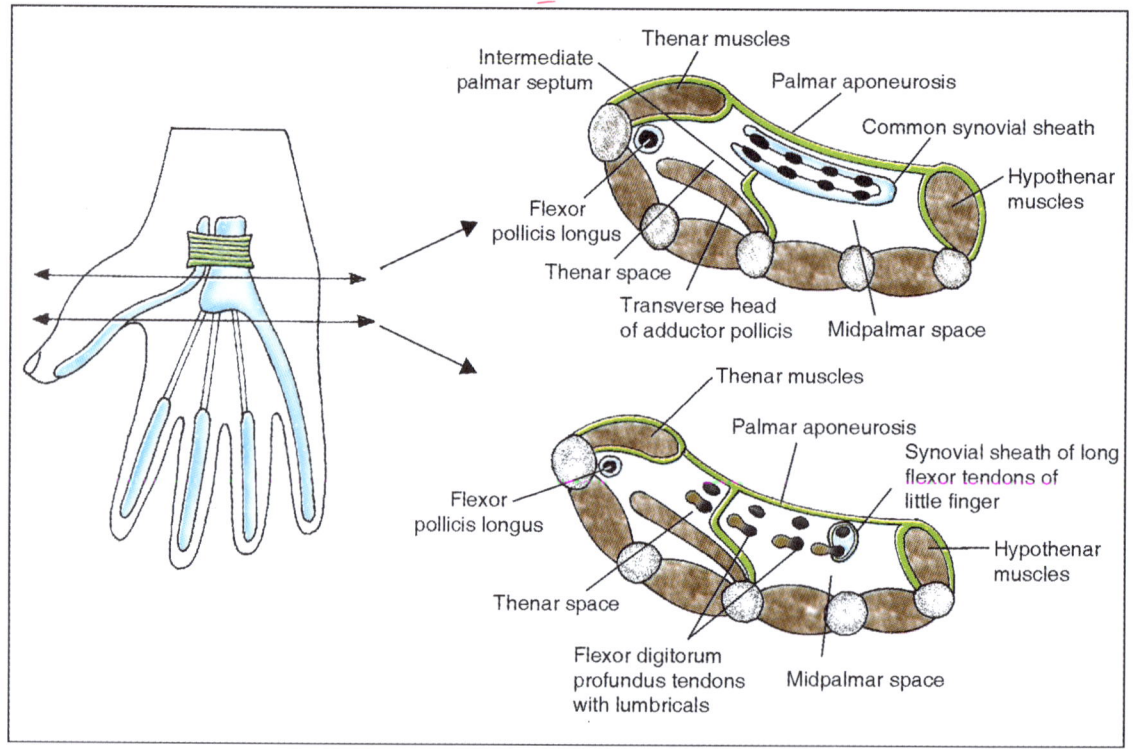

Fig. 19.3 Fascial compartments of palm

DORSAL SPACES OF HAND

Both dorsal subcutaneous and subaponeurotic spaces are triangular in shape with apex at the wrist and base at knuckles. The spaces continue with subcutaneous tissue of adjacent area i.e. proximally with forearm, distally with web of fingers, medially and laterally with the palm.

Pulp space

It is the space between skin and phalanges. It consists of fat in tight compartments of fibrous septa in relation to corresponding phalanges. These are named as terminal, middle and proximal pulp spaces.

Fascial compartments of thenar and hypothenar muscles

These are muscular compartments containing muscles of the corresponding eminence covered with the layer of deep fascia of palm.

Applied anatomy

- Infection of terminal pulp space is common and potentially serious. The digital pulps are subjected to relatively more pricks. The terminal pulp is separated from the rest of the finger by a fascial septum at the level of epiphysial line of the terminal phalanx. Therefore when infected, tension within the space becomes extreme and leads to thrombosis and necrosis of soft tissue and the terminal phalanx.
- The abscess in the middle pulp space spreads to distal flexion crease while that of proximal pulp space spreads to the web space.
- Infection of thenar space gives rise to the typical 'ballooning' of thenar eminence.
- Mid-palmar space infection can result from bursting of an undrained infected flexor tendon sheath of middle, ring or little finger. Cocavity of the palm is obliterated in this condition.
- Midpalmar and thenar spaces can also be involved due to infection of fingers involving lumbrical sheaths.
- Pus in the midpalmar and thenar spaces can be successfully drained by incising the relevant lumbrical sheath.
- The most frequent causes of dorsal space infection are a boil of the overlying skin and a penetrating wound.
- Infection of dorsal subcutaneous space is fairly common but that of subaponeurotic space is rare.

20

Elbow Joint

DISSECTION STEPS: ELBOW JOINT

Separate the muscles from the epicondyles and reflect them distally. Divide the biceps, brachialis and triceps about 3-4 cm proximal to the elbow and turn them distally. Separate the surrounding muscles from the fibrous capsule of the elbow joint retaining the brachial vessels and nerves (median, radial and ulnar). Make a transverse incision through the anterior and posterior parts of the fibrous capsule and identify the synovial membrane.

Classification

Hinge, synovial.

Articular surfaces

Elbow joint has two components,

1. *Humero-ulnar.* Between trochlea of humerus and trochlear notch of ulna.
2. *Humero-radial.* Between capitulum of humerus and capitular surface of head of radius.

Note *Elbow joint and superior radioulnar joint share common cavity and together constitute **cubital articulation**.*

Capsule

Proximally it is attached to the lower end of humerus. On medial and lateral sides it is attached to the articular margins. Anteriorly it encloses radial and coronoid fossae while posteriorly it is attached to the middle of olecranon fossa.

Distally capsule gets attached to articular margin of ulna medially and superior margin of annular ligament of radius laterally.

Synovial membrane

It lines the interior of capsule and also covers the intracapsular parts of ***humeral*** fossae.

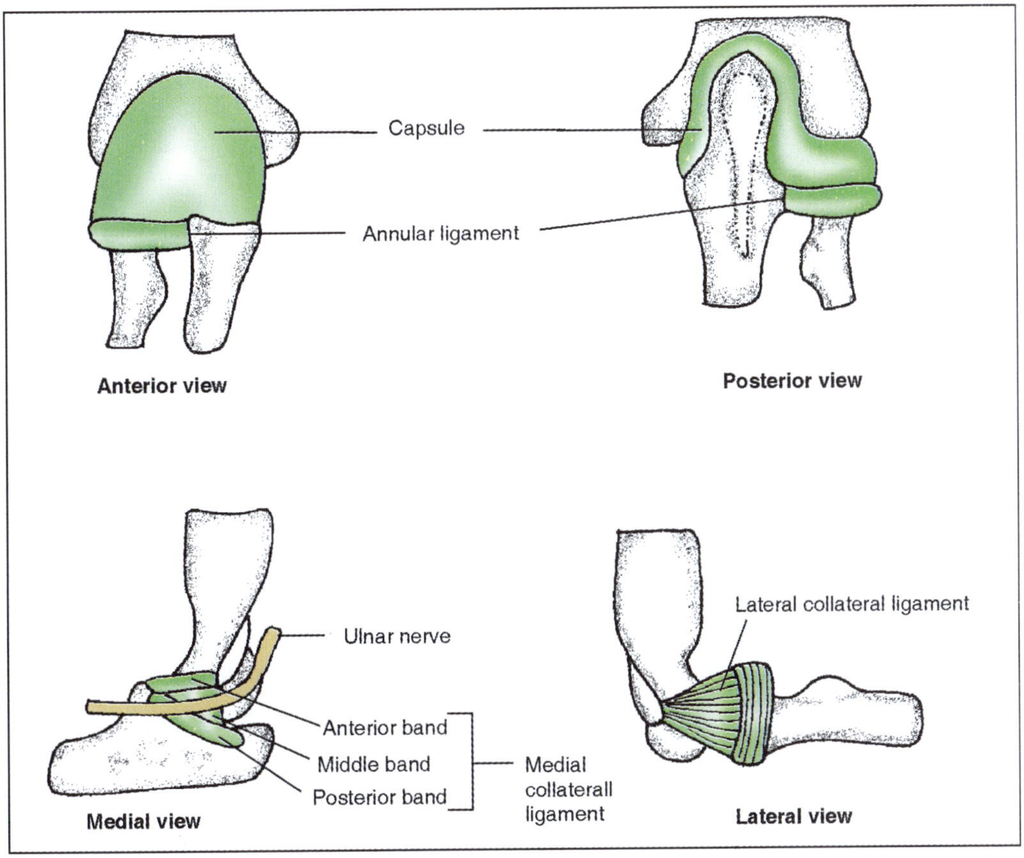

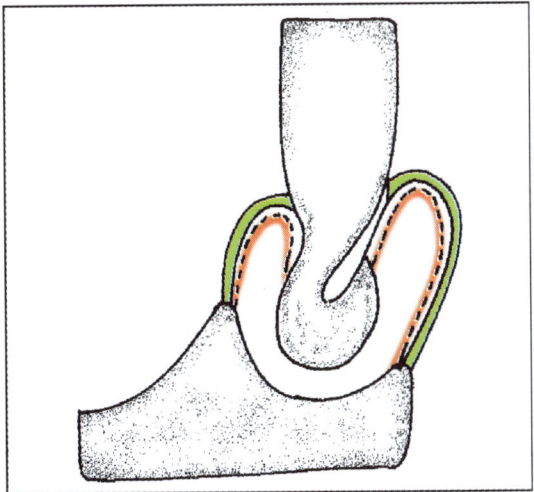

Fig. 20.1 Elbow joint

Anterior view

Posterior view

Capsule

Annular ligament

Ulnar nerve

Anterior band

Middle band

Posterior band

Medial collaterall ligament

Medial view

Lateral collateral ligament

Lateral view

Fig. 20.2 Synovial membrane of the elbow joint

Ligaments

Capsule is thickened medially and laterally, named as ulnar and radial collateral ligaments respectively. Radial collateral ligament extends from the lateral epicondyle to annular ligament of superior radio-ulnar joint. Ulnar collateral ligament has three bands-anterior, posterior and middle. Anterior band extends from medial epicondyle to coronoid process, posterior from olecranon to coronoid process while the middle band bridges between the two bands. Middle band is crossed by the ulnar nerve.

Nerve

All main nerves of upper limb (median, ulnar, musculocutaneous and radial) supply elbow joint.

Arteries

Elbow receives arteries from the anastomoses around it.

Movements

Being uniaxial, the only movements possible are flexion and extension. Range of the former is approximately 140°. Long axis of extended forearm forms an angle of 170° with the long axis of the arm. This is called carrying angle. This is due to downward projection of medial flange of trochlea (about 6 mm) compared to the lateral flange. Angulation of forearm is more (reducing the carrying angle) in female. Carrying angle allows the limb to swing slightly away from the body.

Applied anatomy

- In case of arthritis of elbow joint, patient prefers to flex at 90° as well as pronate the forearm, as this is the position of greatest ease.
- Three bony points, tip of olecranon, the medial epicondyle and lateral epicondyle, form an equilateral triangle when the elbow is flexed at 90°. In extended forearm, three bony points come to lie in one horizontal line. In dislocation of elbow this relationship is altered. While it is maintained in supracondylar fracture of humerus.
- The carrying angle may become altered by fracture or injury to the epiphysis of the lower end of the humerus. If decreased, the condition is known as cubitus varus; when increased, the condition is called cubitus valgus.

  (*Note*. Clinicians consider the lower angle as carrying angle, which is described as 10° in male and 20° in female. The above description applies to same angle).
- Improtance of cubitus valgus lies in the fact that it causes ulnar nerve to become very much stretched and unduly exposed to trauma.
- Effusion of elbow joint first manifests itself by the fullness of the concavity on each side of the olecranon, because here the synovial cavity is nearest to the surface and the posterior ligament is thin and lax.
- In case of loose bodies in the elbow joint, there is always history of locking.
- *Tennis elbow* (*epicondylitis*). This condition is due to sprain in the region of lateral epicondyle. Interestingly, very few of numerous sufferers play tennis.

- *The elbow tunnel syndrome.* In this case, ulnar nerve is involved close to elbow. A tight band of fibrous arch joining the two heads of flexor carpi ulnaris might compress the ulnar nerve and cause the syndrome.
- Dislocation of elbow joint occurs as a result of fall on outstretched hand, since the olecranon is displaced, the bony triangle is no more equilateral.
- Fracture of of olecranon occurs as a result of direct or indirect violence.
- Fracture of coronoid process, less frequent to occur, is usually associated with dislocation.
- An incision on the lateral side of elbow should not be extended lower than the head of radius to avoid damage to the posterior interosseous nerve.
- Aspiration from the elbow joint should be done from the lateral side to avoid injury to ulnar nerve on the medial side.

21

Radioulnar Joints

These have three components, proximal, middle and distal.

PROXIMAL (SUPERIOR) RADIOULNAR JOINT

Classification

Pivot type of synovial joint.

Articular surfaces

It is the circumference of head of radius which articulates with the radial notch of ulna and inner surface of annular ligament. Articular surfaces are lined by hyaline cartilage.

Ligaments

Annular ligament: It encircles the head and gets attached to anterior and posterior margins of radial notch of ulna. This ligament receives attachment of capsule of elbow to its superior border. It is free from radial neck and allows protrusion of synovial membrane beyond its lower border.

Quadrate ligament: It connects the inferior border of radial notch of ulna to the medial aspect of neck of radius.

Nerve

Musculocutaneous, median and radial nerves.

MIDDLE RADIOULNAR UNION (SYNDESMOSIS)

It is the *interosseous membrane* which connects the opposing interosseous borders of two bones of forearm i.e. medial border of radius and lateral border of ulna. Direction of fibres in it is downwards and medially. It performs following functions.

1. Holds two bone together
2. Transmits the force from radius to ulna during thrust on hand.

3. Provides area for muscular attachment.
4. Supports the course of anterior and posterior interosseous nerves and vessels.

Oblique cord. It is an oblique band of fibres connecting the ulnar tuberosity to radius just below its tuberosity.

DISTAL (INFERIOR) RADIOULNAR JOINT

Classification

Pivot type of synovial joint.

Articular surfaces

Head of ulna articulates with ulnar notch of radius and the articular disc.

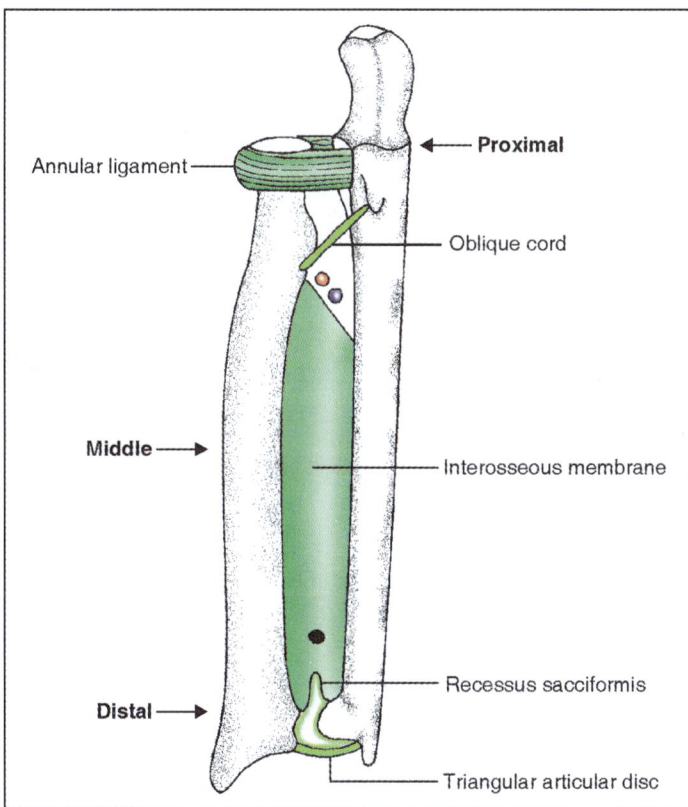

Fig. 21.1 Radioulnar joints

Articular disc

It is a triangular fibrocartilage with its base to the lower margin of ulnar notch of radius and apex to the fossa at the base of ulnar styloid process.

Capsule

It covers the joint anteriorly, posteriorly and superiorly. Its upper part is lax and makes an upward extension in front of interosseous membrane called *recessus sacciformis*.

Nerve

Anterior and posterior interosseous nerves.

MOVEMENTS AT RADIOULNAR JOINTS

Being uniaxial, the joint allows pronation and supintion. Forearm in anatomical position is said to be fully supinated. During pronation the lower end of radius along with hand rotates in such a way that at the end of movement palm faces backwards. Reverse of this movement is called supination. Axis of pronation and supination passes through the center of head of radius above and base of ulnar styloid process below.

Applied anatomy

- *Subluxation of head of radius (pulled elbow)*. When a child's arm is pulled forcibly, it results into subluxation of radial head through the annular ligament.
- *Galieazzi fracture*. This is a fracture–dislocation of the lower end of radius with dislocation of inferior radioulnar joint. The mechanism seems to be fall on hand with a rotational force superimposed on it. Associated ulnar nerve lesion is quite common in this condition.

Wrist Joint

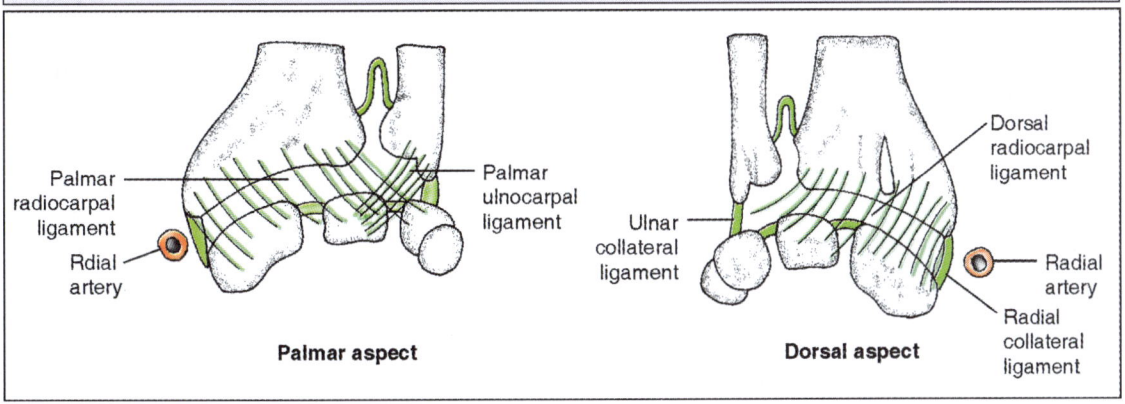

Fig. 22.1 Wrist (Radiocarpal) joint

Classification

Ellipsoid (biaxial) type of synovial joint.

Articular surfaces

Proximal concavity: It is provided by the inferior surface of lower end of radius and articular disc of inferior radioulnar joint.

Distal convexity: It is produced by the superior surfaces of scaphoid, lunate and triquetral and the interosseous ligaments between them.

Ligaments

1. *Capsule.* It is attached to the margins of articular surfaces, articular disc and interosseous ligament.
2. *Palmar radiocarpal ligament.*
3. *Palmar ulnocarpal ligament.*
4. *Dorsal radiocarpal ligament.*

    2, 3 and 4 are thickenings on the palmar and dorsal aspects of capsule. Their names indicate their attachments.

5. *Radial collateral ligament.* It is thickening of capsule laterally extending from radial styloid process to scaphoid. It is crossed by the radial artery.
6. *Ulnar collateral ligament.* It is thickening of capsule medially connecting ulnar styloid process with triquetral.

Nerves

Anterior and posterior interosseous nerves.

Movements

Being biaxial, it allows flexion, extension, abduction and adduction. Flexion and extension movements simultaneously take place in midcarpal joints. Total range of flexion is 85°, of which greater proportion occurs at the midcarpal joint. Total range of extension is also 85°, but its major proportion occurs at the wrist joint itself. Abduction is limited to 15° only due to the downward projection of radial styloid process. Range of adduction is upto 45°.

Applied anatomy

- Both *osteoarthritis* and *rheumatoid arthritis* are common in wrist joint. *Chronic arthritis* produces swelling, tenderness and limitation of movements.

- *Carpal tunnel* is one the important region adjacent to wrist commonly involved. Carpal tunnel syndrome denotes a compressive neuropathy of the median nerve as it passes through the carpal tunnel. The syndrome is occasionally secondary to narrowing of tunnel after **Colles' fracture** or rheumatoid arthritis.

- *Ganglion.* It is the result of myxomatous degeneration occurring in the connective tissue of capsule of joint. Its most common location is dorsum of wrist over the scaphoid-lunar articulation.

- *Fracture of radial styloid process* is caused by forced radial deviation of wrist on falling.

- *Fracture of scaphoid* results from a fall on outstretched hand. This is because of the fact that scaphoid opposes extension of wrist and when intercarpal joint is excessively extended, it breaks. Swelling and tenderness in the anatomical snuff box are most marked signs.

- *Dislocation of lunate*. Normally the lunate occupies the hollow that can be felt on the back of the wrist immediatedly distal to radius in the line of middle finger. When bone is dislocated, this hollowness becomes more concave than normal. Usually, this is a sign of carpal tunnel compression.

- The surgical approach to wrist is on its dorsal aspect between tendon of extensor pollicis longus laterally and tendon of extensor digitorum and indicis medially. There are no major nerve and vessels in this region.

- The best way to indicate the joint line is to palpate the radial styloid process in the anatomical snuff box.

23

Joints of Hand

INTERCARPAL, CARPOMETACARPAL AND INTERMETACARPAL JOINTS

Pisifrom joint

It is an independent plane type of synovial joint between dorsal surface of pisiform and palmar aspect of triquetral. Pisohamate and pisometacarpal ligaments connect the pisiform to the back of hamate and base of 5th metacarpal bone respectively. Both are said to be continuation of the tendon of flexor carpi ulnaris.

Carpometacarpal joint of thumb

It is a saddle type of synovial joint between trapezium and base of 1st metacarpal. It is different from the rest of carpometacarpal joints due to being independent and very movable (1st metacarpal is functional).

Movements of thumb

It is complex phenomenon. Thumb moves at carpometacarpal, metcarpophalangeal and interphalangeal joints. The degree of mobility increases from distal to proximal, being minimum at interphalangeal (flexion and extension), moderate at metcarpophalangeal (flexion, extension, adduction and abduction) and maximum at the carpometacarpal joint (flexion, extension, adduction and abduction as well as rotation). Since, the plane of thumb is perpendicular to that of palm, flexion and extension occur in coronal plane (plane of palm) and adduction and abduction occur in sagittal plane (perpendicular to plane of palm). Medial rotation brings the pulp of the thumb against the palm. A combination of abduction, flexion and medial rotation, in that sequence, brings the pulp of thumb against the slightly fixed fingers' pulp. This is called opposition. Reverse of opposition is reposition which includes lateral rotation, extension and adduction.

Range of flexion of thumb
1. At the interphalangeal joint – 80°.
2. At the metacarpophalangeal joint – 90°.
3. At carpometacarpal joint – 15°.

Range of abduction

1. At carpometacarpal joint – 70°.
2. At metacarpophalangeal joint – 25°.

Main joint complex

Rest of the intercarpal, carpometacarpal and intermetacarpal joints share single cavity called main joint complex.

Bones are held together by palmar, dorsal, and interosseous ligaments. Midcarpal joint is the junction between proximal and distal rows of carpal bones. Midcarpal joint is closed medially and laterally by the collateral ligaments.

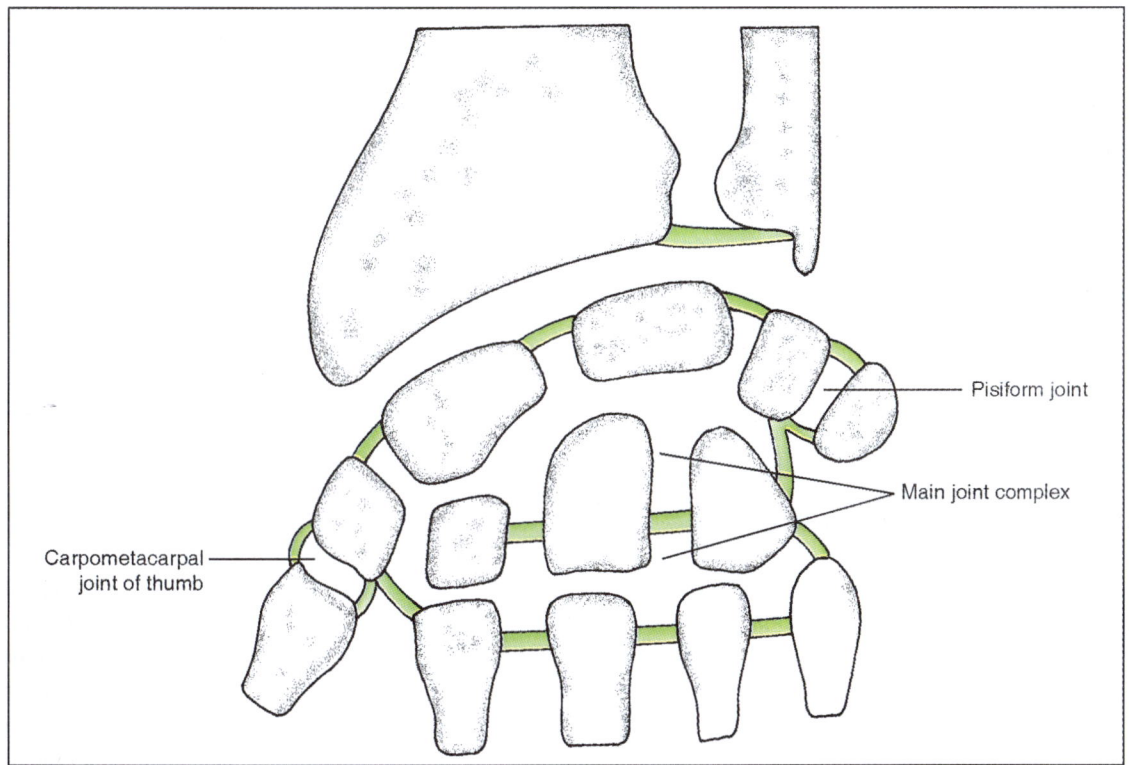

Fig. 23.1 Small joints of hand

Metacarpophalangeal joints

Each of them is an *ellipsoid type* of synovial joint between the head of metacarpal and base of proximal phalanx. The capsule is thickened medially and laterally forming medial and lateral *collateral ligaments* respectively. Thickening on the palmar aspect constitute *palmar ligament*. Margins of adjacent palmar ligaments of medial 4 metacarpophalangeal joints are connected by transversely running bands of fibres. These constitute three *deep transvese metacarpal ligament*.

Movements

Being biaxial, it allows flexion, extension, abduction and adduction.

Range of movements

Flexion – 90°

Abduction and adduction – 30° each

Extension – Few degrees only.

Applied anatomy

- Metacarpophalangeal joint is a common site for rheumatoid arthritis. In the first stage there is only hypertrophy of synovial membrane (*pannus*). The sencond stage is characterized by the ulnar deviation of fingers at the metacarpophalangeal joints

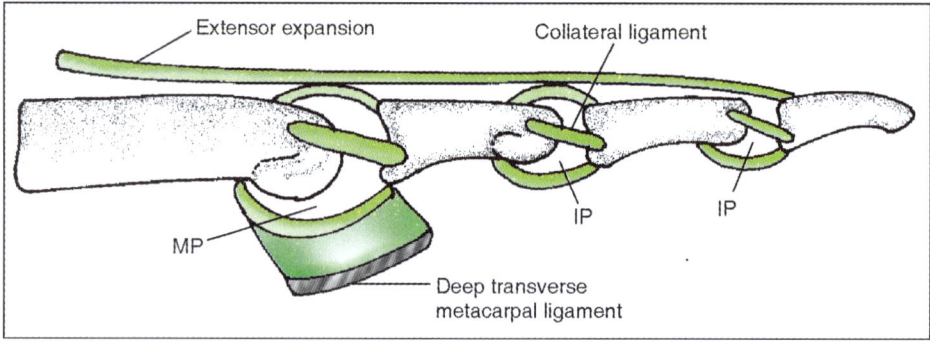

Fig. 23.2 Metacarpophalangeal (MP) and interphalangeal (IP) joints

INTERPHALANGEAL JOINTS

These are *hinge type* of synovial joints between heads and bases of adjacent phalanges.

Its *capsule* is strengthened medially and laterally by medial and lateral *collateral ligaments* respectively. *Palmar ligament* is thickening of capsule on palmar aspect. Being hinge, allows only flexion and extension.

Applied anatomy

- Sprain of an interphalangeal joint is a common occurrence. It gives rise to a spindle-shaped swelling of the digit.

Part-III
Lower Limb

Subdivisions of Lower Limb

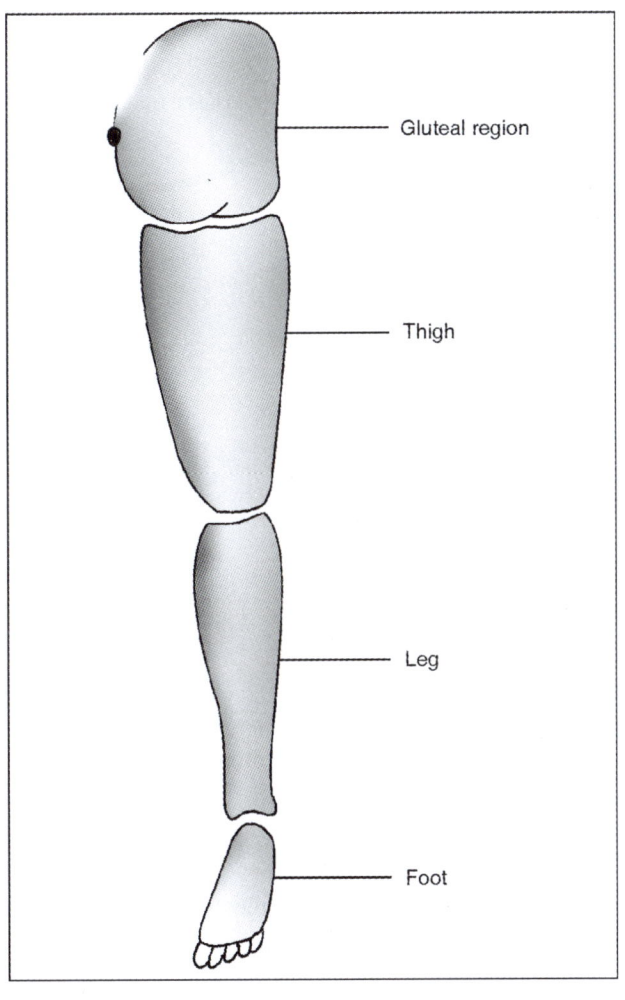

Fig. 24.1 Subdivisions of lower limb

Front of Thigh

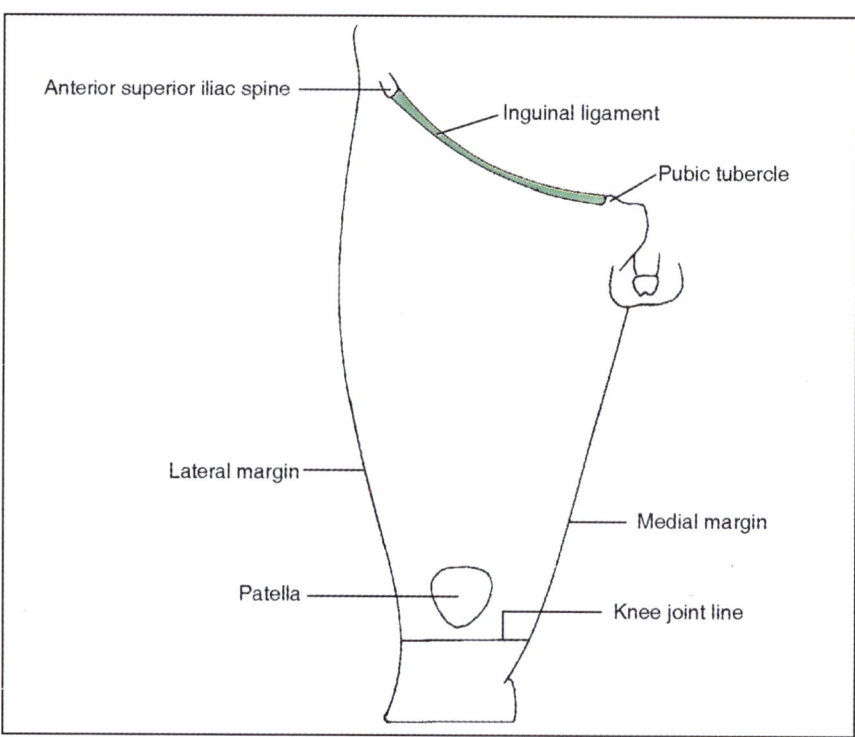

Fig. 25.1 Boundaries of front of thigh

MEMBRANOUS LAYER OF SUPERFICIAL FASCIA

Deep layer of the superficial fascia in the lower part of the anterior abdominal wall is membranous in nature. This is named as the fascia of Scarpa. It descends into the thigh and gets attached to the deep fascia of the thigh along the Holden's line. This line is 8 cm in length and extends laterally from the pubic tubercle.

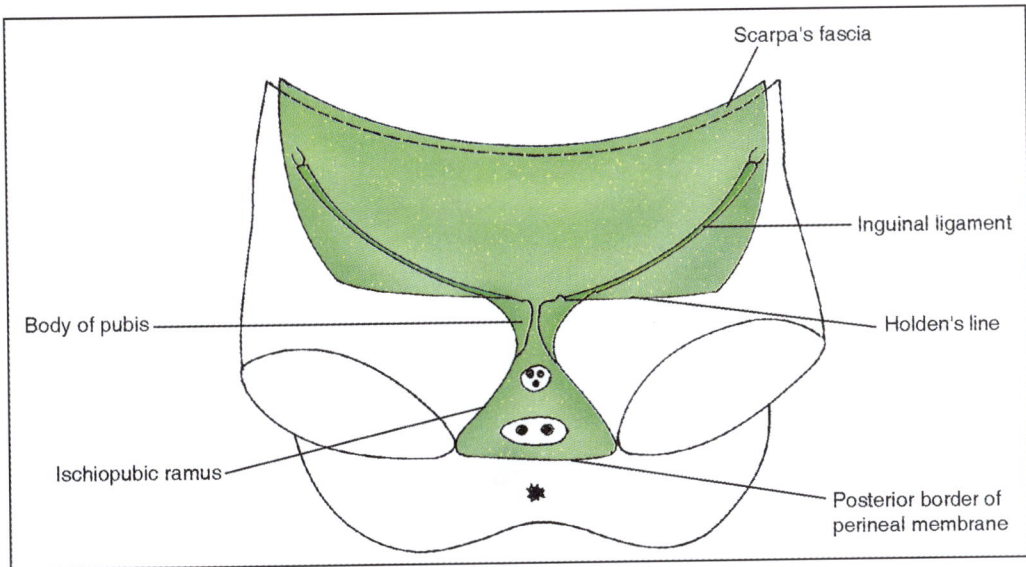

Fig. 25.2 Scarpa's fascia

Applied anatomy

- Extravasation of urine due to the rupture of penile urethra leads to swelling in the upper thigh, urogenital region and lower abdomen. The lower limit of the swelling in the thigh is the Holden's line.

SAPHENOUS OPENING

It is a vertically oval area of weakness in the deep fascia of thigh located 3 cm below and lateral to the pubic tubercle. The opening is 3 cm long and 1.5 cm wide. Its membrane is perforated by lymphatic and blood vessels, which pass through it. It is therefore called as cribriform fascia. Superior, lateral and the inferior margins of the saphenous opening are well defined and named as the falciform margin. The structures passing through the saphenous opening are:

- *Great saphenous vein*
- *Lymphatics*
- *Superficial arteries*
  1. *superficial epigastric artery.*
  2. *superficial external pudendal artery,*
  3. *deep external pudendal artery.*

Applied anatomy

- Contents of the femoral hernia pass through the femoral canal and then push the cribriform fascia forward to ascend up in the subcutaneous fat, thus making a typical 'U' shaped hernia.

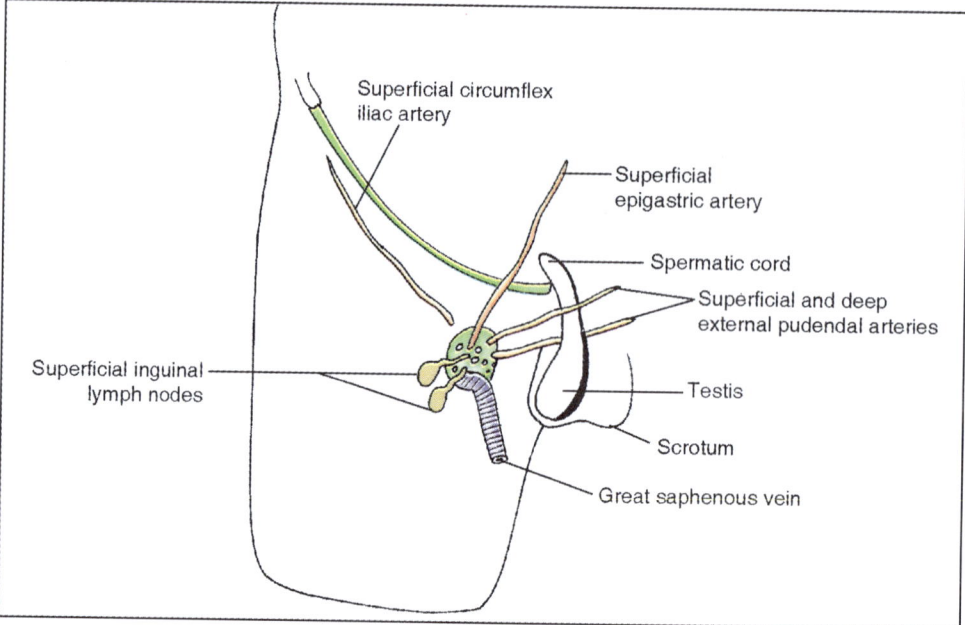

Fig. 25.3 Saphenous opening

SUPERFICIAL INGUINAL LYMPH NODES

These form a 'T' shaped pattern just below the inguinal ligament. It consists of a horizontal chain of lymph nodes which is further divided into the medial and lateral groups. The vertical chain forms the vertical limb of 'T'.

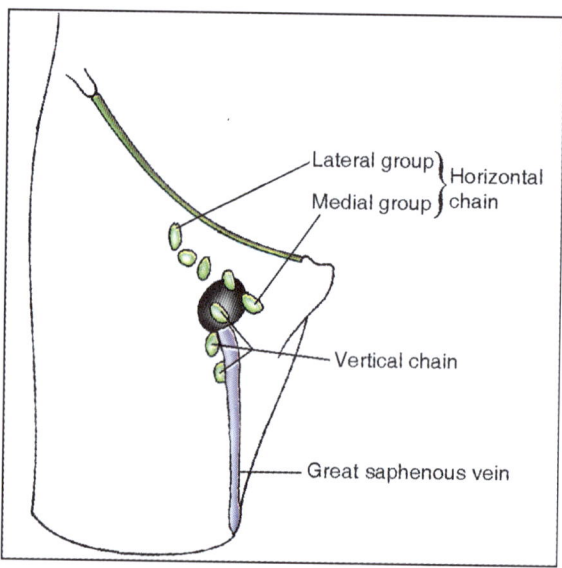

Fig. 25.4 Superficial inguinal lymph nodes

SUPERFICAL ARTERIES

Superficial arteries appear in the upper part of the front of thigh, majority of which pass through the cribriform fascia. The only artery which pierces the deep fascia lateral to the saphenous opening is the *superficial circumflex iliac artery*. It runs towards the anterior superior iliac spine. *Superficial epigastric artery* ascends towards the anterior abdominal wall. *External pudendal arteries* run medially and are two in number, i.e., superficial and deep. The former passes superficial to while the latter deep to the spermatic cord in male or round ligament of uterus in female.

DISSECTION STEPS: FRONT OF THIGH

Make incisions 9 and 10 (Fig. 3.13) and reflect the skin flaps laterally. *Because of the paucity of the superficial fascia at the knee care must be exercised if the patellar plexus of cutaneous nerve is to be preserved.* Identify the inguinal ligament, great saphenous vein and trace it to the saphenous opening. Identify the various structures piercing the cribriform fascia. Expose the deep fascia and identify the femoral sheath with its contents (femoral vein, femoral artery and deep inguinal lymph node in the femoral canal). Clean and define the muscles of the front of the thigh, namely sartorius crossing the front of thigh, quadriceps forming the bulk of the thigh, tensor fasciae latae and iliopsoas.

CUTANEOUS NERVES

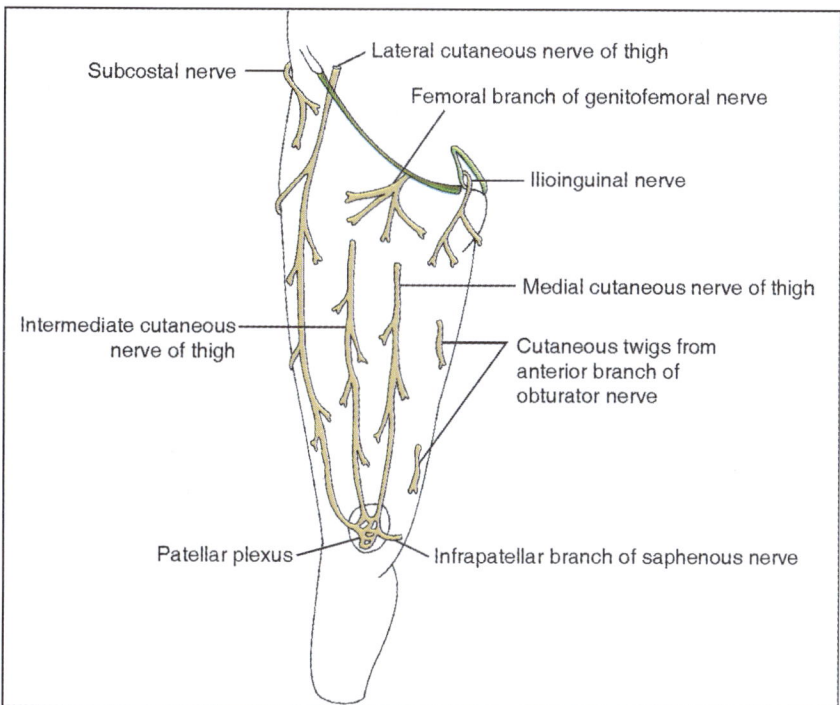

Fig. 25.5 Cutaneous nerves of the front of thigh

DERMATOMES

Axial lines form junction between the adjacent discontinuous segments. There is no overlapping of the dermatomes across the axial lines, an information of great clinical importance. Anaesthesia should be tested across the axial lines. The anterior axial line begins at the external genitalia, turns immediately backwards along the medial aspect of thigh and then descends on the back of thigh and leg to reach a point at the lower margin of the medial malleolus. The posterior axial line on the other hand, begins on the back between the 4th and 5th lumbar spines. After taking a bold convexity, this line descends to reach the middle of the calf. The segmental arrangement of areas of skin supplied by single spinal nerve (dermatomes) are shown in the following diagram.

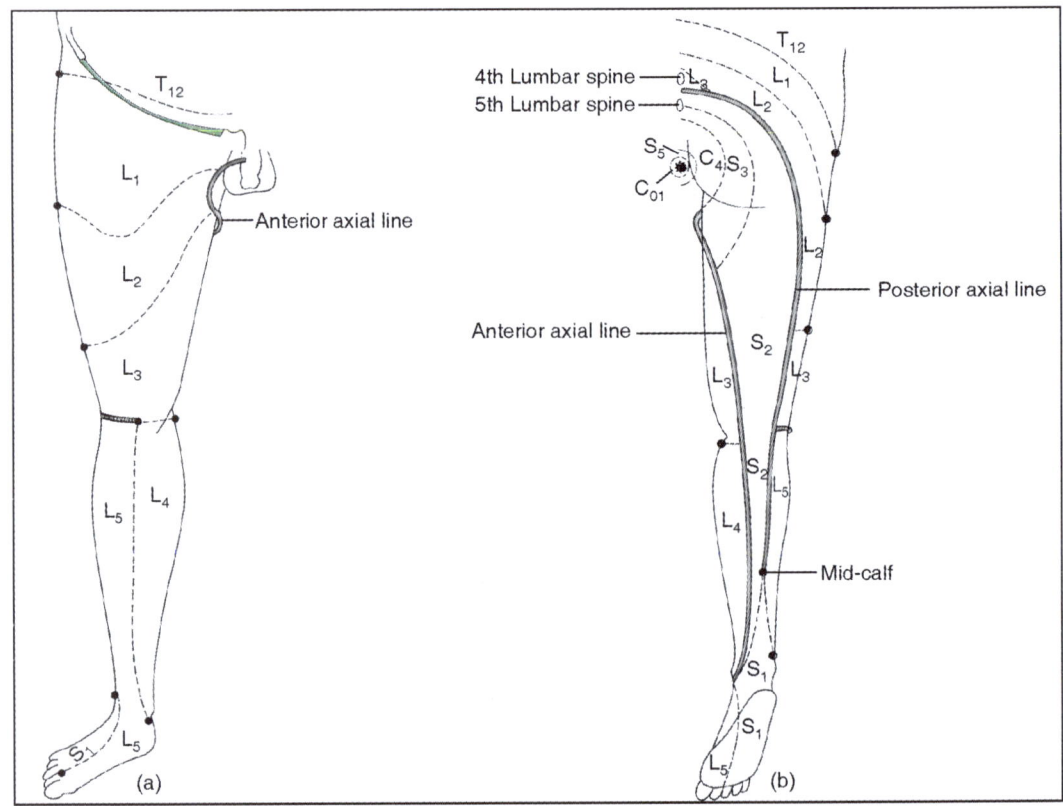

F ig. 25.6 Dermatomes of lower limb (a) Anterior view (b) Posterior view

SUPERFICIAL VEINS

Superficial veins begin on the dorsum of the feet as dorsal venous arch. Its medial and lateral ends continue upwards as great and small saphenous veins respectively. Small saphenous vein ascends on the back of the lateral malleolus and middle of the calf to reach the level of knee where it pierces the deep fascia (roof of the popliteal fossa) to join the popliteal vein.

Great saphenous vein

It is continuation of medial end of the dorsal venous arch. It courses upwards in front of the medial malleolus, medial to leg, posteromedial to the knee and anteromedial to the thigh. Reaching the saphenous opening this vein pierces the cribriform fascia and femoral sheath to terminate into the femoral vein.

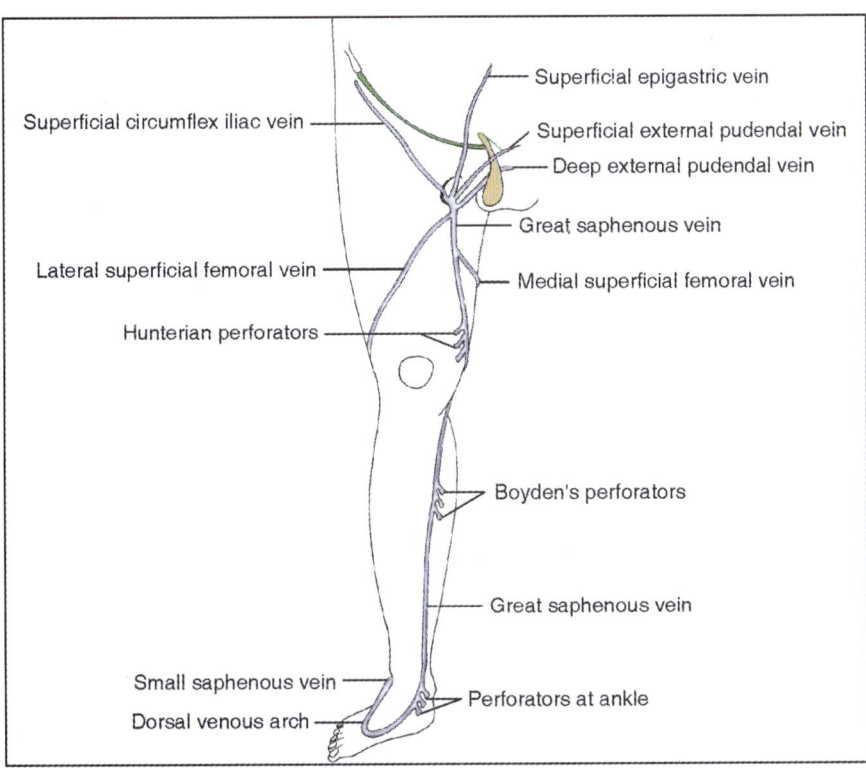

Fig. 25.7 Great saphenous vein

Tributaries

- *Superficial and deep external pudendal veins.* These veins run laterally superficial and deep to the spermatic cord in male (round ligament of uterus in female) to join the terminal part of the great saphenous vein.
- *Superficial circumflex iliac vein.* It runs medially from the region of the anterior superior iliac spine below and parallel to the inguinal ligament.
- *Medial and lateral superficial femoral veins.* These drain the corresponding sides of the thigh.
- *Communicating veins.*
  - Accessory femoral (or saphenous) vein. It connects great saphenous with the small saphenous vein.
  - Perforators. These connect great saphenous vein with deep veins. These are present in the region of thigh (Huntarian perforators), calf (Boyd's perforators) and ankle.

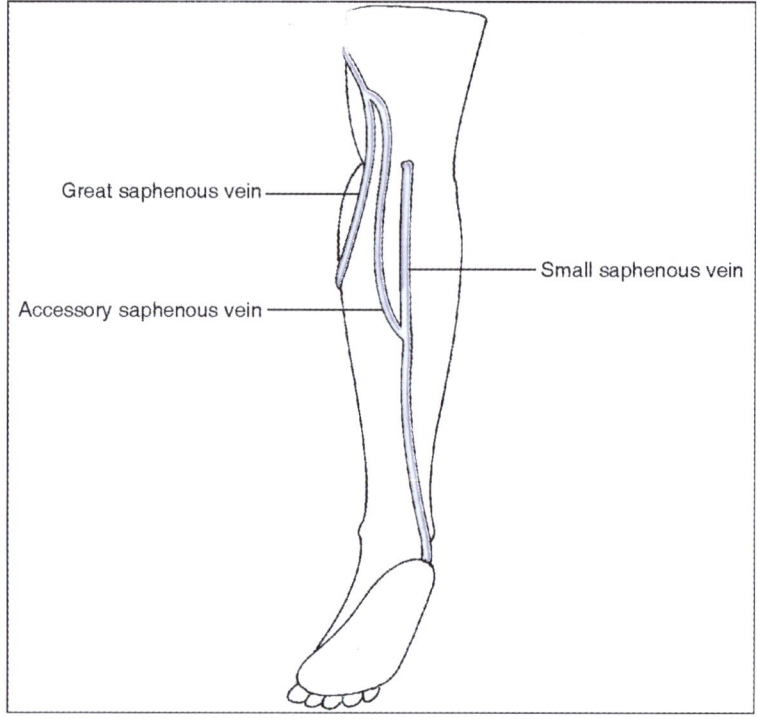

Fig. 25.8 Small saphenous vein

Valves

About 10-20 valves in the great saphenous vein divert the blood flow in an upward direction. Valves are also located in the perforators which direct the blood from the superficial to the deep veins.

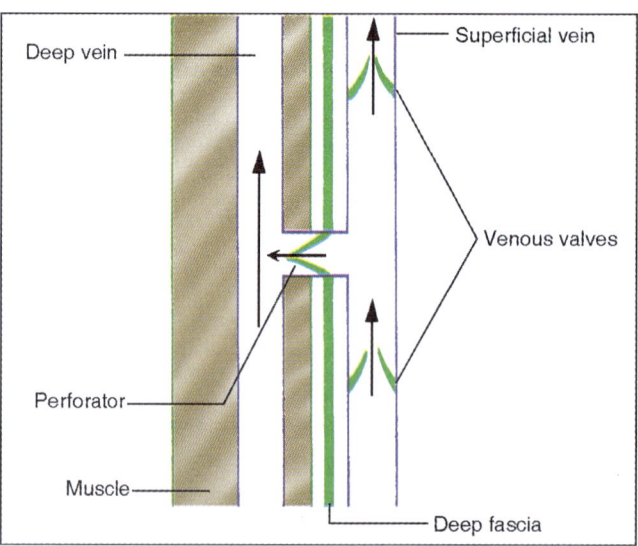

Fig. 25.9 Venous valves and directions of blood flow

Applied anatomy

- *Cut open or cut down operation or venipuncture.* Because of constant anterior relation of the great saphenous vein with the medial malleolus, the former is selected for the cut open operation in cases of dehydration when other veins are invisible. Its purpose is to put needle into the vein for hydration therapy.

- *Coronary bypass.* Great saphenous vein is preferably selected for coronary bypass surgery because of its long course and convenient accessibility. During vascular surgery, the lower end of venous segment is always put upwards to avoid risk of blood flow being hampered by the venous valves.

- *Varicose veins.* Varicosity is defined as dilatation and tortuosity of veins. Great saphenous vein is commonly involved. Treatment of varicose vein ranges from ligation of perforators (to prevent reverse flow of blood from deep to superficial vein due to valvular incompetence) to excision and removal of the great saphenous vein.

DEEP FASCIA OF THIGH (FASCIA LATA)

Deep fascia of the lower limb is like stocking where the upper free margin gets attached to the iliac crest, sacrum, sacrotuberous ligament, ischial tuberosity, ischiopubic ramus, body of pubis, pubic tubercle and the inguinal ligament.

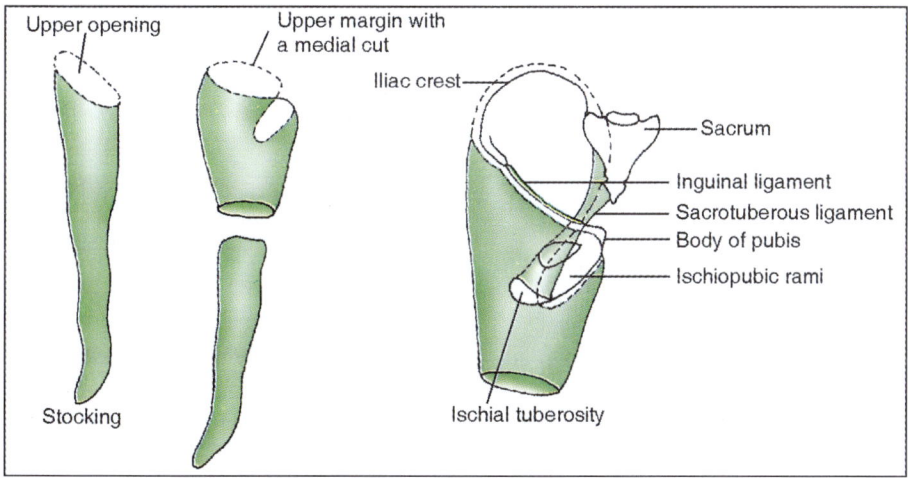

Fig. 25.10 Deep fascia of thigh

Iliotibial tract

It is the lateral part of fascia lata which is thickened and extends from the iliac crest to the front of the lateral condyle of tibia. In the upper part it splits to enclose or in other words receives insersions of two muscles, tensor fasciae latae and gluteus maximus. Only three fourth of the latter gets attached to iliotibial tract (deep half of the lower half of it gets attached to the gluteal tuberosity of femur). Primary function of the iliotibial tract is to maintain the slightly flexed knee in position.

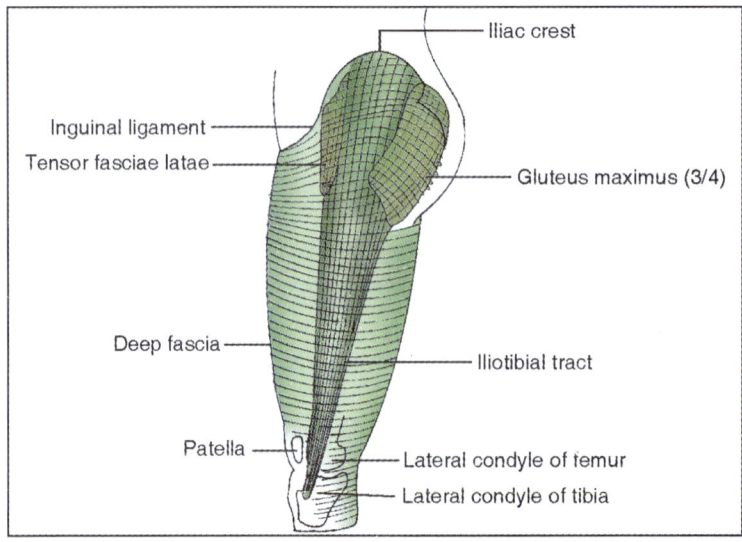

Fig. 25.11 Iliotibial tract

Intermuscular septa

Three intermuscular septa (medial, posterior and lateral) connect the deep surface of fascia lata with the linea aspera of femur, thus dividing the thigh into three compartments.

1. Extensor compartment.
2. Adductor compartment.
3. Flexor compartment.

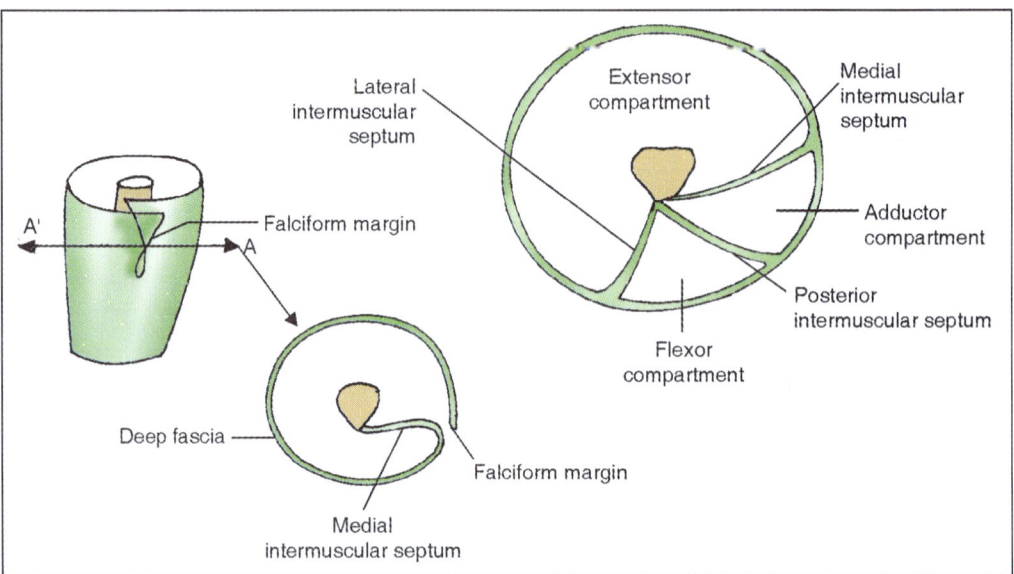

Fig. 25.12 Intermuscular septa of thigh

FEMORAL TRIANGLE

Boundaries

Base. Inguinal ligament.

Medial margin. Medial border of adductor longus.

Lateral margin. Medial border of sartorius.

Apex. Where two margins meet. Some consider the junction of medial border of sartorius and lateral border of adductor longus as apex of the femoral triangle.

Roof. Deep fascia.

Floor. From medial to lateral; adductor longus, pectineus, psoas major and iliacus.

Contents

1. Femoral sheath.
2. Femoral artery
3. Femoral vein.
4. Femoral nerve.
5. Deep inguinal lymph nodes.

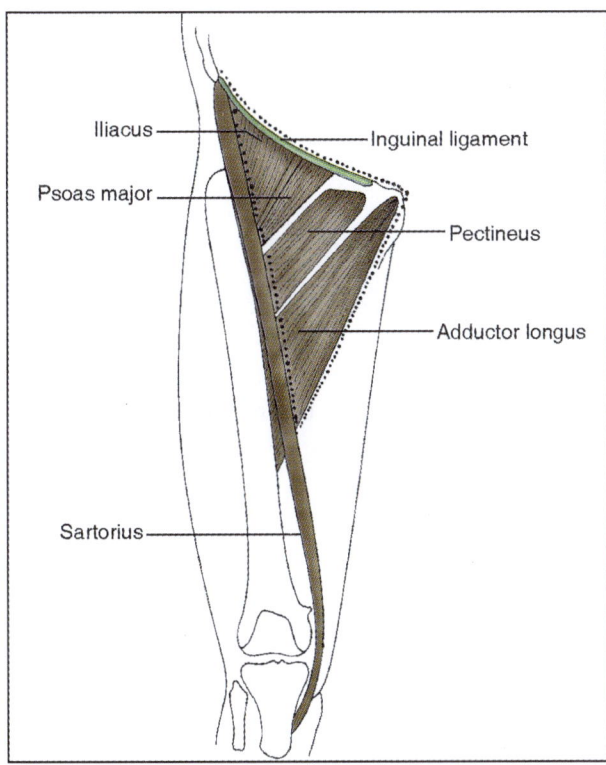

Fig. 25.13 Boundaries of femoral triangle

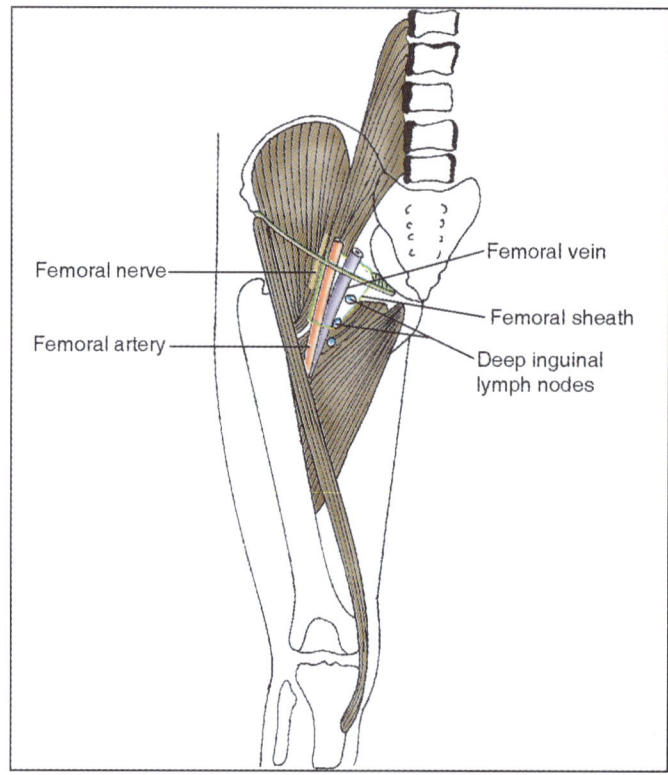

Fig. 25.14 Contents of femoral triangle

1. Femoral sheath

It is a tubular sheath around the proximal parts of femoral vessels. It measures about 2.5 to 4 cm in length. It is formed by the continuity of the fascia transversalis and fascia iliaca from abdomen into the proximal part of the thigh. These two contribute to its anterior and prosterior walls respectively. Two vertical septa divide the femoral sheath into three compartments (lateral, intermediate and medial).

Lateral compartment. It lodges;

- Femoral artery.
- Femoral branch of the genitofemoral nerve.

Intermediate compartment. It contains the femoral vein.

Medial compartment or femoral canal. It lodges:

- *Lymph node of Cloquet.*
- *Loose connective tissue.*
- *Lymphatics.*

Femoral ring: It is the upper opening of the medial compartment of femoral sheath. It is covered by the extraperitoneal fat called femoral septum.

Boundaries of the femoral ring.

Medial. *Lacunar ligament.*

Lateral. *Femoral vein.*

Anterior. *Inguinal ligament.*

Posterior. *Pectineal ligament.*

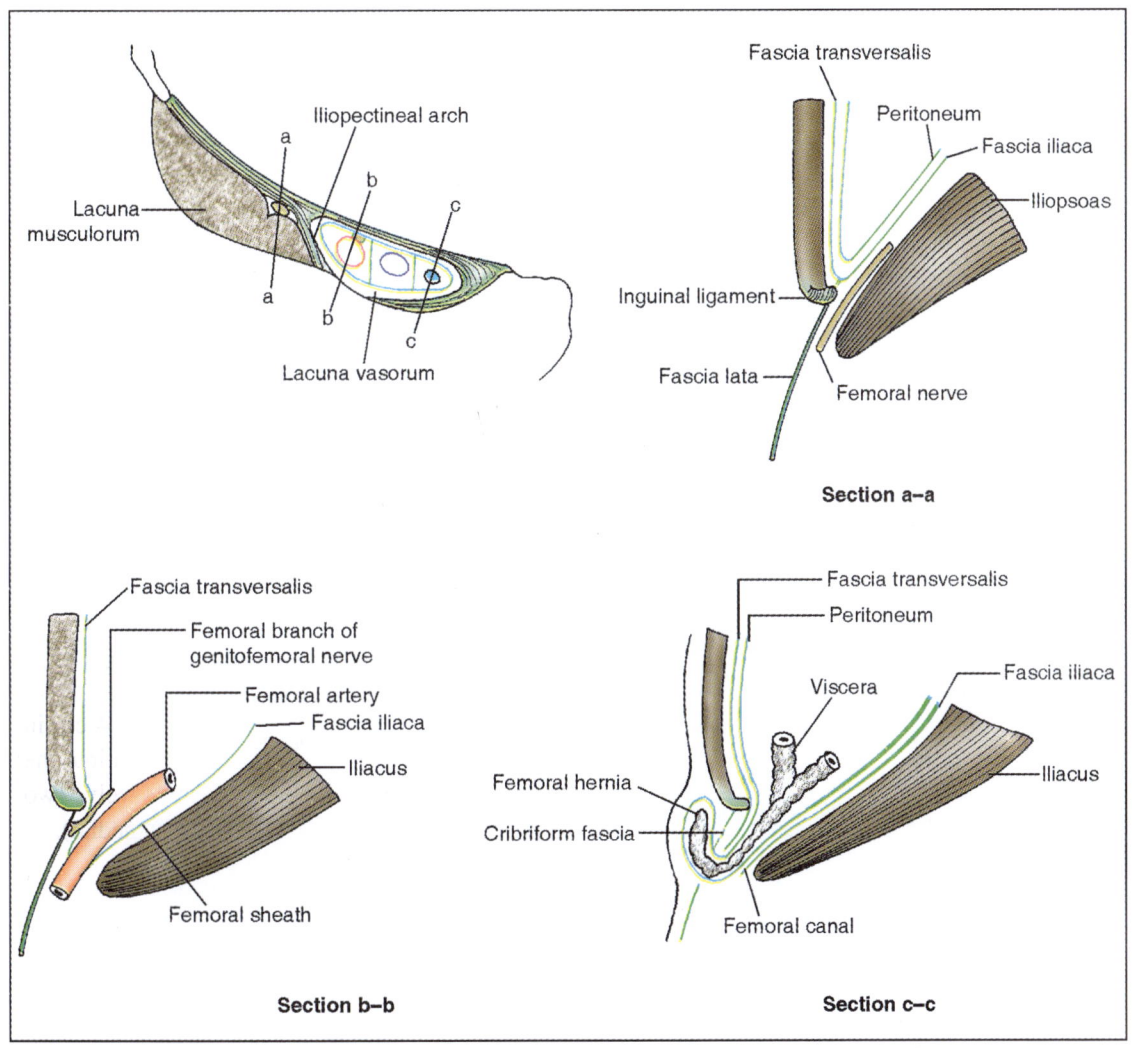

Fig. 25.15 Space between inguinal ligament and hip bone

Applied anatomy

- Abdominal viscera may pass through the weak point of the femoral sheath (femoral canal) to form a swelling below and lateral to the pubic tubercle. This is called the femoral hernia.

DISSECTION STEPS: FEMORAL TRIANGLE

Define the boundaries of the femoral triangle by cleaning the fat from the upper 1/3rd of the thigh. Superiorly, the inguinal ligament forms the base of the femoral triangle. It is bounded laterally and medially by sartorius and adductor longus respectively and its apex is the meeting of lateral and medial boundaries. Clean the femoral triangle and identify its contents: femoral nerve and its two branches, femoral artery, profunda femoris, femoral vein and opening of great saphenous vein in the femoral vein, and deep inguinal lymph nodes. Clean the muscular floor of the triangle formed by iliacus, psoas major, pectineus, and adductor longus.

2. Femoral artery

Course. Femoral artery is the continuation of external iliac artery beyond the inguinal ligament. It itself continues as the popliteal artery through the hiatus in the adductor magnus at the junction of upper 2/3rd with the lower 1/3rd of thigh. Its upper half is located in the femoral triangle while lower half is situated in the adductor canal.

Relaltions with the femoral vein and saphenous nerve
Femoral vein is lateral to its lower end. It then ascends to become posterior at its middle and lastly medial at its commencement in the femoral sheath.

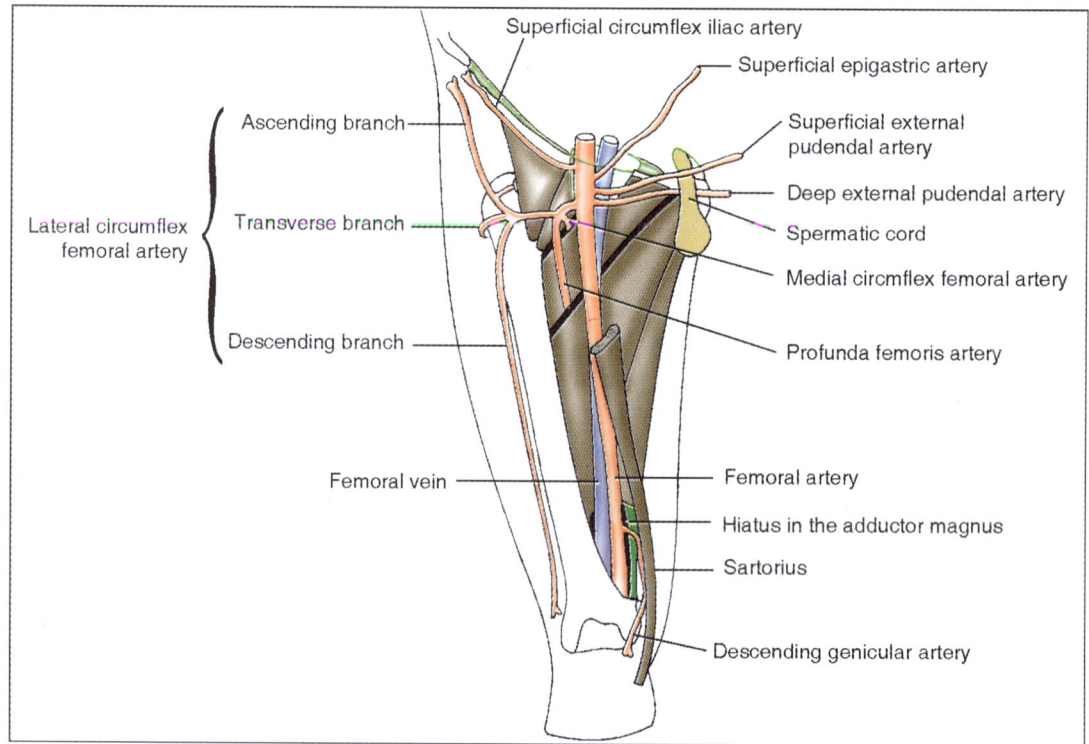

Fig. 25.16 Femoral artery

Saphenous nerve, a branch of the femoral nerve, descends in front of the artery from lateral to medial. It is interesting to note that through out its course, femoral artery is sandwiched between the femoral vein and the saphenous nerve.

Branches

- *Four superficial branches,*
    1. *Superficial circumflex iliac artery.*
    2. *Superficial epigastric artery.*
    3. *Superficial external pudendal artery.*
    4. *Deep external pudendal artery.*
- *Muscular branches*: Several branches from the femoral artery supply the adjacent muscles of the thigh.
- *Profunda femoris artery*: It is the largest branch of femoral artery. It originates from the lateral aspect of femoral artery about 3.5 cm below the inguinal ligament. It descends in the floor of femoral triangle and disappears by passing in the cleft between the pectineus and adductor longus. Following branches arise from the profunda femoris artery;
    1. *Muscular branches.*
    2. *Medial circumflex femoral artery*. This artery disappears by passing in the cleft between the psoas and pectineus.
    3. *Lateral circumflex femoral artery*. It runs laterally between the anterior and posterior divisions of femoral nerve. After passing deep to sartorius and rectus femoris, it splits into three branches, each participating in the formation of arterial anastomoses as shown below.

Branch		Anastomoses
• Ascending branch	:	Iliac anastomosis
		Trochanteric anastomosis
• Transverse branch	:	Cruciate anastomosis
• Descending branch	:	Anastomoses around knee

- *Descending genicular artery*: It originates from the terminal part of the femoral artery close to the hiatus in the adductor magnus. The artery descends in relation to the medial aspect of the knee and helps in the formation of anstomoses around knee.

Applied anatomy

- Femoral pulsation can be felt against the head of the femur.
- Femoral artery is commonly selected for left cardiac angiography.
- Due to its superficial position, the artery is commonly involved in cases of gun shot wound leading to its laceration.

- Femoral artery is one of the arteries in the body which is prone to narrowing (stenosis) as well as dilatation (aneurysm). The site of involvement is usually its lower part in the adductor canal.
- It is the artery of choice for infusion of embalming fluid (for preservation of dead body).

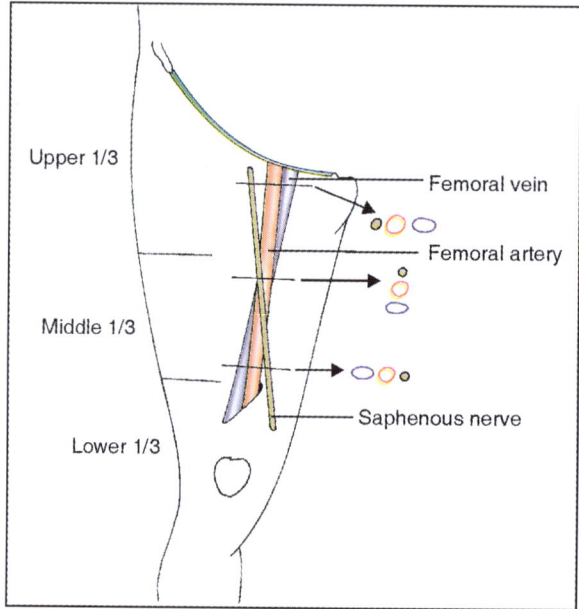

Fig. 25.17 Interrelationships between femoral vessels and saphenous nerve

3. Femoral vein

It is continuation of the popliteal vein at the opening in the adductor magnus. It ascends behind the inguinal ligament as the external iliac vein. During its course it passes behind the femoral artery from lateral to the medial side.

Applied anatomy

- Femoral vein is used for the right cardiac angiography.
- Femoral vein is equally prone to gun shot wound due to its superficial position along with the femoral artery.

4. Femoral nerve

Route value

Dorsal divisions of $L_{2, 3, 4}$ roots of lumbar plexus.

Location

Groove between the psoas major and iliacus.

Termination

About 1" below the inguinal ligament, femoral nerve splits into anterior and posterior divisions between which passes the lateral circumflex femoral artery.

Branches

From anterior division

Two muscular branches:
- Nerve to sartorius.
- Nerve to pectineus

Two cutaneous branches:
- Medial cutaneous nerve of thigh.
- Intermediate cutaneous nerve of thigh.

From the posterior division

Four muscular branches to the four heads of the quadriceps femoris.

One cutaneous branch: Saphenous nerve. This nerve crosses the femoral artery in front from lateral to medial. In the leg and foot it accompanies the great saphenous vein.

Applied anatomy

- Like femoral vessels, the femoral nerve is also prone to the gun shot or stab wound due to its superficial location.

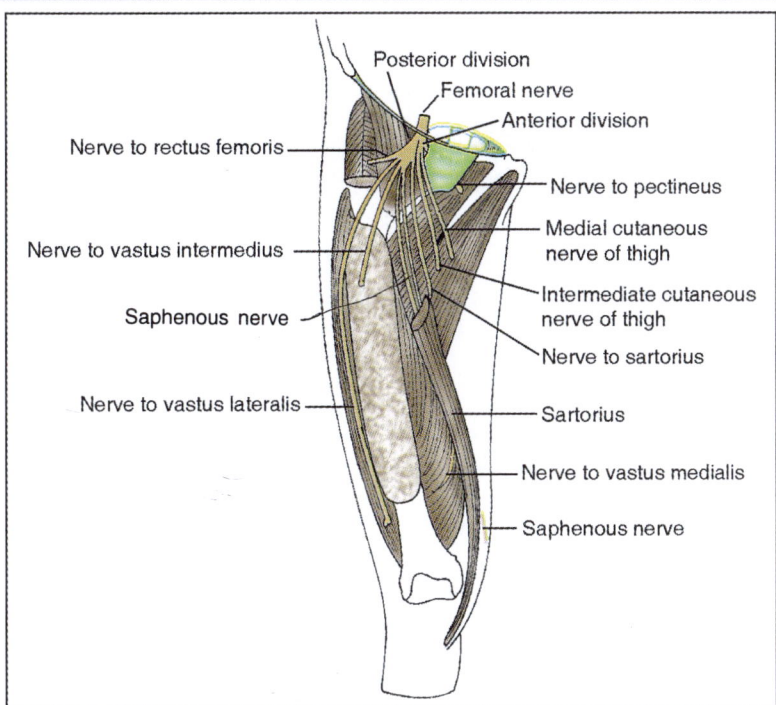

Fig. 25.18 Femoral nerve

5. Deep inguinal lymph nodes

These are two to three in number located medial to the femoral vein. It receives afferents from the deep tissues of the lower limb and from the superficial inguinal lymph nodes. Its efferents reach the external iliac group of lymph nodes.

Applied anatomy

- Lesions of the superficial lymph nodes due to disease or injury in the area of drainage may secondarily involve deep inguinal lymph nodes.
- Deep inguinal lymph nodes may be directly implicated in diseases of injury of deeper tissue of the lower limb.
- Inguinal lymph nodes can be easily visualized by lymphangiography by injecting ultrafluid lipidol into lymph vessels on the dorsum of foot.

SARTORIUS

Origin. Upper 1 cm of the anterior border of the ilium.

Insertion. Upper part of the medial surface of tibia.

Nerve. Femoral nerve.

Actions. Flexion at hip and knee. Abduction and lateral rotation of thigh.

Aforementioned actions bring the lower limb to sitting tailor's position. That is why this muscle is also called tailor's muscle.

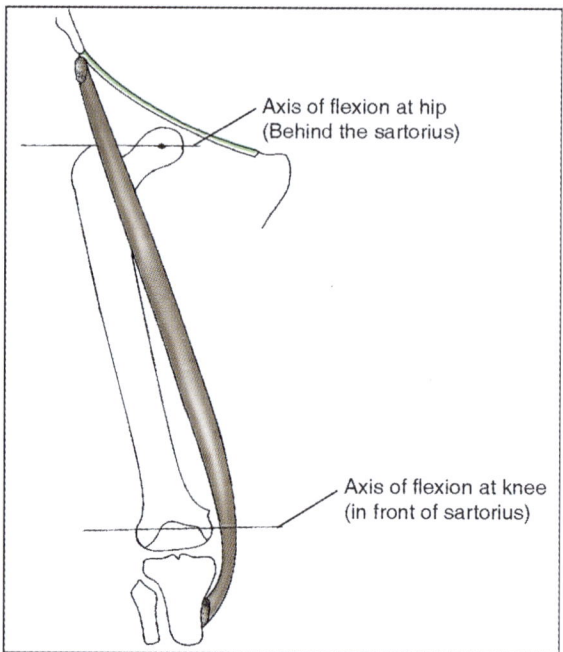

Fig. 25.19 Sartorius

ADDUCTOR CANAL (Subsartorial or Hunter's Canal)

Situation. Deep to the sartorius in the middle 3rd of thigh.

Extent. From the apex of the femoral triangle to the opening in the adductor magnus.

Shape. Triangular in cross section.

Boundaries

Anterior. Vastus medialis.

Posterior. Adductor longus and adductor magnus.

Medial. Aponeurosis deep to the sartorius.

Contents

- *Femoral artery.*
- *Femoral vein.*
- *Saphenous nerve.*
- *Nerve to vastus medialis.*

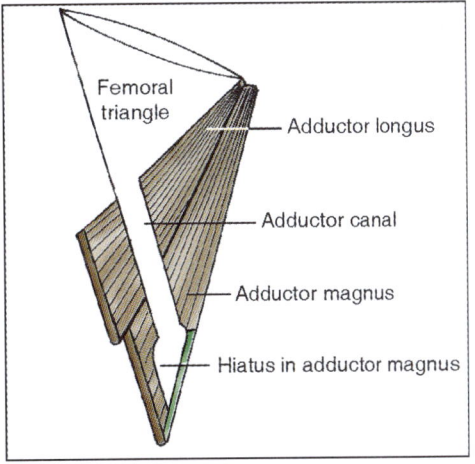

Fig. 25.20 A funnel formed by the femoral triangle and adductor canal

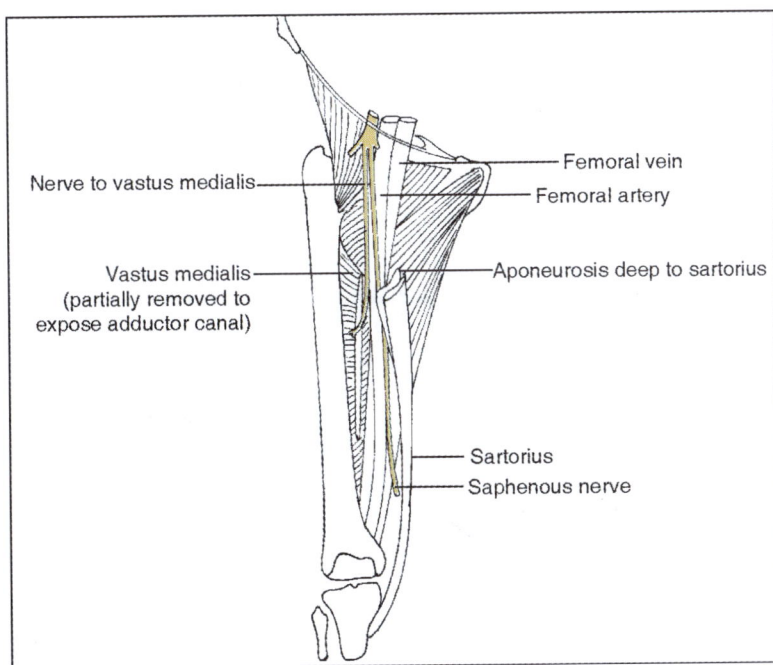

Fig. 25.21 Adductor canal

Applied anatomy

- Femoral artery can be compressed laterally against the shaft of femur in this region to feel the pulsation of femoral artery or to apply a tourniquet for surgical operation on the distal part of the limb.

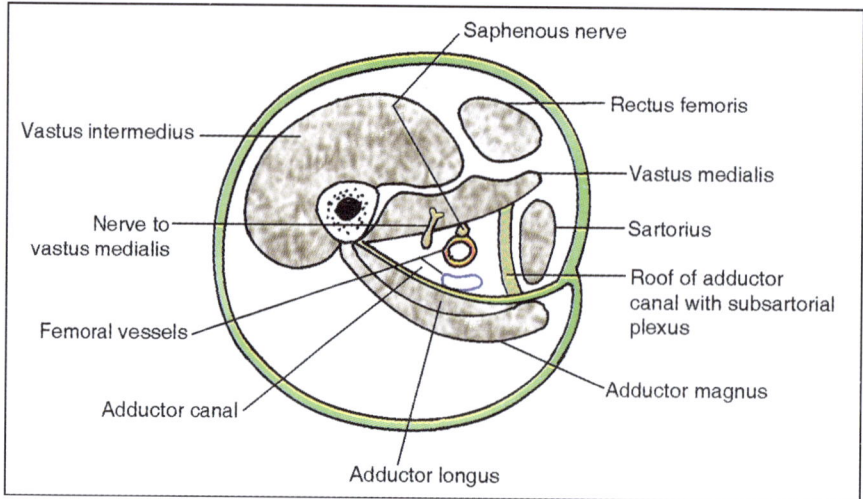

Fig. 25.22 Cross section of adductor canal

QUADRICEPS FEMORIS

Origin

There are four heads of this muscle, i.e., rectus femoris, vastus lateralis, vastus intermedius and vastus medialis. Rectus femoris arises by two heads from the ilium while vasti arise from large area of femoral shaft as follows:

Rectus femoris
Straight head. Anterior inferior iliac spine.
Reflected head. Depressed area just above the acetabulum.

Vastus lateralis
- Upper part of the intertrochanteric line
- Greater trochanter.
- Lateral margin of the gluteal tuberosity.
- Lateral lip of linea aspera.
- Upper 2/3rd of the lateral supracondylar line.

Vastus intermedius
- Upper 2/3rd of front and lateral surface of shaft of femur.

Vastus medialis
- Lower part of the intertrochanteric line.
- Spiral line
- Medial lip of linea aspera.
- Medial supracondylar line.
- Tendon of adductor magnus.

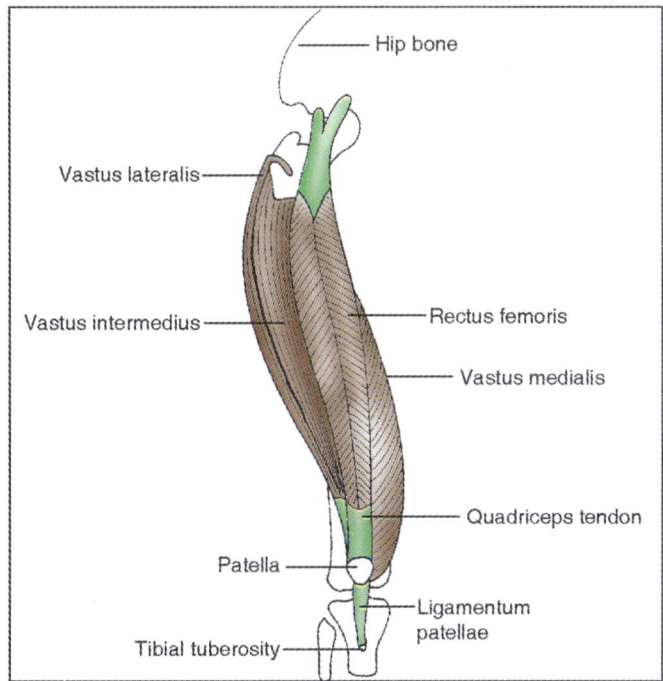

Fig. 25.23 Quadriceps femoris

Insertion

A trilaminar quadriceps tendon is formed of which the anterior lamina is contributed by the rectus femoris, the intermediate lamina by the vastus lateralis and the posterior lamina by the vastus intermedius. Trilaminar quadriceps tendon gets attached to the base (superior border) of patella. Muscular fibres of the vastus medialis gets inserted directly to the medial margin of posterior and anterior lamina of quadriceps tendon and patella.

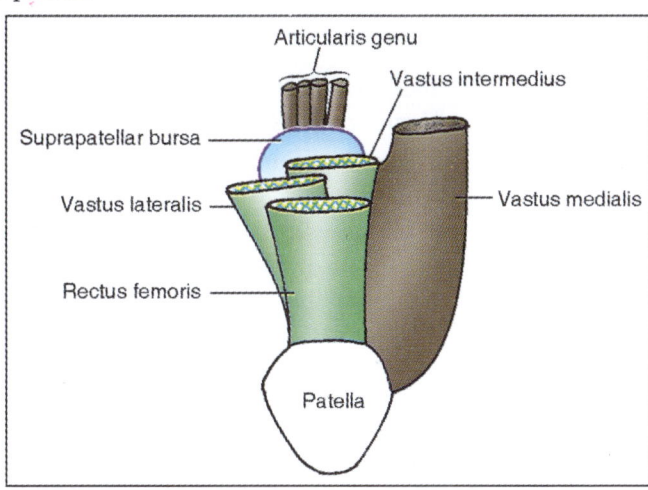

Fig. 25.24 Trilaminar quadriceps tendon

Some of the lower fibres of the vastus intermedius get attached directly to the superior margin of the supra patellar bursa. These constitute the *articularis genu*.

Patellar ligament connects the apex (lower pointed end) of patella to the tibial tuberosity.

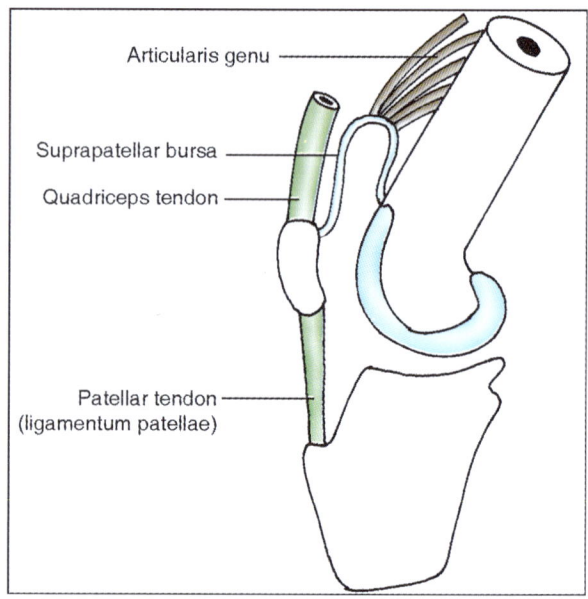

Fig. 25.25 Suprapatellar bursa and articularis genu

Nerve

Femoral nerve.

Actions

1. Extension at knee.
2. Articularis genu protects the suprapatellar bursa from being caught between patella and femoral condyles during extension at knee.
3. Vastus medialis prevents lateral displacement of patella.

Applied anatomy

Knee jerk or patellar tendon reflex. Patient is asked to sit on the table with legs hanging free. A gentle tap on the patellar tendon causes reflex contraction of the quadriceps which can be easily palpated by hand. The test confirms the integrity of 2nd, 3rd, and 4th lumbar segments of spinal cord. A brisk jerk is the sign of upper motor neuron paralysis.

STABILITY OF PATELLA

The pull of qudriceps tendon is upwards and lateral while that of patellar tendon is downwards and therefore patella tends to be displaced laterally.

Three factors prevent lateral displacement of patella and therefore stabilize it.

1. *Bony factor.* Lateral condyle of femur projects more forward than the medial condyle.
2. *Ligamentous factor.* Medial patellar retinaculum exerts a downwards and medial pull over the patella.
3. *Muscular factor.* Lower fibers of vastus medialis get attached to the medial margin of patella and thus pull it medially during extension at the knee.

26

Medial Side of Thigh

MUSCLES

Pectineus

Origin. Anterior surface of the superior pubic ramus.

Insertion. Upper part of the posteror surface of shaft of femur.

Nerve. Obturator nerve.

Actions. Adduction and flexion of thigh.

Adductor longus

Origin. Upper part of anterior surface of pubis.

Insertion. Posterior surface of middle 3rd of the shaft of femur.

Nerve. Obturator nerve.

Actions. Adduction and medial rotation of thigh.

Adductor brevis

Origin. Front of lower part of body and inferior ramus of pubis.

Insertion. Back of shaft of femur.

Nerve. Obturator nerve.

Action. Adduction of thigh.

Adductor magnus

Origin. Anterior surface of ischiopubic rami and inferolateral part of ischial tuberosity.

Insertion. Posterior aspect of shaft of femur along a line extending from the level of lesser trochanter to the adductor tubercle.

Nerve. Obturator nerve.

Actions. Adduction and medial rotation of thigh.

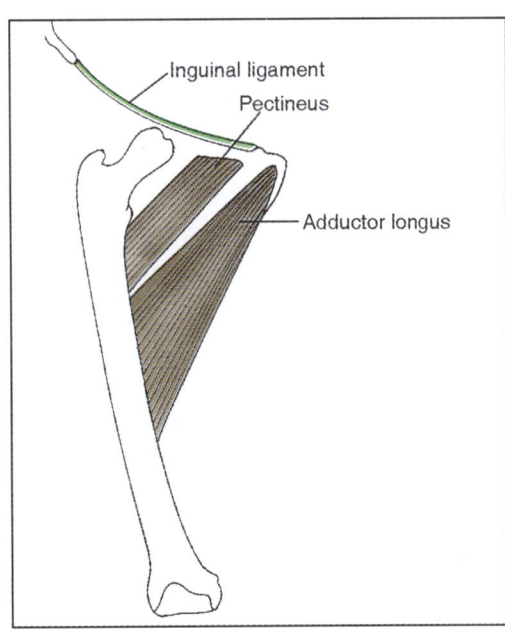

Fig. 26.1 Pectineus and adductor longus

155

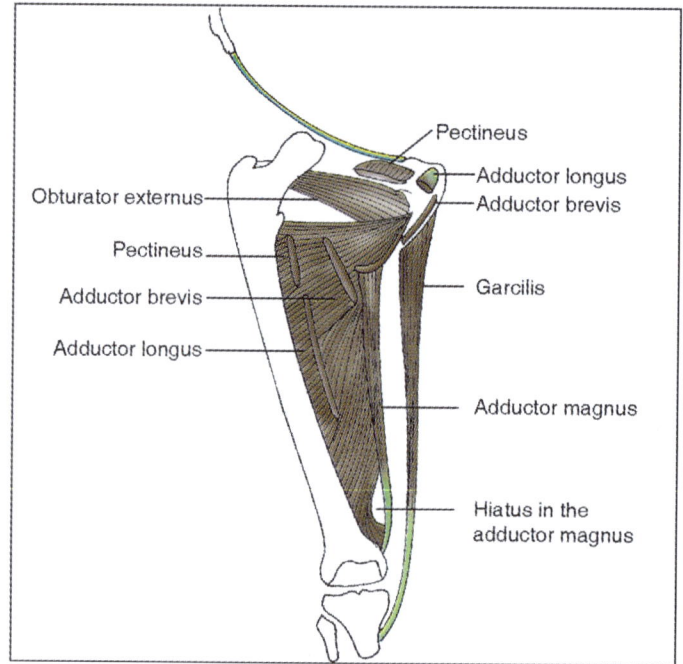

Fig. 26.2 Muscles of the adductor compartment of thigh

Gracilis

Origin. Just medial to the origin of adductor brevis.

Insertion. Upper part of the medial surface of shaft of tibia.

Nerve. Obturator nerve.

Actions. Adduction of thigh and flexion and medial rotation of leg.

Obturator externus

Origin. External surface of the obturator membrane and adjacent bone.

Insertion. Trochanteric fossa on the medial aspect of the greater trochanter of femur.

Nerve. Obturator nerve.

Actions. Flexion and lateral rotation of thigh. Acts as an extensile ligament of hip.

NERVES

Obturator nerve

Root value. Ventral divisions of the ventral rami of 2nd, 3rd, and 4th lumbar nerves.

Course and branches. Obturator nerve appears along the medial border of psoas major at the inlet of the pelvis. After running over the obturator internus on the lateral wall of the pilvis, it splits into anterior and posterior branches at the obturator canal.

Anterior branch. It passes over the obturator externus and then descends between the adductor longus and adductor brevis. Following branches emerge from it.

- *Articular branch* to the hip joint.
- *Muscular branches* to pectineus, adductor longus, adductor brevis and gracilis.
- *Cutaneous branch* to the subsartorial plexus.
- *Vascular branch* to the femoral artery.

Posterior branch. It passes through the obturator externus and then descends between the adductor brevis and adductor magnus. It gives following branches.

- *Muscular branches* to the obturator externus, adductor brevis (inconsistent) and adductor magnus.
- *Articular branch* to the knee joint.

Applied anatomy

- Since the obturator nerve supplies both the hip and knee joints, pain arising from one joint may be referred to the other joint.

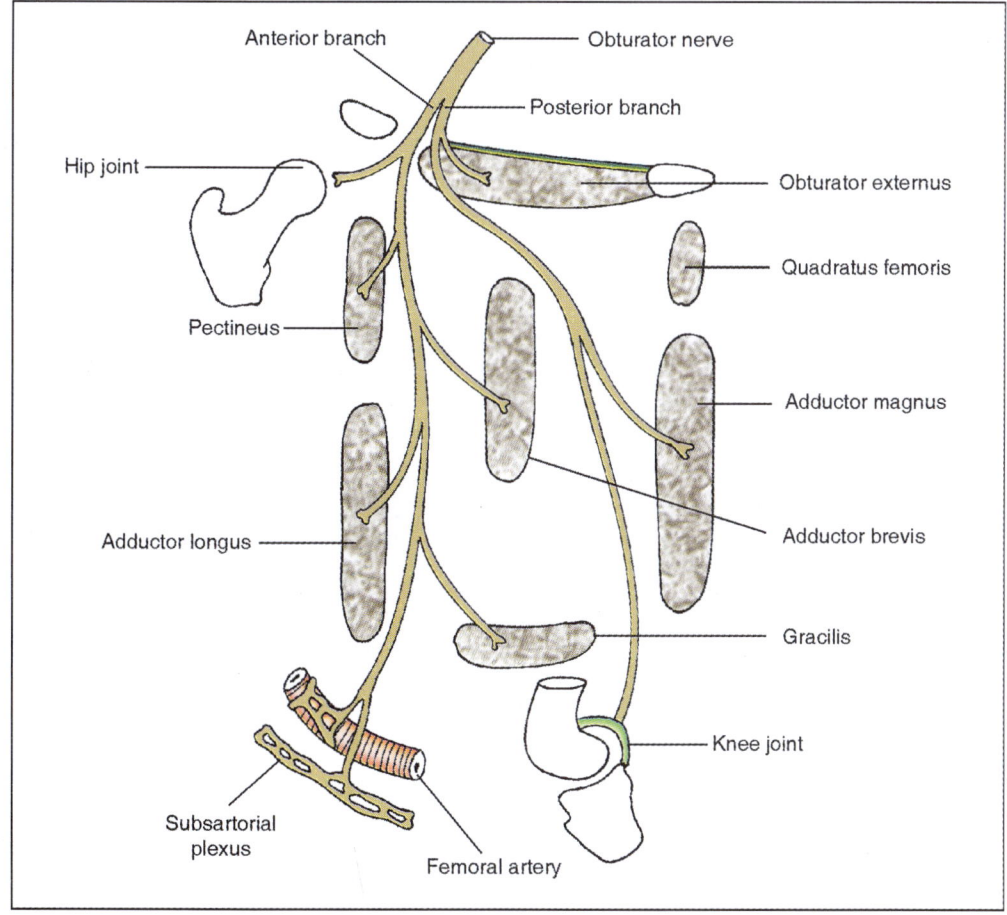

Fig. 26.3 Obturator nerve

- Anterior division of obturator nerve is sometimes severed to reduce the spasticity of the adductor muscles.

Accessory obturator nerve

- It is present in 9% of cadavers.
- This nerve arises from the dorsal divisions of ventral rami of 3rd and 4th lumbar nerves. Its better name could have been accessory femoral nerve.
- The nerve passes above the suprior ramus of pubis and deep to the pectineus.
- It supplies pectineus and the hip joint.
- It finally joins anterior division of obturator nerve.

ARTERIES

Obturator artery

It is a branch of internal iliac artery. It passes through the obturator canal and immediately splits into *anterior* and *posterior branches*. It is the posterior branch which gives rise to an *acetabular branch*. The latter passes under the transverse acetabular ligament and accompanies the round ligament of head of femur to the fovea capitis.

Applied anatomy

- In about 20-30% cases the obturator artery originates from the inferior epigastric artery. This is called abnormal (aberrant) obturator artery. This artery runs over the femoral ring and thus may be endangered during surgical reduction of hernia.

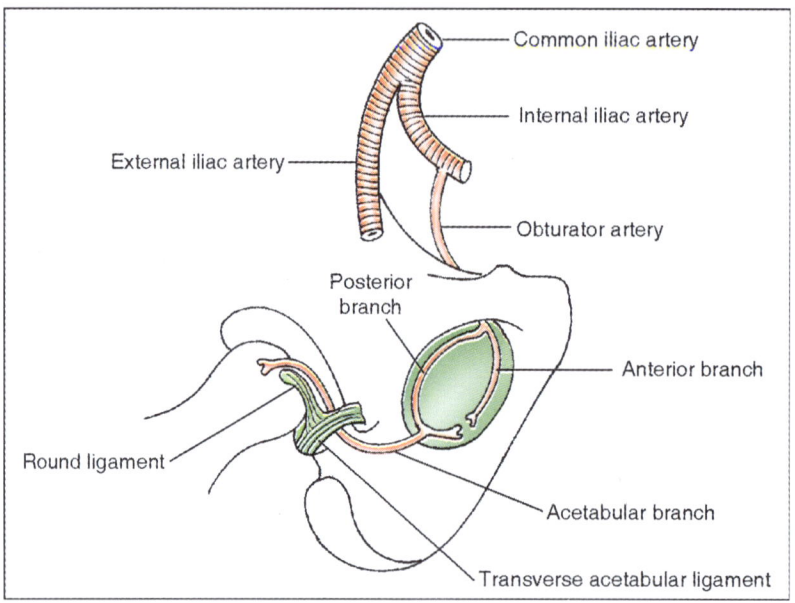

Fig. 26.4 Obturator artery

DISSECTION STEPS: ADDUCTOR COMPARTMENT OF THIGH

Remove the fat and fascia from the medial side of thigh and identify the muscles of adductor compartment namely, adductor longus, gracilis and pectineus. Cut the adductor longus about 2-3 cm from its origin and turn it downwards. Detach the pectineus from its origin and turn it laterally to identify the structures deep to adductor longus viz, anterior division of obturator nerve and adductor brevis. Also note the various muscular branches of the obturator nerve. Now detach adductor brevis close to its origin and define its attachment. Identify the posterior division of obturator nerve, adductor magnus and obturator externus. Now, remove the obturator externus from origin and turn it laterally and identify the obturator artery and its branches.

Profunda femoris artery

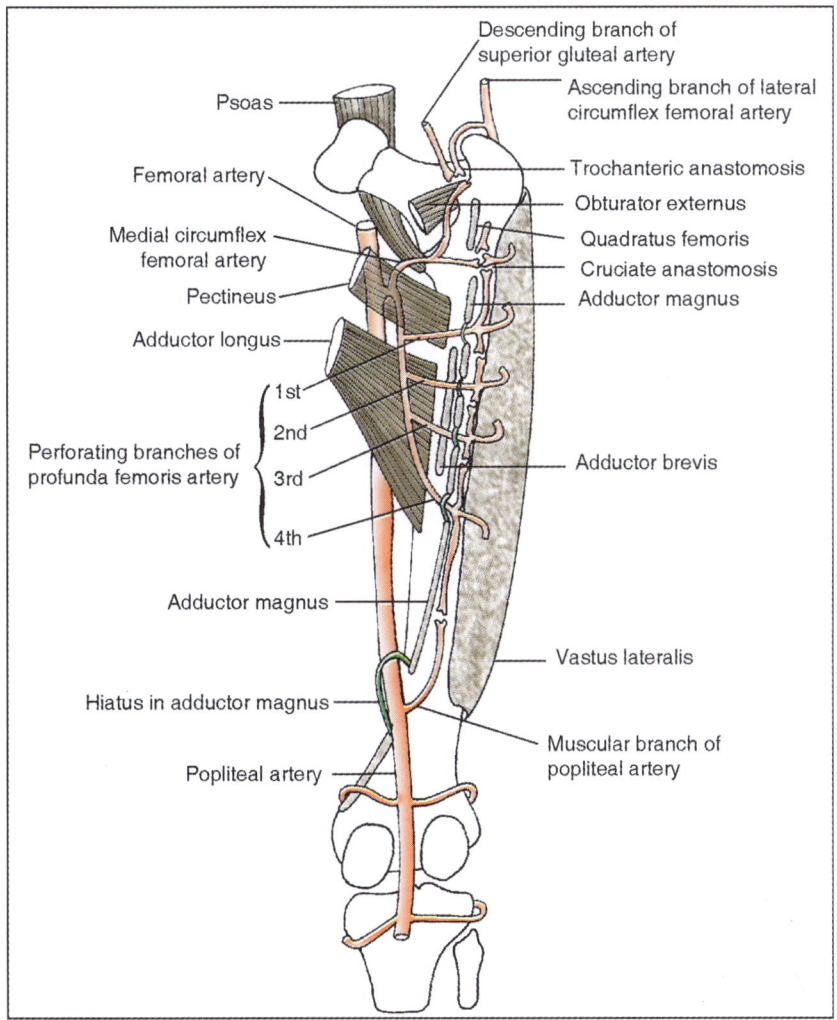

Fig. 26.5 Profunda femoris artery

This artery originates from the lateral aspect of the femoral artery, about 3.5 cm below the inguinal ligament. Its terminal branch continues as the 4th perforating artery.

The artery disappears in the femoral triangle by passing between the pectineus and adductor longus. It then descends between the adductor longus and adductor brevis. Following branches emerge from the profunda femoris artery.

- *Lateral cicumflex femoral artery.*
- *Medial circumflex femoral artery.* It passes first between the pectineus and psoas and then between adductor brevis and obturator externus. It divides into an ascending branch and a transverse branch. The former contributes to the trochanteric anastomosis. The latter traverses between the adductor magnus and quadratus femoris to participate in the formtion of cruciate anastomosis.
- *Muscular branches.*
- *Perforating arteries.* There are four perforating arteries arising from the profunda femoris artery. The first passes above, the 2nd and 3rd through and the 4th perforating artery passes below the adductor brevis. These are called perforating arteries because they pass through the insertion of adductor magnus and end in the vastus lateralis muscle.

27

Gluteal Region

Gluteal region extends vertically from the iliac crest to the gluteal fold and horizontally from the natal cleft to a line between anterior superior iliac spine to the greater trochanter.

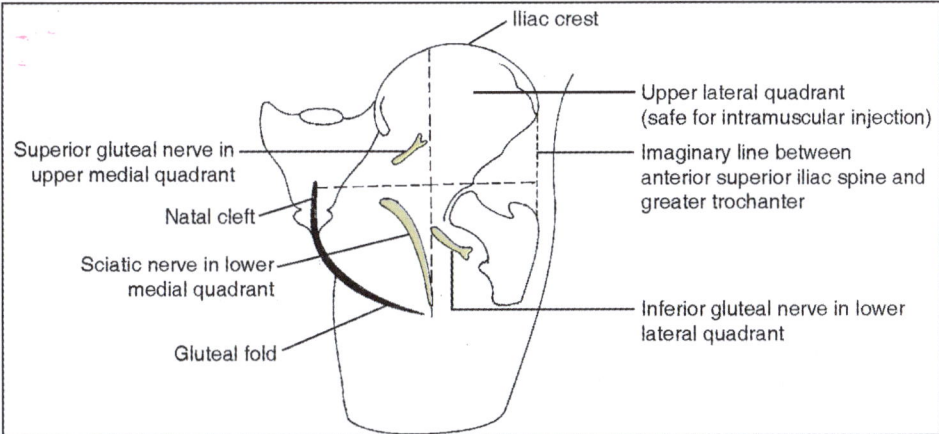

Fig. 27.1 Extent of gluteal region

CUTANEOUS NERVES

Cutaneous nerves converge to gluteal region from all sides.

Quadrants	Cutaneous nerves	Root value
Upper lateral	Lateral cutaneous branches of,	
	1. Subcostal nerve	T12
	2. Iliohypogastric nerve	L1
Lower lateral	Branch from lateral cutaneous nerve of thigh	L2, 3
Lower medial	Recurrent branch from posterior cutaneous nerve of thigh.	S2, 3
	Perforating cutaneous nerve	S2, 3
Upper medial	Posterior rami of upper three lumbar and sacral nerves	L1, 2, 3
		S1, 2, 3

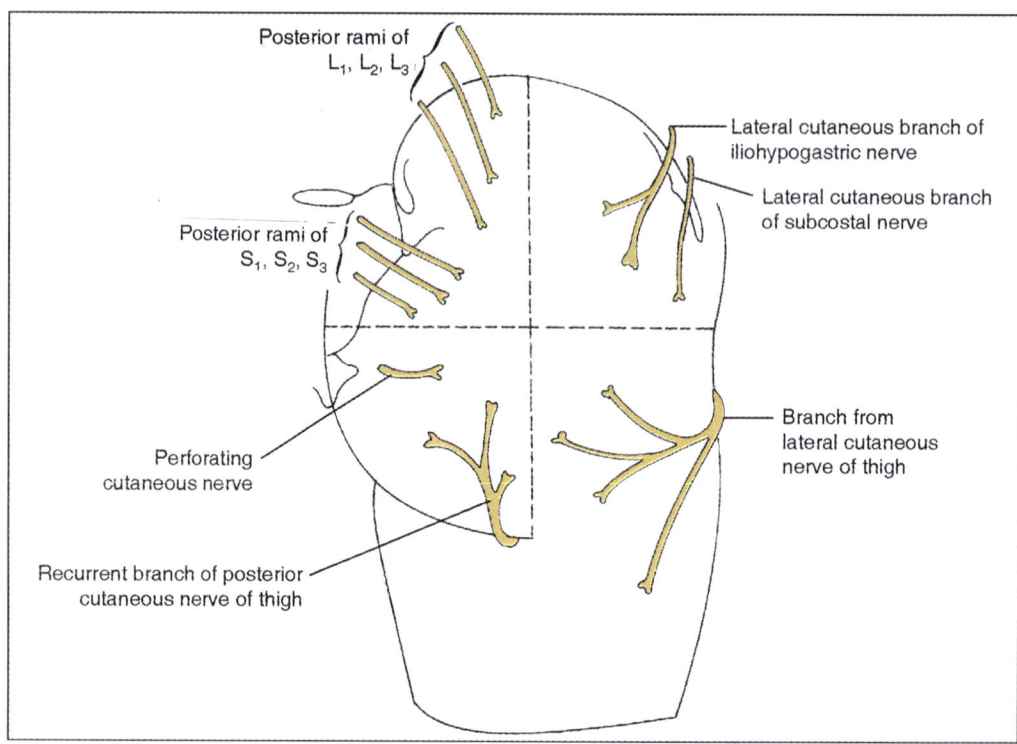

Fig. 27.2 Cutaneous nerves of the gluteal region

GLUTEUS MAXIMUS

Origin
- Gluteal surface of ilium behind the posterior gluteal line.
- Dorsal surface of sacrum.
- Gluteal surface of sacrotuberous ligament.

Insertion
- Deep half of lower half go to the gluteal tuberosity of femur.
- Rest of the muscle (3/4), is inserted via iliotibial tract to smooth facet on the front of lateral tibial condyle.

Nerve
Inferior gluteal nerve. L_5, $S_{1, 2}$.

Actions
- At the hip. Most active during extremes of extension.
- At the knee. Maintains slightly flexed knee.

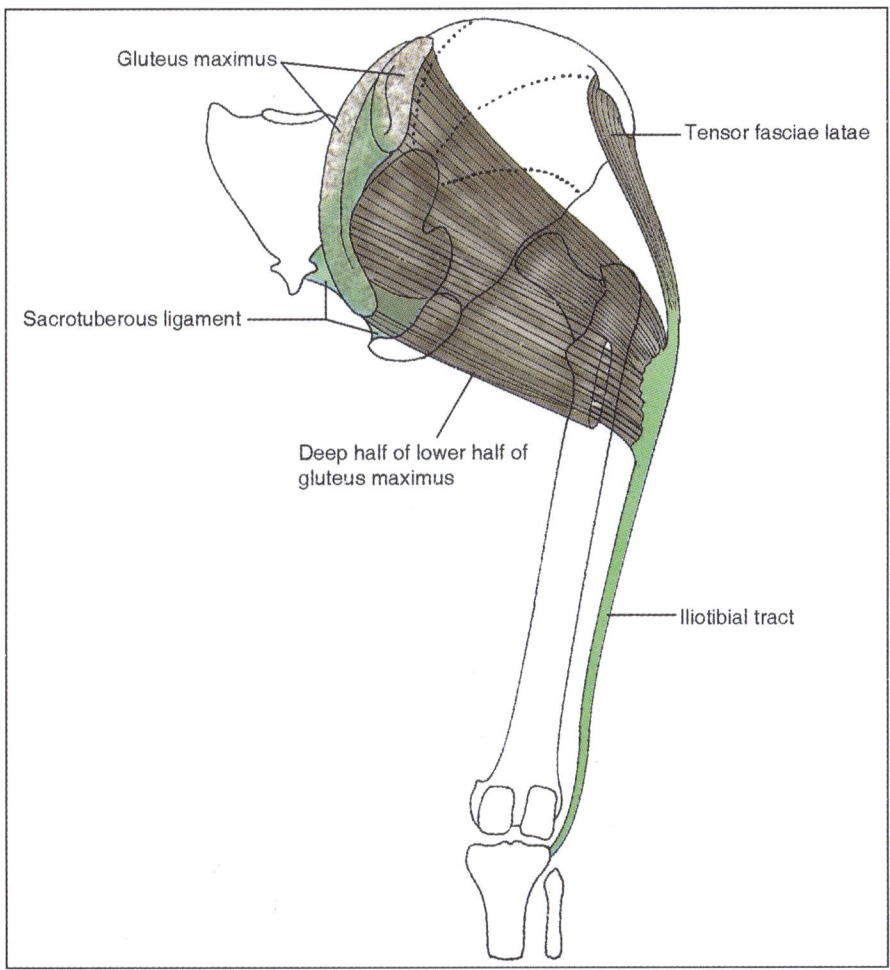

Fig. 27.3 Gluteus maximus

STRUCTURES UNDER THE COVER OF GLUTEUS MAXIMUS

Bones

- Gluteal surface of ilium.
- Ischial tuberosity.
- Greater trochanter.

Ligaments

1. *Sacrotuberous ligament.* It extends from the medial margin of ischial tuberosity to the posterior border of ilium and sides of scrum and coccyx.

2. *Sacrospinous ligament.* It is a triangular ligament corresponding to the triangular posterior surface of ischiococcygeus muscle. Its apex faces laterally and is attached to the ischial spine. While the medial base gets attached to the side of the lower sacrum and upper coccyx.

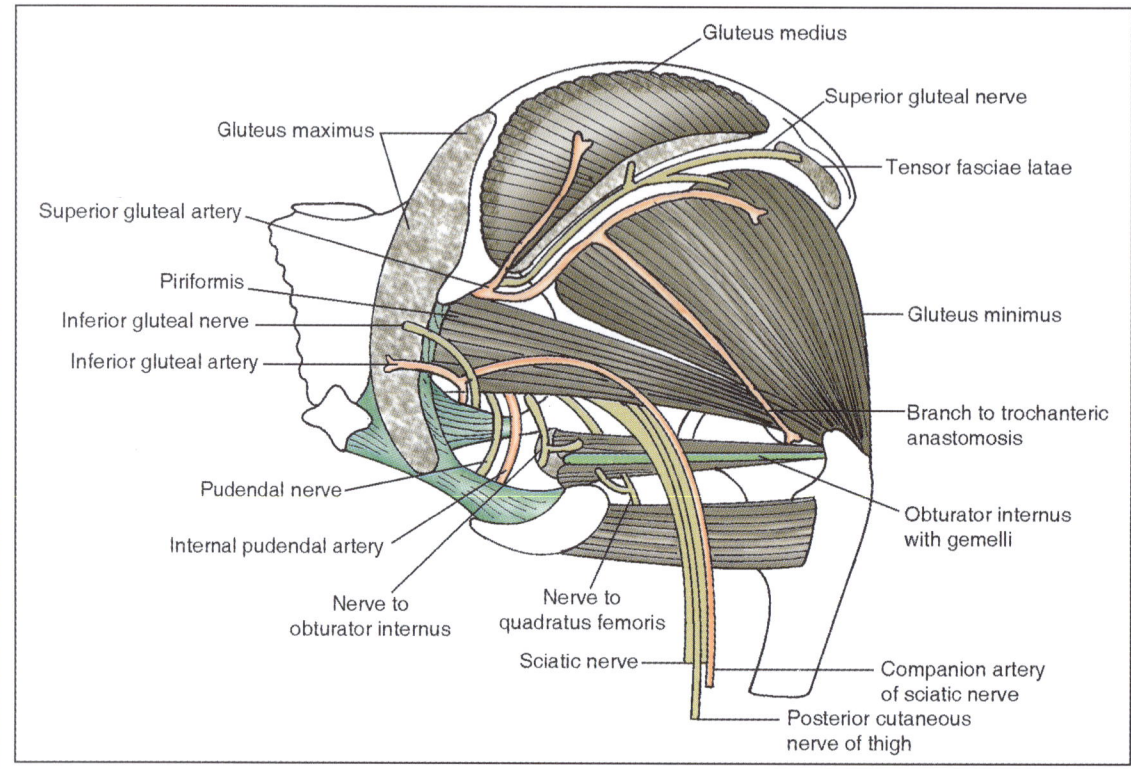

Fig. 27.4 Structures under the cover of gluteus maximus

Scarotuberous and sacrospinous ligaments together convert the greater and lesser schiatic notches into foramina.

MUSCLES

Gluteus medius

Origin. Gluteal surface of ilium between the anterior and posterior gluteal lines.

Insertion. Lateral surface of greater trochanter.

Nerve. Superior gluteal nerve ($L_{4, 5}$, S_1).

Action. Abduction at hip.

Gluteus minimus

Origin. Gluteal surface of ilium between the anterior and inferior gluteal lines.

Insertion. Front of greater trochanter.

Nerve. Superior gluteal nerve ($L_{4, 5}$, S_1).

Action. Abduction at hip.

Pirifiormis

Origin. Anterior (pelvic) surfaces of the middle 3 pieces of sacrum.

Insertion. Superior margin of greater trochanter.

Nerve. Nerve to piriformis ($S_{1, 2}$) from sacral plexus.

Action. Stabilizes the hip joint.

Obturator internus with gemelli

Origin. Obturator internus takes origin from the pelvic surface of bturator membrane and adjacent bones (fan shaped). Two gemelli (surperior and inferior) arise from the corresponding margins of the lesser sciatic notch.

Insertion. Upper medial part of greater trochanter of femur.

Nerve. Obturator internus and superior gemellus are supplied by the nerve to obturator internus (L_5, $S_{1, 2}$). While the inferior gemellus receives its innervation from the nerve to quadratus femoris ($L_{4, 5}$, S_1).

Action. Helps in the stability of the hip joint.

Quadratus femoris

Origin. Lateral margin of the ischial tuberosity.

Insertion. Quadrate tubercle of femur.

Nerve. Nerve to quadratus femoris ($L_{4, 5}$, S_1).

Action. Helps in the stability of the hip joint.

DISSECTION STEPS: GLUTEAL REGION

Place the cadaver in prone position and make skin incision numbers 16 and 17 (Fig. 3.13). Reflect the skin flap laterally. After identifying the cutaneous nerves of the gluteal region remove the fat and fascia. Expose and define the attachments of gluteus maximus. Now, pass a forceps deep to the gluteus maximus and cut it from its lower border about 2-3 cm medial to its insertion on the femur. Reflect the two part of gluteus maximus medially and laterally. Identify the structures lying deep to the gluteus maximus viz, gluteus medius and minimus, obturator internus, gemelli, quadratus femoris, piriformis, origin of hamstring muscles, sciatic nerve, sacrotuberous and sacropinous ligaments. Try also to identify the nerve to quadratus femoris, superior gluteal nerve and vessels, inferior gluteal nerve and vessels, posterior cutaneous nerve of thigh, pudendal nvere and nerve to obturator internus. Cut across the gluteus medius about 5 cm above the greater trochanter and reflect it to identify the gluteus minimus.

NERVES AND VESSELS

All nerves and vessels originate in the pelvis and pass through the greater sciatic notch to enter the gluteal region. Depending upon their course and distribution, these are divided into three groups.

Structures confined to the gluteal region

- *Superior gluteal nerve* ($L_{4, 5}$, S_1). It passes first above the piriformis and then runs under the cover of gluteus medius and minimus and ends by supplying the tensor fasciae latae.
- *Superior gluteal artery*. It passes above the piriformis and divides into superficial and deep branches, passing superficial and deep to the gluteus medius respectively. The latter accompanies the superior gluteal nerve and splits into superior and inferior rami. Superior ramus contributes to the iliac anastomosis while the inferior ramus descends to participate in the trochanteric anastomosis.
- *Inferior gluteal nerve* (L_5, $S_{1, 2}$). It passes below the piriformis and enters the deep surface of gluteus maximus to supply it.
- *Inferior gluteal artery*. It follows the inferior gluteal nerve.
- *Nerve to quadratus femoris* ($L_{4, 5}$, S_1). It passes below the piriformis and then descends deep to the obturator internus and gemelli to reach the deep surface of the quadratus femoris. It supplies quadratus femoris as well as inferior gemellus.

Structures which enter the perineum by passing through the lesser sciatic foramen

These are as follows from medial to lateral.

- *Pudendal nerve* ($S_{2, 3, 4}$). It crosses the base of ischial spine.
- *Internal pudendal vessels*. These cross the tip of ischial spine.
- *Nerve to obturator internus* (L_5, $S_{1,2}$). It crosses the sacrospinous ligament and enters the substance of obturator inturnus to supply it. This nerve also supplies the superior gemellus.

Structures descending into the thigh

- *Sciatic nerve* ($L_{4, 5}$, $S_{1, 2, 3}$). It is the thickest nerve of the body. It enters the thigh below the piriformis and descends between the ischial tuberosity and greater trochanter.
- *Posterior cutaneous nerve of thigh* ($S_{2, 3}$). This nerve enters the gluteal region along with the sciatic nerve and descends in the middle of the back of thigh deep to the deep fascia. It becomes subcutaneous at the level of knee by piercing the roof of the popliteal fossa. Its branches supply the skin of gluteal region, back of thigh and the perineal region.
- *Companion artery of the sciatic nerve*. It is a branch of the inferior gluteal artery. It accompanies the sciatic nerve and is the remnant of the axis artery of developing lower limb.

Applied anatomy

- Upper lateral quadrant is the safest area in the gluteal region for deep intramuscular injection.
- Paralysis of the gluteus medius and minimus (abductors of hip) leads to sagging of the pelvis when standing on the affected side (+ve Trendelenberg's sign) and is responsible for lurching gate.

28

Hip Joint

Hip joint is a ball and socket type of synovial joint in which concave acetabulum (socket) of hip bone articulates with the head (ball) of femur. Acetabulum shows a notch (acetabular notch) in its lower part and a non-articular circular area (acetabular fossa) in the central part leaving a semilunar articular surface (lunate surface) in its periphery. The head is more than half of a sphere whose lateral surface is non-articular with multiple foramina for vessels. A little below the centre of the head, a small non-articular depression (fovea capitis) receives the attachment of round ligament of head.

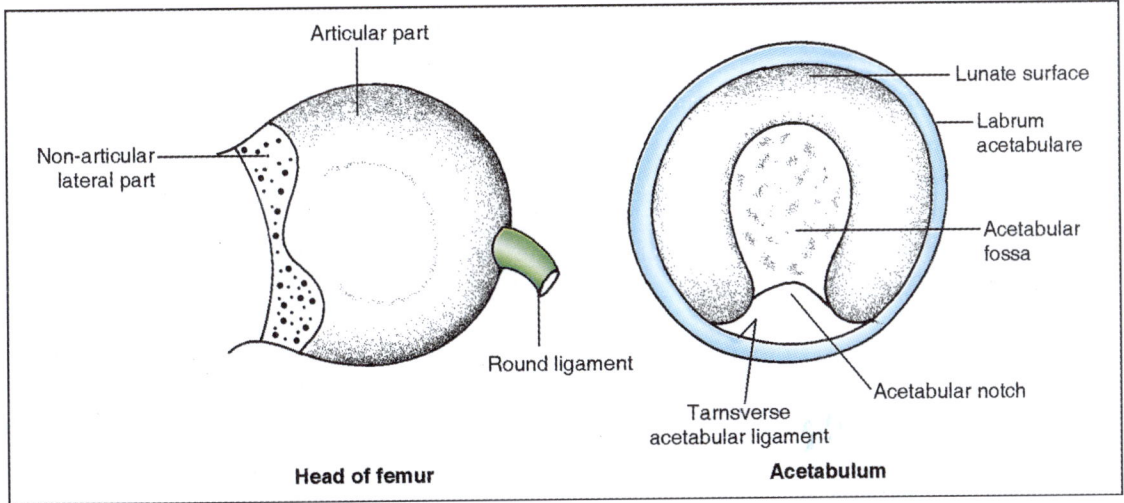

Fig. 28.1 Articular surfaces of hip joint

Ligaments

- *Capsule*. It is attached medially to the peripheral margin of the lunate surface and transverse acetabular ligament. Laterally it is attached to the intertrochanteric line of femur anteriorly (making whole of the anterior surface of neck intracapsular) and middle of the neck of femur posteriorly (making the lateral half of posterior surface of neck extracapsular). Some of the deeper fibers encircle the capsule and constitute the zona orbicularis. Retinacula are the capsular fibres which reflect from its deep surface to the intracapsular neck. These fibres support the arteries which enter the neck to supply the head of femur.

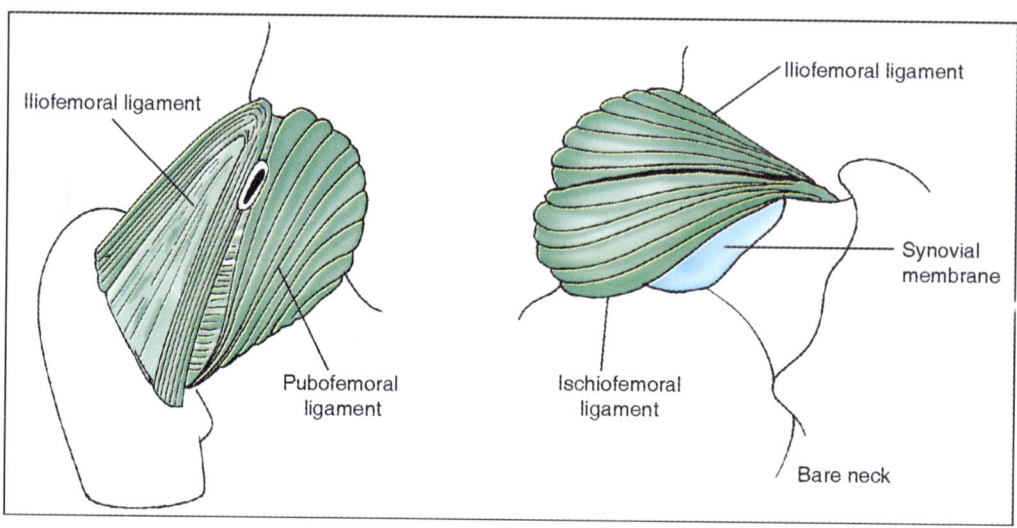

Fig. 28.2 Capsule of the hip joint with thickenings (ligaments).

- *Iliofemoral ligament.* It is a triangular thickening in the capsule whose apex is attached to the lower part of anterior inferior iliac spine of hip bone and base is attached to the intertrochanteric line of femur. It is the strongest ligament of this joint.
- *Pubofemoral ligament.* It is also a thickening in the capsule in its front and inferiorly. Between the pubofemoral ligament and iliofemoral ligament there is a small opening which connects psoas bursa with the joint cavity.
- *Ischiofemoral ligament.* It is a thickening in the posterior and lower part of the capsule.

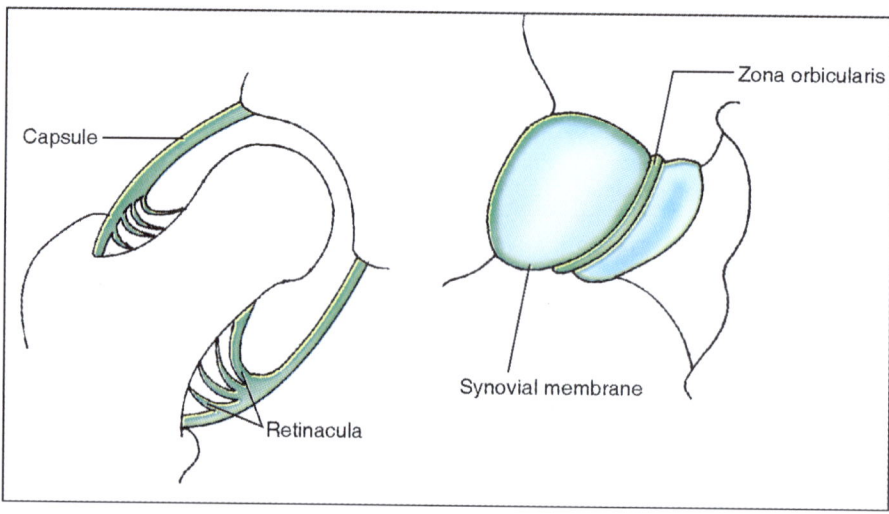

F ig. 28.3 Deep fibres of the capsule of hip joint

- *Transverse acetabular ligament.* It bridges the acetabular notch.
- *Labrum acetabulare*. It is a rim of fibrocartilage attached to the acetabular margin and transverse acetabular ligament.
- *Ligament of head of femur*. It is also called round ligament or ligamentum teres which connects the transverse acetabular ligament with the fovea capitis.

Synovial sheath

It lines the capsule and covers the intracapsular part of neck, non-articular part of head and acetabular fossa. It provides a tubular sheath around the ligamentum teres.

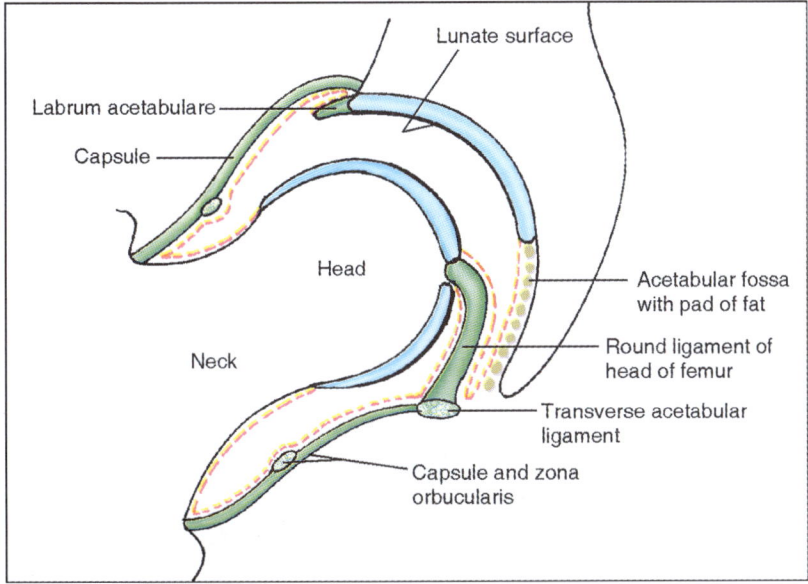

Fig. 28.4 Synovial membrane (red) of the hip joint

Relations

Anterior

- *Rectus femoris.*
- *Iliopsoas.*
- *Pectineus.*
- *Femoral nerve and vessels.*

Superior

- *Reflected head of the rectus femoris.*
- *Gluteus medius and minimus.*

Inferior

- *Pectineus*

- *Obturator externus.*
- *Medial circumflex femoral artery.*

Posterior

- *Piriformis.*
- *Obturator internus with gemelli.*
- *Quadratus femoris.*
- *Nerve to quadratus femoris.*
- *Ascending branch of medial circumflex femoral artery.*
- *Sciatic nerve.*

Arteries

- *Circumflex femoral arteries (medial and lateral).*
- *Gluteal arteries (superior and inferior).*

Nerves

- *Nerve to rectus femoris.*
- *Nerve to quadratus femoris.*
- *Anterior branch of obturator nerve.*
- *Sciatic nerve.*

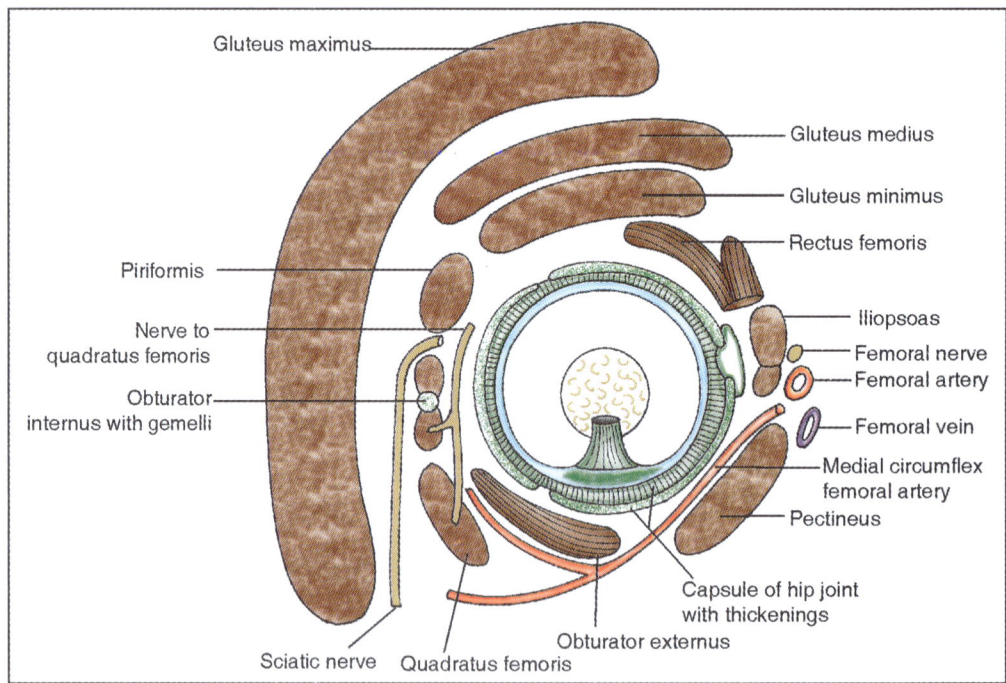

Fig. 28.5 Relations of the hip joint

DISSECTION STEPS: HIP JOINT

Cut femoral vessels just below the inguinal ligament. Cut sartorius and rectus femoris 5 cm below their origin and turn them downwards. Cut iliopsoas near its insertion and turn it up wards. Now, identify the ligaments of hip joint and fibrous capsule; define their attachments. Cut the capsule and expose the head of femur. Identify the labrum acetabulare, transverse acetabular ligament, and also the ligament of head of femur. Now, disarticulate the lower limb from trunk by cutting anteriorly through the adductors and ischio-pubic ramus. On the posterior aspect detach the gluteus minimus, and cut through the origin of hamstrings, short muscles, sciatic nerve finally the posterior part of capsule.

Movements

Type	Axis	Range (From anatomical position	Muscles
Flexion	*Transverse*; passing through centres of heads of the two femora	When knee is flexed -120° When knee is extended - 90°	Sartorius, iliopsoas, pectineus, rectus femoris.
Extension	do	15°	Gluteus maximus, hamstring muscles.
Abduction	*Antero-posterior*; through centre of head of femur	50°	Gluteus medius, gluteus minimus
Adduction	do	0°	Adductor longus, adductor brevis, adductor magnus, pectineus and gracilis
Medial rotation	*Vertical*; through centre of head and lateral condyle of femur	25°	Adductors (longus, brevis magnus); anterior fibres of gluteus medius and minimus
Lateral rotation	do	60°	Gluteus maximus, posterior fibres of gluteus medius and minimus, piriformis, obturator internus, gemelli and quadratus femoris

Stability

(a) *Bony factors*. Deep acetabular concavity, further increased by the labrum acetabulare, receiving relatively small spheroidal head makes the joint more stable.

(b) *Ligaments*. These are very strong and thus can bear the forces of different kinds without allowing much displacement.

(c) ***Muscles***. As compared to the shoulder joint where the muscles play key role in the stability of the joint, their role in the stability of hip joint is limited.

(d) ***Atmospheric pressure***. Being a closed compartment, the articular surfaces can not be separated due to negative pressure generated in such an attempt.

(e) ***Lower range of movement***

(f) ***Gravity***. Hip joint is a weight transmitting joint and therefore during standing posture, the gravity keeps the articular surfaces together with great force.

Applied anatomy

- ***Dislocation.*** It is relatively common.
  - *Congenital*. It is bilateral due to deficient upper acetabular rim. Waddling gait and positive Trendelenberg's sign are the characteristic features.
  - *Acquired.* This condition is rare. The displacement of the head is usually inferomedial. Depending upon the force, it may be anterior or posterior.
- ***Osteoarthritis***. It is due to the inflammation of the joint. It is a painful condition. Pain is very much increased when the patient stands on the side of the lesion as the pressure between the two articular surfaces becomes four times that of the body weight. This is due to the fact that contraction of gluteus medius and minimus produces a pressure which is three times that of body weight.
- *Pain* of the hip joint is often *referred* to the knee and vice-versa due to common nerve supply i.e., by the obturator nerve.

29

Back of The Thigh

POSTERIOR CUTANEOUS NERVE OF THE THIGH

Root value ($S_{2, 3}$).

Course. This nerve descends in the middle of the back of thigh deep to the deep fascia till it reaches the level of the knee in the popliteal fossa where it pierces the deep fascia to bcome subcutaneous. It terminates in the middle of back of leg.

Branches

- *Gluteal branch*. It winds round the lower border of gluteus maximus and then ascends to supply to the gluteal skin.
- *Perineal branch*. It runs medially to supply the perineal skin.
- *Cutaneous branches*. These supply the back of thigh and upper half of leg.

MUSCLES OF THE FLEXOR COMPARTMENT OF THIGH

These are also called the ***hamstring*** muscles because of cord like tendons (ham; back of upper leg, string; cord like). Muscles possessing following properties are included in this list.

1. Origin from the ischial tuberosity.
2. Insertion to one of the two bones of the leg.
3. Nerve supply from the tibial component of the sciatic nerve.

Muscles included in this list are;

- Long head of biceps femoris.
- Semitendinosus.
- Semimembranosus.
- Dorsal portion (*hasmstring component*) of adductor magnus.

Recently, it was proposed to divide the hamstring muscles into two groups;

1. *Lateral hamstring*. Biceps femoris.
2. *Medial hamstring*. Semitendinosus and semimembranousus.

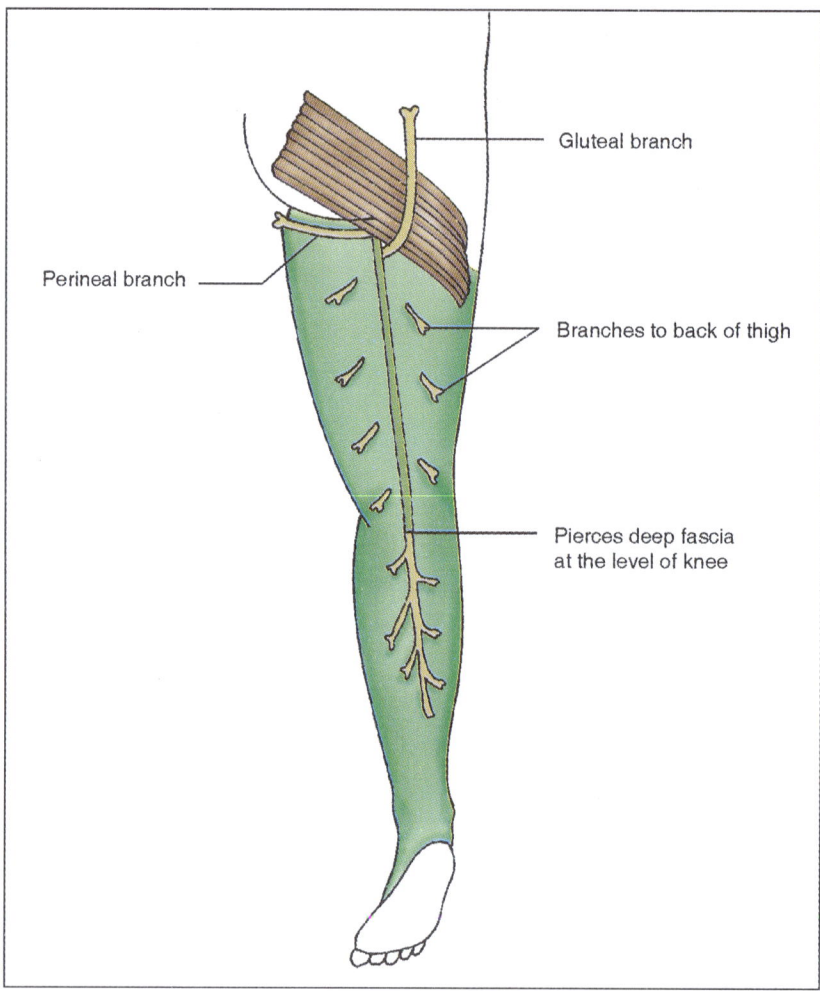

Fig. 29.1 Posterior cutaneous nerve of thigh

Biceps femoris
Origin

Long head. Upper medial part of the ischial tuberosity.

Short head. Lateral lip of linea aspera and upper part of the lateral supracondylar line.

Insertion. Two heads join and form a tendon in the lower part of the thigh. Tendon descends downwards and laterally to reach the head of fibula where it splits to enclose the fibular collateral ligament before inserting into it.

Nerves

Long head. Tibial component of the sciatic nerve.

Short head. Common peroneal component of the sciatic nerve.

Actions. Flexion at knee and intermediate part of extension at hip.

Semitendinosus

Origin. Upper medial part of ischial tuberosity (along with the long head of biceps femoris).

Insertion. Muscle is replaced by a rounded tendon in its lower half which gets attached to the upper part of the medial surface of tibia.

Nerve. Tibial component of sciatic nerve.

Actions. Flexion at knee and intermediate part of extension at hip.

Semimembranosus

Origin. Upper lateral part of the ischial tuberosity.

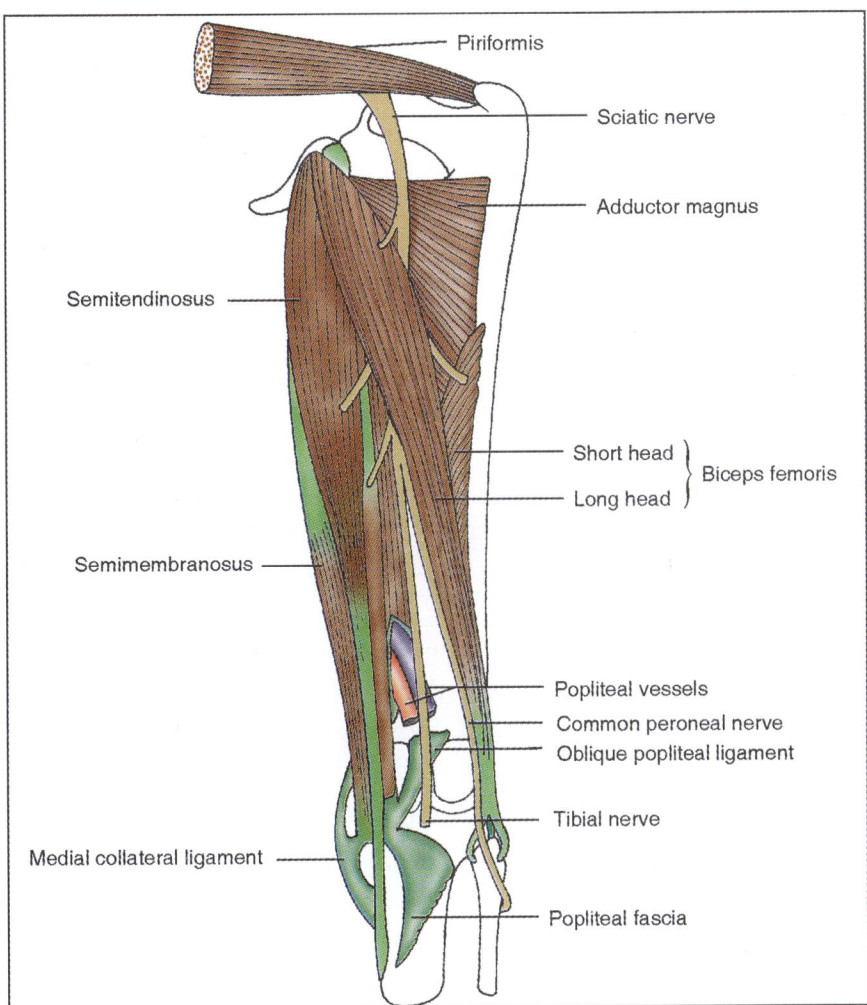

Fig. 29.2 Muscles of the flexor compartment of thigh

Insertion. The muscle lies deep to the semitendinosus and is in the form of a flattened tendon in the upper half replaced by muscular belly in the lower half. The tendinous lower end of the muscle is attached into the deep groove on the back of medial condyle of tibia. Three expansions extend from its insertion;

1. *Oblique popliteal ligament.*
2. *Popliteal fascia.*
3. *Contribution to the tibial (medial) collateral ligament* of knee.

Nerve. Tibial component of the sciatic nerve.

Actions. Flexion at knee and intermediate part of extension at hip.

ARTERIES OF THE BACK OF THIGH

Branches supplying the back of the thigh originate from the following main arteries.

- **Internal iliac artery**

  Its gluteal branches (*superior and inferior gluteal arteries*) supply the upper part. Inferior gluteal artery gives a branch to the sciatic nerve.

- **Femoral artery**

  It provides profunda femoris artery which plays most important role in supplying the region.

- **Popliteal artery**

  Its muscular branches help in supplying the lower part.

Anastomoses on the back of thigh

Branches appearing from the aforementioned arteries help in the formation of series of anastomoses on the back of thigh as follows:

1. **Trochanteric anastomosis.**

   It is located in the trochanteric fossa and is formed by the contribution of the following arteries;
   - *Descending branch of superior gluteal artery.*
   - *Ascending branch of medial circumflex femoral artery.*
   - *Ascending branch of lateral circumflex femoral artery.*

2. *Cruciate anastomosis*

   It is located at the level of lesser trochanter of femur. It receives following arteries from four sides.
   - Transverse branch of medial circumflex femoral artery from medial side.
   - Transverse branch of lateral circumflex femoral artery from the lateral side.
   - Descending branch of inferior gluteal artery from above.
   - Ascending branch of 1st perforating branch of profunda femoris artery from below.

3. *Vertical anastomoses*

It is located along the linea aspera on the back of thigh and it is formed by the contributions from ascending and descending branches of four perforating arteries.

4. *Genicular anastomosis*

It is located around knee. It receives contribution from the descending branch of 4th perforating artery which anastomoses with the superior muscular branches of popliteal artery.

DISSECTION STEPS: BACK OF THIGH

Make a median vertical skin incision on the back of thigh extending from the middle of incision 17 (Fig. 3.13). Turn skin flaps and remove superficial fascia and divide the deep fascia vertically. Remove fascia from back and define the muscles of back and sciatic nerve. Identify hamstrings e.g., semimembranosus, semitendinosus, biceps femoris and ischial head of adductor magnus and also the posterior cutaneous nerve of thigh. Try to identify the muscular branches from sciatic nerve to the hamstrings. Now, detach hamstrings from ischial tuberosity and turn aside to expose the insertion of adductor magnus. Note the adductor hiatus and the popliteal vessels emerging from it. Try to identify the perforating branches of profunda femoris passing through the adductor magnus.

SCIATIC NERVE

Root value. $L_{4, 5}, S_{1, 2, 3}$

Course

The nerve originates in the pelvis and enters the gluteal region by passing through the greater sciatic foramen below the piriformis. It descends over the back of adductor magnus deep to the long head of biceps femoris. It consists of two components (tibial and peroneal) which separate at the upper angle (apex) of the popliteal fossa.

Branches

Terminal branches

Sciatic nerve terminates in the middle of the thigh into following two branches;

1. *Tibial nerve* ($L_{4, 5}, S_{1, 2, 3}$). It descends vertically in the midline.
2. *Common peroneal nerve* ($L_{4, 5}, S_{1, 2,}$). It accompanies the biceps tendon to reach the head and neck of the fibula where it terminates into superficial peroneal and deep peroneal nerves.

Muscular branches

Most of the branches appear from its medial side i.e., from its tibial component to supply the hamstring muscles. Only one branch arises from its lateral side i.e., from its common peroneal component to supply the short head of biceps.

Anomalies

Some times the sciatic nerve terminates inside the pelvis. In such cases its tibial component follows the course of sciatic nerve, i.e. passes below the piriformis. The common peroneal component passes either through the obturator internus (12.2%) or above it (0.5%).

Applied anatomy

- Pulled hamstring is a common problem in players. It is due to the spasm of hamstring muscles.
- Contracture of hamstring tendons may result from the diseases of the knee joint.
- Involvement of sciatic nerve anywhere leads to neuralgia along its distribution. This condition is called 'Sciatica'
- Extensive anastomoses on the back of the thigh provide an opportunity for collateral circulations during obstruction of main arteries.

Popliteal Fossa

30

It is a depressed area on the back of the knee and also extending into the lower thigh and upper leg. It is diamond shaped and therefore having four sides. Its upper angle is also called the apex of the popliteal fossa.

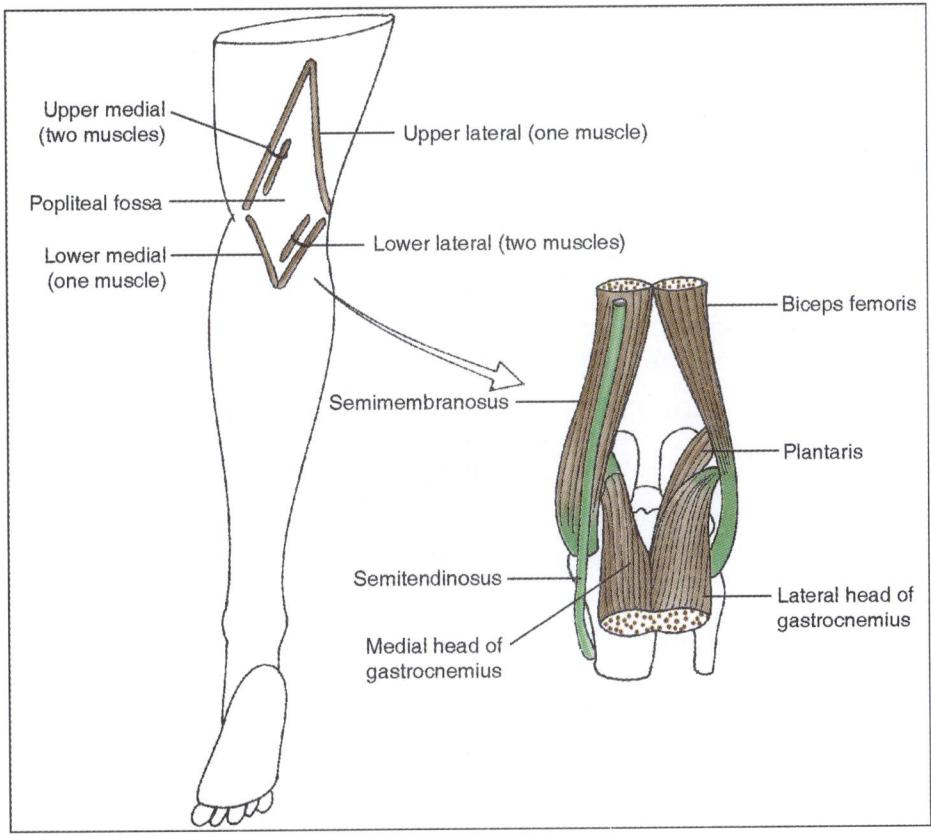

Fig. 30.1 Boundaries of the popliteal fossa

Boundaries

Upper lateral	*Biceps femoris.*
Upper medial	*Semitendinosus and semimembranosus.*
Lower medial	*Medial head of gastrocnemius.*
Lower lateral	*Plantaris and lateral head of gastrocnemius.*

Roof

Formed by the deep fascia. It is pierced by the following structures.

- *Posterior cutaneous nerve of thigh.*
- *Peroneal communicating nerve.* It connects common peroneal nerve with sural nerve.
- *Lateral cutaneous nerve of calf.* It arises from the common peroneal nerve.
- *Small saphenous vein.* It drains into the popliteal vein.

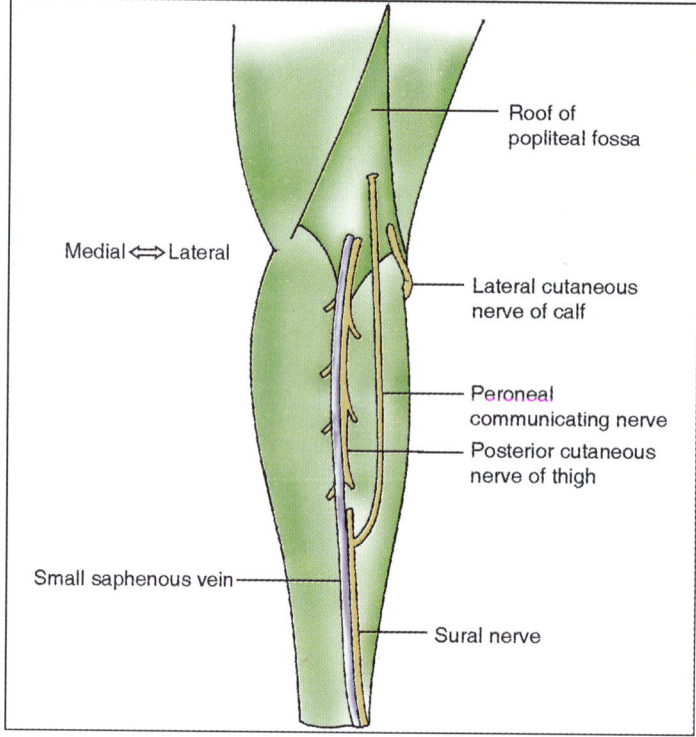

Fig. 30.2 Roof of the popliteal fossa

Floor

It is formed by the following structures from above downwards.

- *Popliteal surface of femur.*
- *Posterior part of capsule of knee.*

- *Oblique popliteal ligament.* It is pierced by the following structures.
  - Middle genicular vessels.
  - Middle genicular nerve.
  - Articular branch of the posterior branch of obturator nerve.
- *Fascia over the popliteus.*

Contents

It includes the following structures.

- *Tibial (medial popliteal) nerve.*
- *Common peroneal (lateral popliteal) nerve.*
- *Popliteal artery.*
- *Popliteal vein.*
- *Popliteal lymph nodes.*

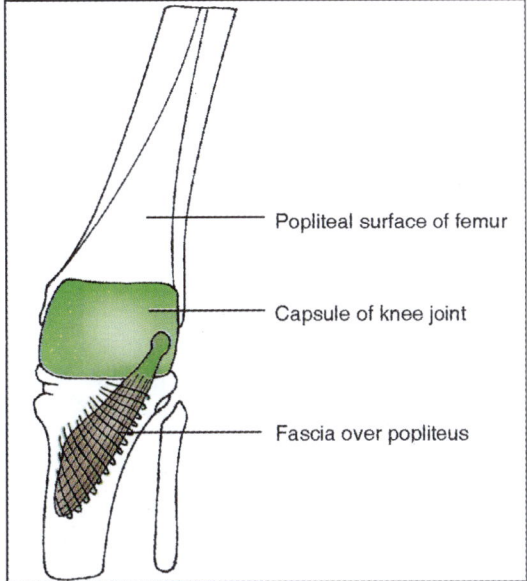

Popliteal surface of femur

Capsule of knee joint

Fascia over popliteus

Fig. 30.3 Floor of the popliteal fossa

TIBIAL NERVE

Root value. $L_{4, 5}$, $S_{1, 2, 3}$.

Course. It arises as a terminal branch at the apex of the popliteal fossa and descends almost upto the flexor retinaculum at the ankle. In the popliteal fossa it extends from its apex to the lower margin of the popliteus muscle.

Branches

Muscular branches to;

- Plantaris.
- Gastrocnemius (both heads).
- Soleus.
- Popliteus. This branch also supplies the superior tibiofibular joint and the interosseous membrane.

Articular branches

These supply the knee joint.

- *Upper medial genicular nerve.* It runs medially superficial to the medial head of the gastrocnemius muscle.
- *Lower mdial genicular nerve.* It runs medially deep to the medial collateral ligament at the level of medial tibial condyle.
- *Middle genicular nerve.* It pierces the oblique popliteal ligament.

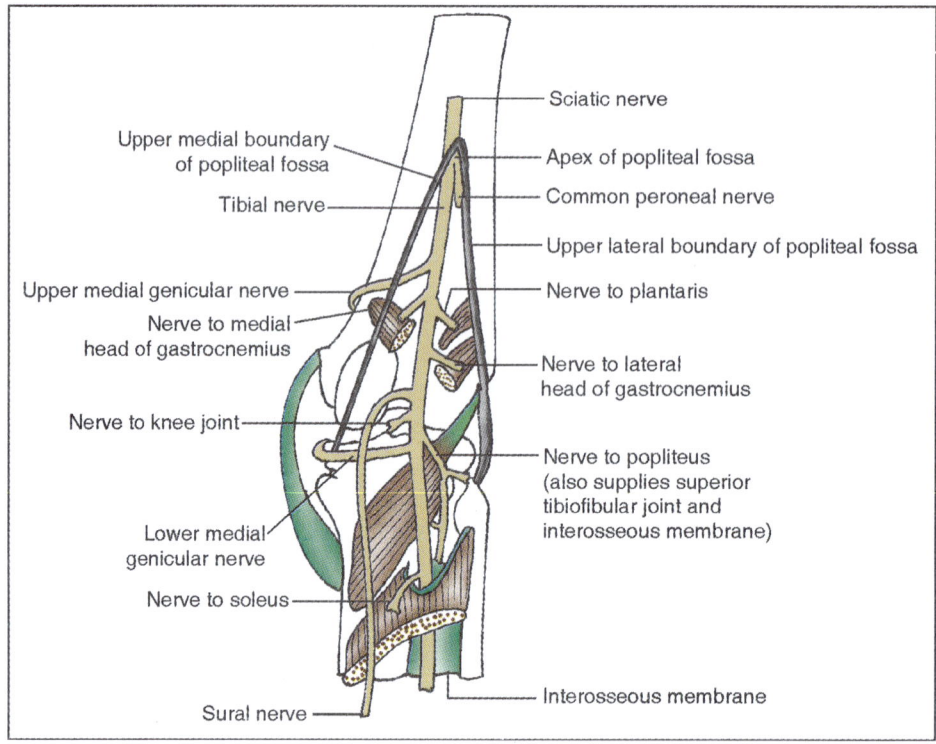

Fig. 30.4 Tibial nerve in the popliteal fossa

Cutaneous branch

This is called the sural nerve $(S_{1, 2})$. It descends deep to the deep fascia till it reaches the middle of leg where it becomes subcutaneous by piercing the deep fascia. It then follows the course of small saphenous ven.

COMMON PERONEAL NERVE

Root value: $L_{4, 5}$, $S_{1, 2}$

Course: it arises as a terminal branch of sciatic nerve at the apex of the popliteal fossa. It follows the tendon of biceps femoris (upper lateral boundary of the politeal fossa) to reach the fibula where it terminates.

Branches

Articular

- *Upper lateral genicular nerve*. It reaches laterally deep to the tendon of biceps femoris just above the lateral femoral condyle.
- *Lower lateral genicular nerve*. It runs laterally deep to the biceps tendon and fibular collateral ligament at the level of lateral tibial condyle.

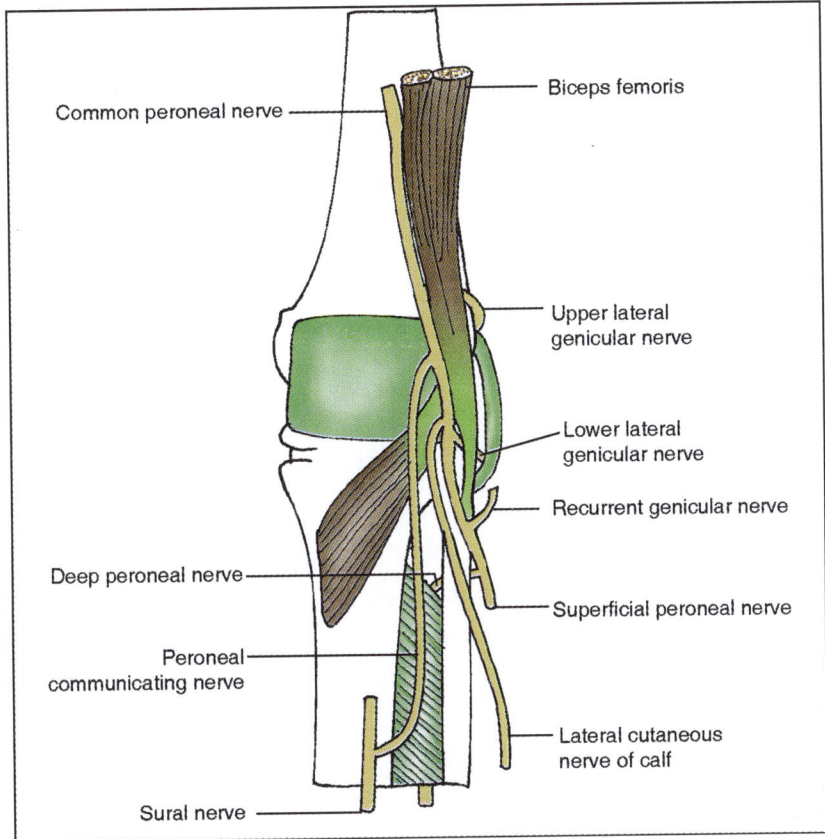

Fig. 30.5 Common peroneal nerve

- *Recurrent genicular nerve.* It arises just proximal to the termination of common peroneal nerve and runs a recurrent course (ascends) to supply the knee joint.

Cutaneous

- *Lateral cutaneous nerve of calf.* It descends at the lateral aspect of leg and supplies its upper part.
- *Peroneal communicating nerve.* It descends and joins the sural nerve on the back of leg.

Terminal

- *Superficial peroneal nerve.*
- *Deep peroneal nerve.*

POPLITEAL ARTERY

Commencement. It is continuation of femoral artery at the tendinous hiatus in the adductor magnus.

Termination. It terminates at the level of tendinous arch for the attachment of soleus.

Relations. While going from superficial to deep, the tibial nerve is most superficial, popliteal vein is next to it and the popliteal artery being the deepest. In the upper part, the tibial nerve is most lateral, and popliteal artery is most medial and popliteal vein is in between the two. While descending downwards, the artery courses from medial to lateral and nerve from lateral to medial making the relations reverse. In all situations, the popliteal vein is always sandwitched between the artery and nerve.

Branches

Muscular. These are also called sural arteries as they supply the superficial muscles of calf.

Articular. Five genicular branches appear from the popliteal artery to participate in the formation of anastomoses around knee.

- *Upper medial genicular artery.*
- *Upper lateral genicular artery.*
- *Middle genicular artery.*
- *Lower medial genicular artery.*
- *Lower lateral genicular artery.*

Genicular arteries follow the courses of genicular nerves.

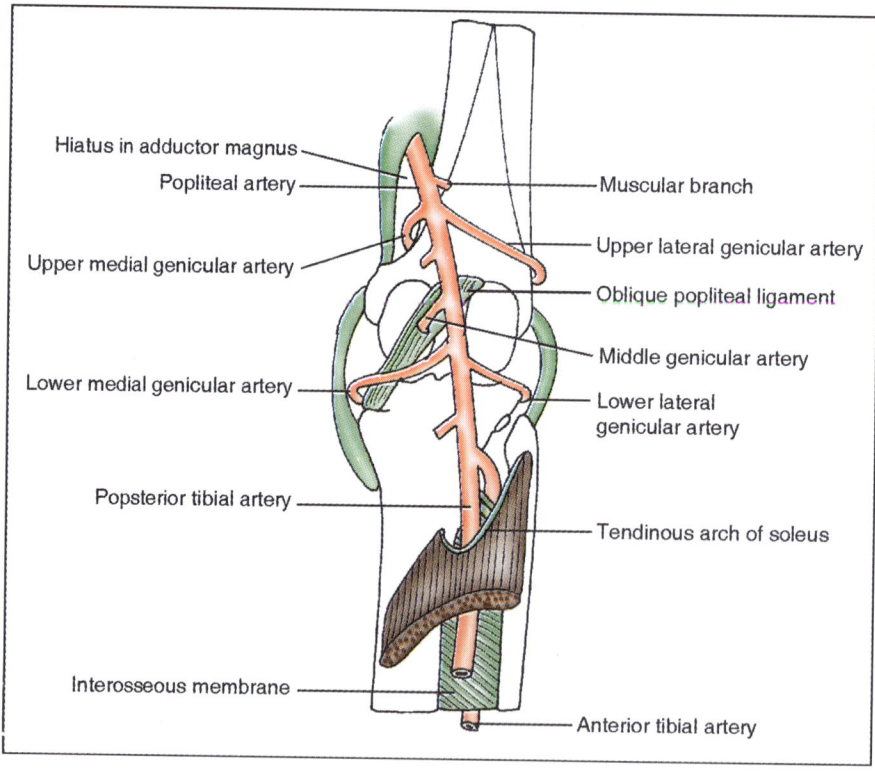

Fig. 30.6 Popliteal artery

Terminal

- *Anterior tibial artery*. It enters the extensor compartment of leg by passing through a passage in the upper part of the interosseous membrane.
- *Posterior tibial artery*. It accompanies the tibial nerve to enter the flexor compartment of leg under the tendinous arch for soleus.

POPLITEAL VEIN

It receives tributaries accompanying the branches of popliteal artery in addition to small saphenous vein.

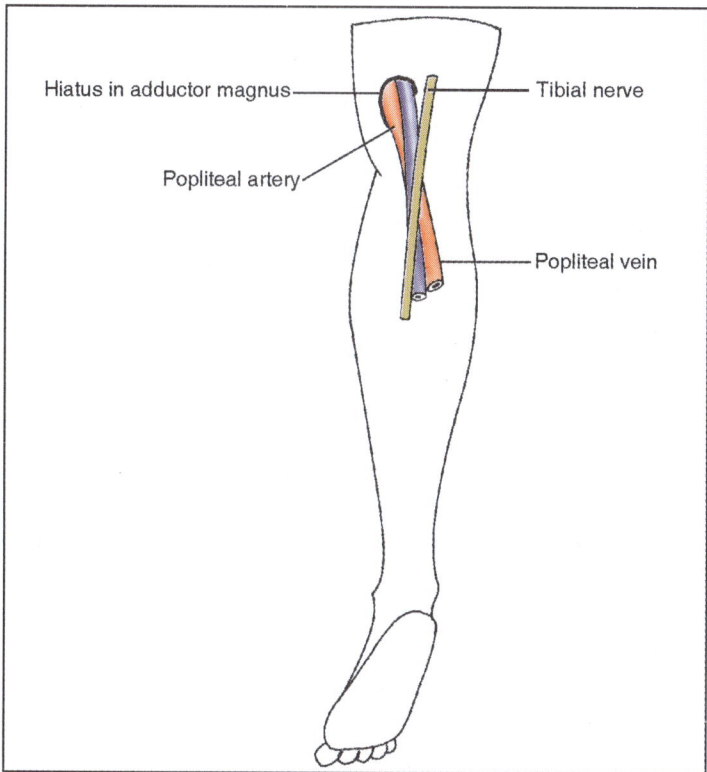

Hiatus in adductor magnus — Tibial nerve

Popliteal artery

Popliteal vein

Fig. 30.7 Interrelationship between popliteal vessels and tibial nerve

POPLITEAL LYMPH NODES

These are deep lymph nodes in relation to the popliteal vein. It receives both superficial and deep afferent lymphatics. Superficial afferents accompany small saphenous vein and drain the lateral margin of foot and back of leg. Deep lymphatics are derived from the deep tissues of leg and foot. Their efferent lymphatics drain into deep inguinal lymph nodes.

DISSECTION STEPS: POPLITEAL FOSSA

Make skin incision No. 18 (Fig. 3.13). Reflect the skin flaps laterally. While reflecting the superficial and deep fascia, identify the small saphenous vein, posterior cutaneous nerve of thigh, sural nerve and lateral cutaneous nerve of calf. Define the muscles forming the boundaries of the popliteal fossa i.e., superomedially by the semimembranosus and semitendinosus; superolaterally by the biceps femoris; inferomedially by the medial head of gastrocnemius and inferolaterally by the lateral head of gastrocnemius and plantaris. Clean and identify its following contents: popliteal artery, popliteal vein, tibial nerve, common peroneal nerve, genicular branch of popliteal artery, nerve to popliteus, popliteal group of lymph nodes and popliteal pad of fat.

Applied anatomy

- Popliteal artery pulsation is easily palpated in the flexed position of knee.
- Semimembranosus bursitis produces a swelling in the upper medial part of the popliteal fossa.
- Swelling in the midline of the popliteal fossa is usually due to the popliteal artery aneurysm. It is pulsatile in nature.
- Some times an inflamed popliteal lymph node may lead to complications like abscess in the region called the popliteal abscess.
- Involvement of common peroneal nerve is because of local injury due to its superficial position or fracture of neck of fibula. If so, it leads to paralysis of muscles of the extensor compartment of leg. In this condition the patient will walk with undue lifting of the foot to clear the dropped foot off the ground.
- Tibial nerve is rarely injured except in open wound. Patient is unable to plantar flex his ankle with loss of sensation in the sole. Since it also supplies the plantar muscles, there will be claw foot also.
- Crossed leg test (Fuchsig's test). Movement of foot of the crossed leg are noticed only when the corresponding popliteal artery is patent.

31

Front of Leg and Dorsum of Foot

CUTANEOUS NERVES

Front of leg

Medial side. Saphenous nerve

Lateral side. Upper 2/3rd, Lateral cutaneous nerve of calf.

Lower 1/3rd, Superficial peroneal nerve.

Dorsum of foot

Medial margin. Saphenous nerve.

Lateral margin. Sural nerve.

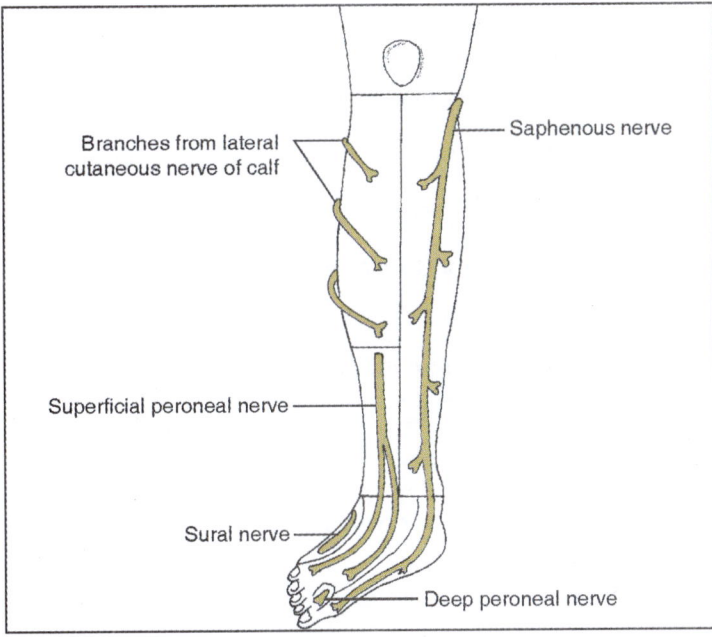

Fig. 31.1 Cutaneous nerves of front of leg and dorsum of foot

Ist interdigital cleft. Deep peroneal enrve.

Rest of the dorsum of foot. Superficial peroneal nerve.

Applied anatomy

- Injury to the cutaneous nerve results into loss of sensation in the area supplied by it, a condition called anaesthesia.

DEEP FASCIA AND INTERMUSCULAR SEPTA

Deep fascia is attached to the medial and anterior border of tibia making its medial surface subcutaneous. It is also attached to both the malleoli. Two intermuscular septa (anterior and posterior) arise from the deep surface of the deep fascia and get attached to the corresponding border of fibula. These fasciae along with the two bones of the leg and interosseous membrane bound three compartments (anterior, lateral and posterior).

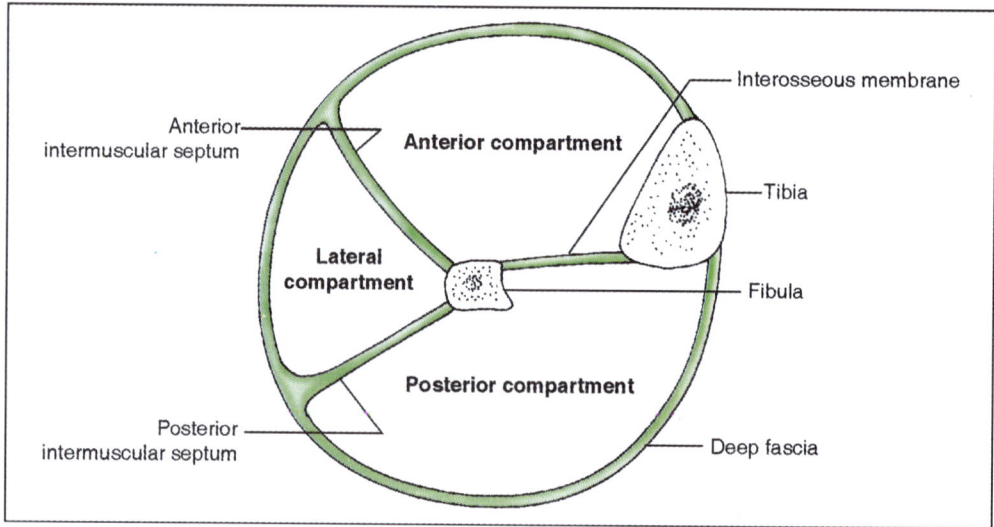

Fig. 31.2 Compartments of leg

Deep fascia is thickened in the region of ankle to form retinacula, holding long tendons of the muscles of different compartment of leg before these enter into the foot. Those holding the extensor tendons derived from the anterior compartment are superior and inferior extensor retinacula.

Superior extensor retinaculum

It extends between the distal ends of the anterior borders of tibia and fibula.

Inferior extensor retinaculum

It is 'Y' shaped. The stem of 'Y' is attached to the anterior part of the superior surface of calcaneum and two limbs of 'Y' are attached to the medial malleolus and deep fascia of sole.

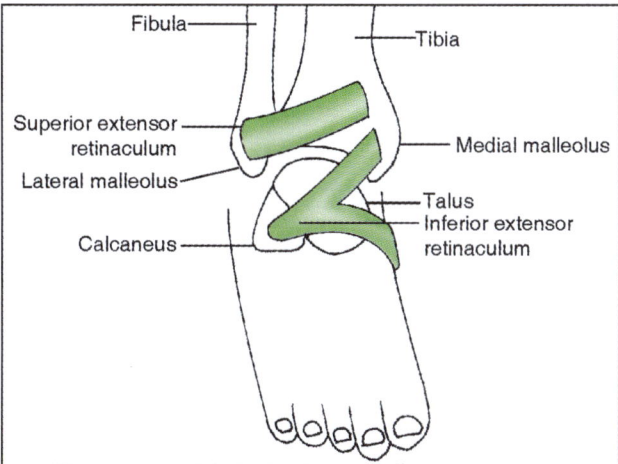

Fig. 31.3 Extensor retinacula

CONTENTS OF THE ANTERIOR COMPARTMENT OF LEG

Muscles

- Tibialis anterior.
- Extensor digitorum longus.
- Extensor hallucis longus.
- Peroneus tertius.

Nerve. Deep peroneal nerve.

Artery. Anterior tibial artery.

Tibialis anterior

Origin. Upper half of the lateral surface of tibia and adjacent interosseous membrane.

Insertion. Mainly to the medial aspect of medial cuneiform, and also to the base of the Ist metatarsal.

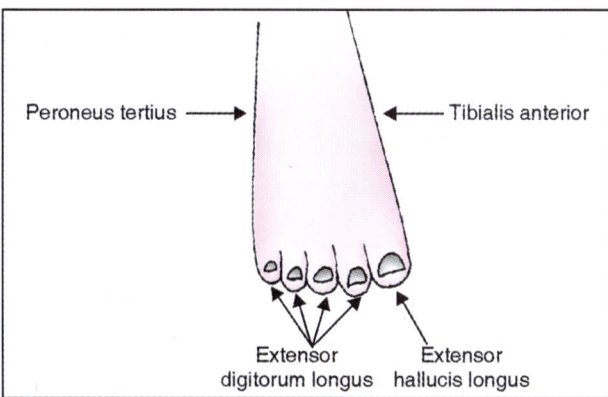

Fig. 31.4 Insertions of muscles of the extensor compartment of leg

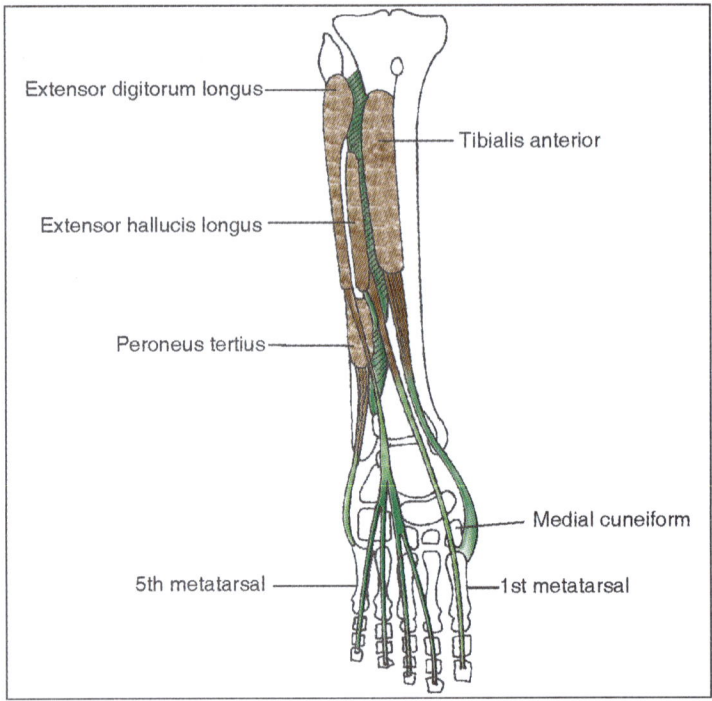

Fig. 31.5 Muscles of the extensor compartment of leg

Nerve. Deep peroneal nerve.

Actions. Dorsiflexion and inversion of foot.

Extensor digitorum longus

Origin. Upper 1/4th and lateral half of middle 2/4th of anterior surface of fibula.

Insertion. The tendon divides into four divisions which extend towards the lateral four toes. Each division joins the base of the dorsal digital expansion of the corresponding toe. Each tendon divides into three slips. The central slip gets attached to the base of middle phalanx. Marginal (collateral) slips reunite and get attached to the dorsal aspect of the base of distal phalanx.

Nerve. Deep peroneal nerve.

Actions. Dorsiflexion of foot and extension of the lateral four toes.

Extensor hallucis longus

Origin. Medial half of middle 2/4th of anterior surface of fibula and adjacent interosseous membrane.

Insertion. Dorsal aspect of the base of the distal phalanx of great toe.

Nerve. Deep peroneal nerve.

Actions. Dorsiflexion and inversion of foot and extension of great toe.

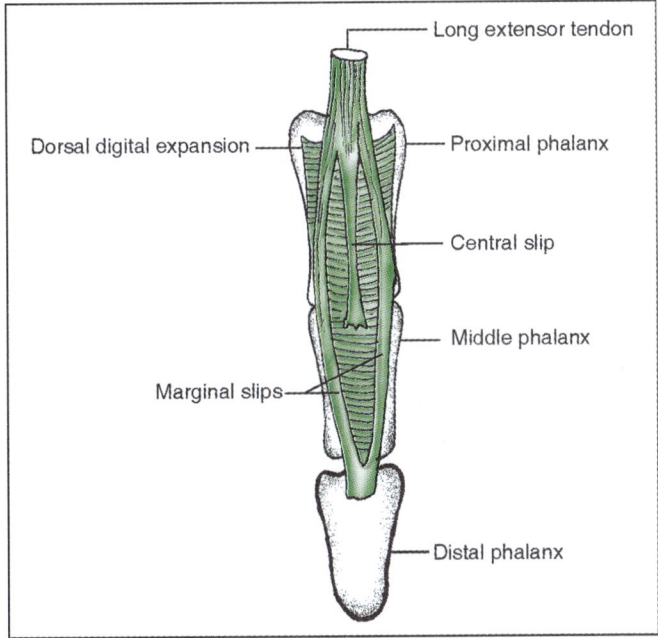

Fig. 31.6 Mode of insertion of extensor digitorum longus tendon

Peroneus tertius

Origin. Lower 1/4th of the medial surface of fibula.

Insertion. Base of the 5th metatarsal.

Nerve. Deep peroneal nerve.

Actions. Dorsiflexion and eversion of foot.

Synovial sheaths of extensor tendons

There are three synovial sheaths enclosing four extensor tendons, the details of which are as under:

Tendons of muscles	Extent	
	From	**To**
1. Tibialis anterior	Upper border of superior extensor retinaculum	Insertion of muscle
2. Extensor hallucis longus	Lower border of superior extensor retinaculum	Base of the proximal phalanx of great toe.
3. Extensor digitorum and peroneus tertius	Lower border of superior extensor retinaculum	Middle of the foot

---

DISSECTION STEPS: FRONT OF LEG AND DORSUM OF FOOT

Make skin incision No. 11 (Fig. 3.13) and a horizontal incision across malleoli and reflect the skin flaps from front of leg and dorsum of foot. Remove the superficial fascia and identify the commencement of great saphenous vein in front of medial malleolus. Also identify the superficial and deep peroneal nerves, saphenous nerve and dorsal venous arch. Remove the deep fascia and identify the muscles of anterior compartment of leg (from medial to lateral these are tibialis anterior, extensor hallucis longus, extensor digitorum longus and peroneus tertius); muscles of the dorsum of foot (extensor hallucis brevis and extensor digitorum brevis). Define the modification of deep fascia near ankle and dorsum of the foot (superior and inferior extensor retinacula respectively) and identify the structures passing deep to it (tibialis anterior, extensor hallucis longus, dorsalis pedis artery, deep peroneal nerve, extensor digitorum longus and peroneus tertius). Clean and trace the structures of the dorsum of foot viz dorsalis pedis artery, extensor hallucis brevis, extensor digitorum brevis and tendon of perorneus longus and brevis.

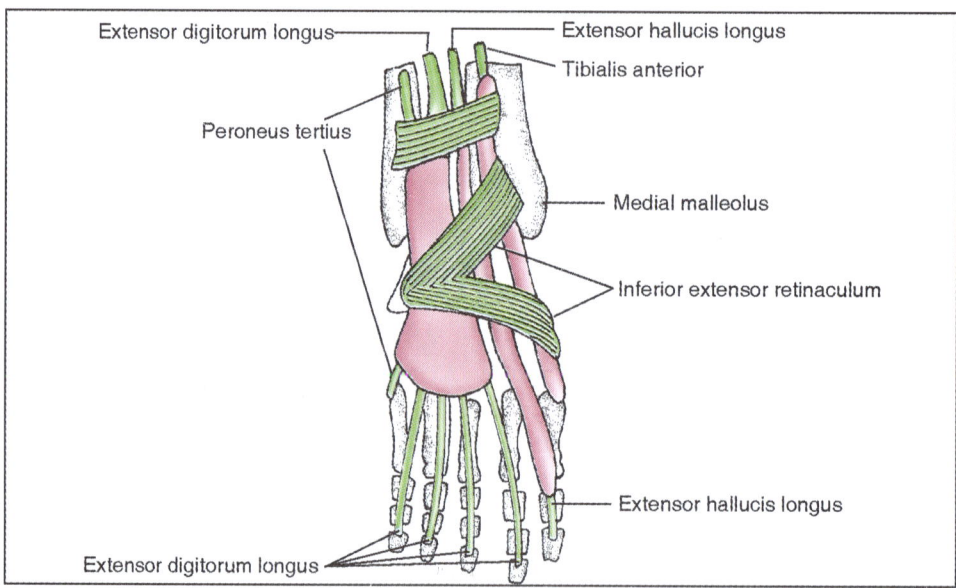

Fig. 31.7 Synovial sheaths of extensor tendons of leg

DEEP PERONEAL NERVE

Commencement. It arises as a terminal branch of the common peroneal nerve on the back of the neck of fibula.

Course. At the origin, it is deep to the peroneus longus. It pierces the anterior intermuscular septum and the extensor digitorum longus to reach the interosseous membrane on which it descends. In the lower part of the leg it crosses the front of lower end of the tibia deep to the superior extensor retinaculum to enter the dorsum of foot.

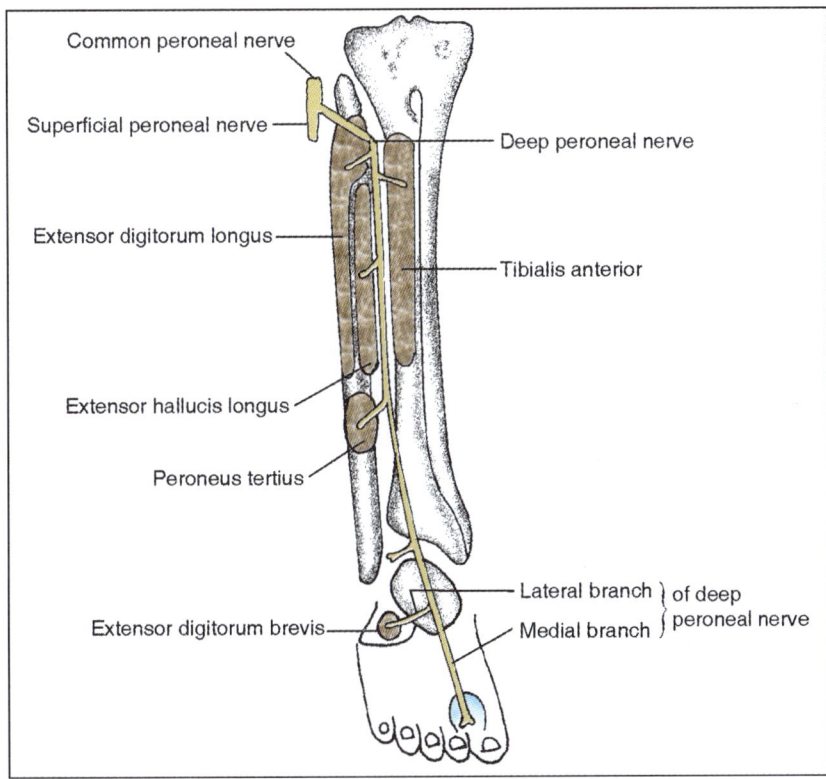

Common peroneal nerve

Superficial peroneal nerve

Deep peroneal nerve

Extensor digitorum longus

Tibialis anterior

Extensor hallucis longus

Peroneus tertius

Lateral branch } of deep
Medial branch } peroneal nerve

Extensor digitorum brevis

Fig. 31.8 Deep peroneal nerve

Termination. Just below the ankle it divides into lateral and medial branches.

- *Lateral branch*. It passes laterally under the extensor digitorum brevis and supplies it.
- *Medial branch*. It courses towards the interdigital cleft between 1st and 2nd toes and supplies the skin there.

Branches. In the leg it supplies all the muscles of the extensor compartment. It also provides twigs to the ankle joint.

Applied anatomy

- Common peroneal nerve is liable to be injured in the fracture of the neck of the fibula. This results into *foot drop* (paralysis of the extensor muscles of the foot) and *talipes equinovarus* deformity (paralysis of peronei).

ANTERIOR TIBIAL ARTERY

Commencement. It is one of the terminal branches of the popliteal artery.

Course. It enters the extensor compartment of the leg from behind through the oval aperture in the proximal part of the interosseous membrane. It then descends on the front of the interosseous membrane close to the deep peroneal nerve.

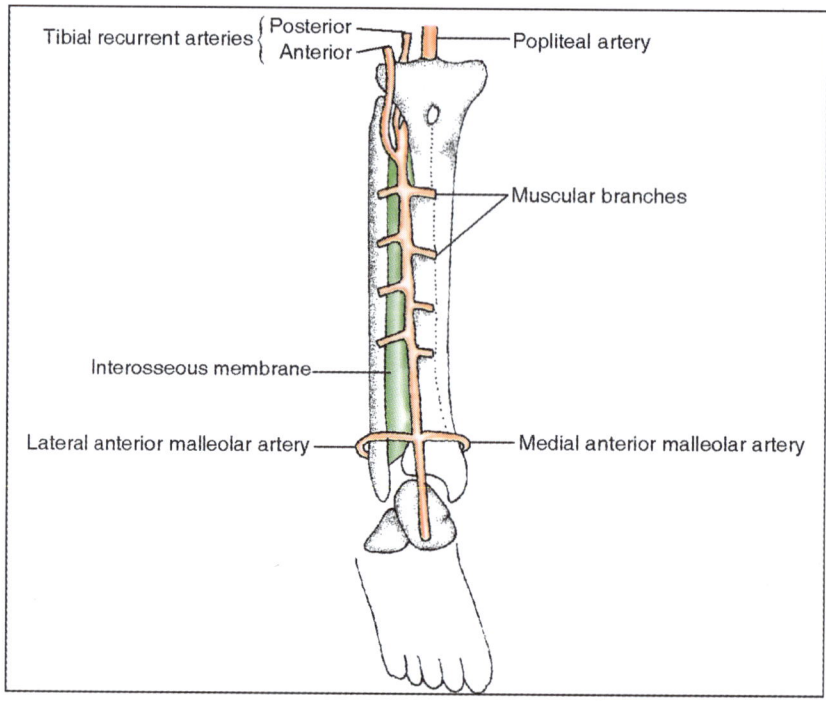

Fig. 31.9 Anterior tibial artery

Termination. At the level of the ankle, anterior tibial artery continues as dorsalis paedis artery.

Branches

- *Tibial recurrent arteries*. Anterior and posterior tibial recurrent arteries arise from its upper part and ascend in front and behind the lateral tibial condyle respectively.
- *Muscular branches*.
- *Anterior malleolar arteries*. Medial and lateral anterior malleolar arteries run in the corresponding direction close to the lower ends of tibia and fibula respectively.

Applied anatomy

- Pulsation of anterior tibial artery is felt anteriorly between two malleoli against the lower end of tibia just above the ankle joint lateral to the tendon of extensor hallucis longus.
- Anterior tibial artery may be occluded partially or completely. Patient complains of intermittent claudication i.e., pain and weakness in the legs on walking.

Extensor digitorum brevis

Origin. Anterior part of the superior surface of calcaneus.

Insertion. The muscle provides 4 tendons for the medial 4 toes. The most medial tendon constitutes the extensor hallucis brevis, which gets attached to the dorsal aspect of the base of the proximal phalanx of great toe. Lateral three tendons extend to the dorsal digital expansion of the middle three toes.

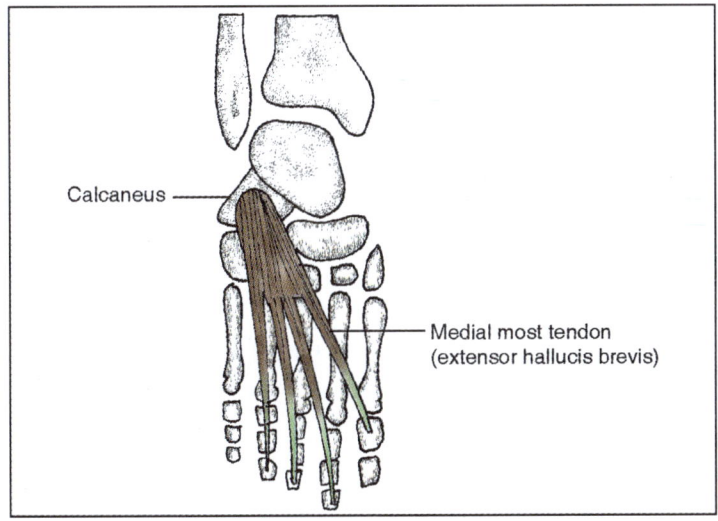

Fig. 31.10 Extensor digitorum brevis

Nerve. Deep peroneal nerve.

Actions. Extension of the corresponding toe.

Dorsalis pedis artery

Commencement. It is continuation of the anterior tibial artery at the level of ankle.

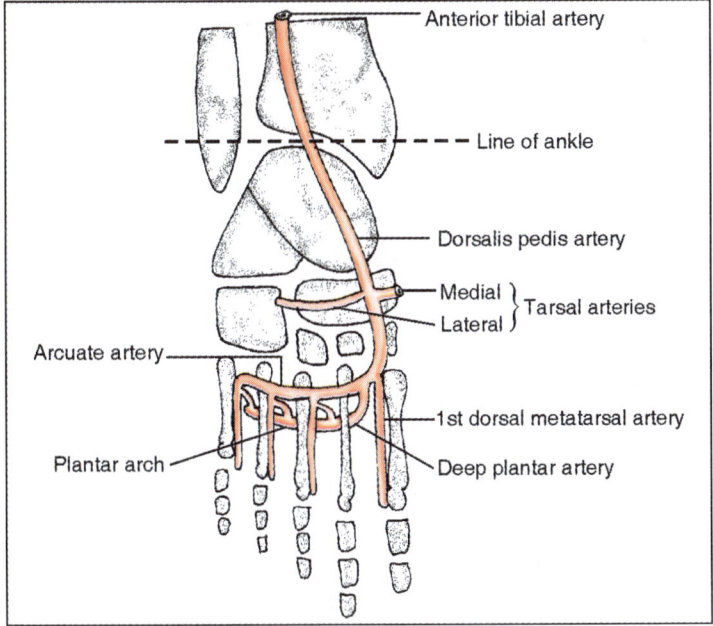

Fig. 31.11 Dorsalis pedis artery

Branches

- *Medial and lateral tarsal arteries.* These run in the corresponding direction across the tarsal bones.
- *Terminal branches*
  - *Ist dorsal metatarsal artery.* It runs forward along the Ist inter-metatarsal space.
  - *Arcuate artery.* It runs laterally across the 2nd, 3rd and 4th metatarsal bases. It gives rise to 2nd, 3rd and 4th dorsal metatarsal arteries, which run forward, along 2nd, 3rd and 4th inter-metatarsal spaces respectively. Proximal ends of these dorsal metatarsal arteries are connected with the plantar arch through proximal perforating arteries. Perforating artery in the Ist inter-metatarsal space connects the medial end of arcuate artery with plantar arch and is called deep plantar artery.

Applied anatomy

- Pulsation of dorsalis paedis artery can be felt just lateral to the tendon of extensor hallucis longus. It is absent in 10% of individuals.

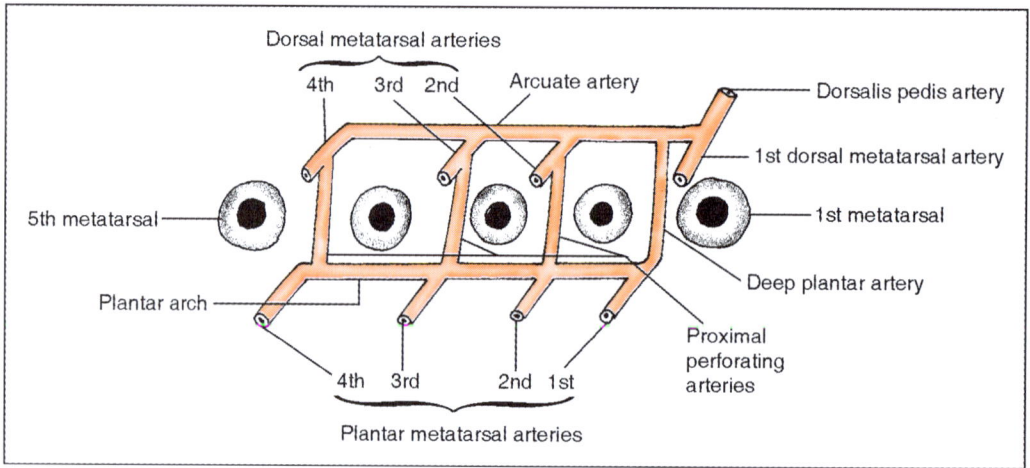

Fig. 31.12 Diagramatic presentation of arcuate artery and plantar arch

32

Medial Side of The Leg

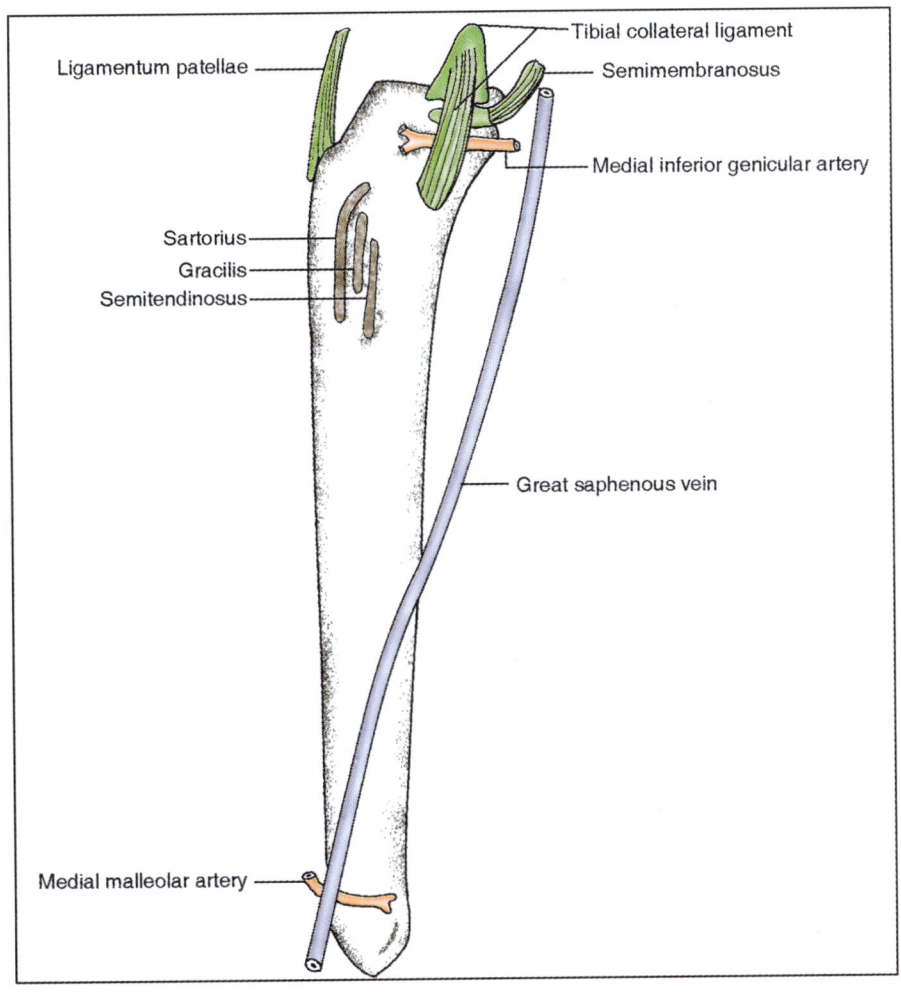

Ligamentum patellae

Sartorius
Gracilis
Semitendinosus

Medial malleolar artery

Tibial collateral ligament
Semimembranosus

Medial inferior genicular artery

Great saphenous vein

Fig. 32.1 Medial side of leg

- It is formed by the subcutaneous, medial aspect of the tibia.
- Three muscles attached to the upper part of the medial surface of the shaft of the tibia (from anterior to posterior) are, sartorius, gracilis and semitendinosus.
- Semimembranosus gets attached to the groove on the posterior aspect of the medial condyle of tibia.
- Tibial collateral ligament (deep and superficial parts) gets attached to the medial aspect of upper end of tibia.
- Medial inferior genicular artery passes forwards deep to the superficial part of the tibial collateral ligament.
- Medial surface of tibia is crossed obliquely by the great saphenous vein.
- Medial malleolar artery crosses the medial aspect of the lower end of tibia.

33

Lateral Compartment of The Leg

Lateral compartment of leg is bound by the lateral surface of fibula, deep fascia of leg and anterior and posterior intermuscular septa. Its contents include two muscles (peroneus longus and peroneus brevis), a nerve (superficial peroneal nerve) and muscular branches of the peroneal artery.

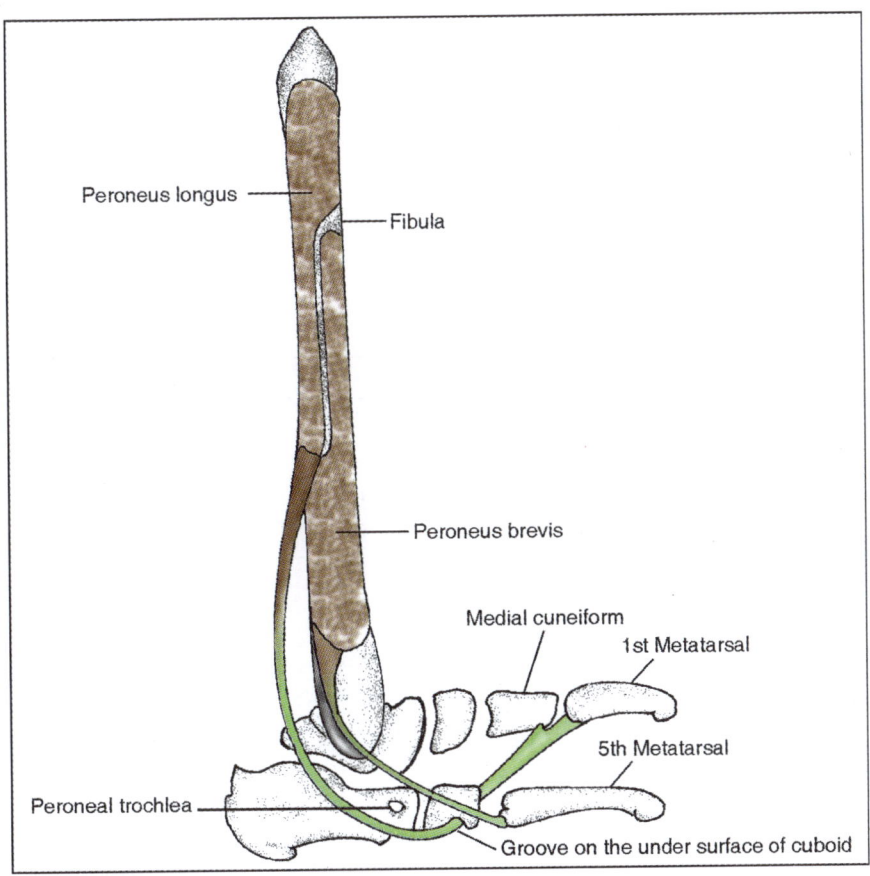

Fig. 33.1 Muscles of the lateral compartment of leg

PERONEUS LONGUS

Origin. Upper 2/3rd of lateral surface of fibula.

Insertion. Tendon of this muscle runs a long course. It passes behind the lower end of fibula (posterior to the tendon of peroneus brevis), runs forward on the lateral aspect of calcaneus (below the peroneal trochlea) and then turns medially to run in the groove on the under surface of cuboid and ultimately reaches the medial margin of the foot to get inserted mainly to the base of Ist metatarsal in addition to the medial cuneiform.

Nerve. Superficial peroneal nerve.

Actions.

- Plantar flexion and eversion of foot.
- To maintain the lateral longitudinal and transverse arches of the foot.

PERONEUS BREVIS

Origin. Lower 2/3rd of lateral surface of fibula.

Insertion. Its tendon grooves the back of the lateral malleolus and passes forwards on the lateral aspect of calcaneus above the peroneal trochlea to get inserted to the base of the 5th metatarsal.

Nerve. Superficial peroneal nerve.

Actions. Plantar flexion and eversion of foot.

PERONEAL RETINACULA

These are thickenings in the deep fascia on the lateral aspect of foot. These are two in number (superior and inferior) and hold the tendons of peronei.

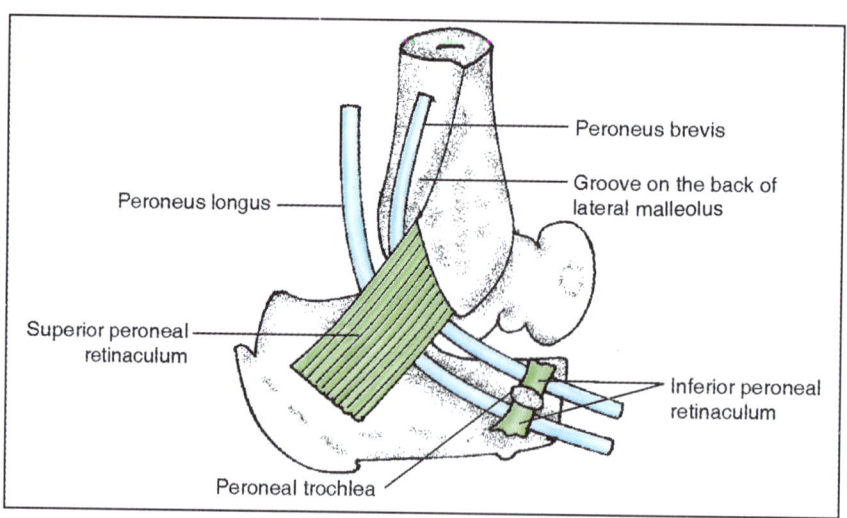

Fig. 33.2 Peroneal retinacula

Superior peroneal retinaculum. It extends between the posterior margin of lateral malleolus and lateral aspect of calcaneus.

Inferior peroneal retinaculum. It is attached just above and below the peroneal trochlea on the lateral aspect of calcaneus. It is also attached to the peroneal trochlea leading to the formation of compartments. Upper compartment is meant for peroneus brevis tendon while the lower one for the peroneus longus tendon.

SYNOVIAL SHEATH

There is a common synovial sheath for both the tendons under the superior peroneal retinaculum. It becomes double deep to the inferior peroneal retinaculum enclosing the corresponding tendon of peronei.

SUPERFICIAL PERONEAL NERVE

Commencement. It is one of the terminal branches of the common peroneal nerve at the level of neck of fibula.

Course. It descends in the lateral compartment of leg.

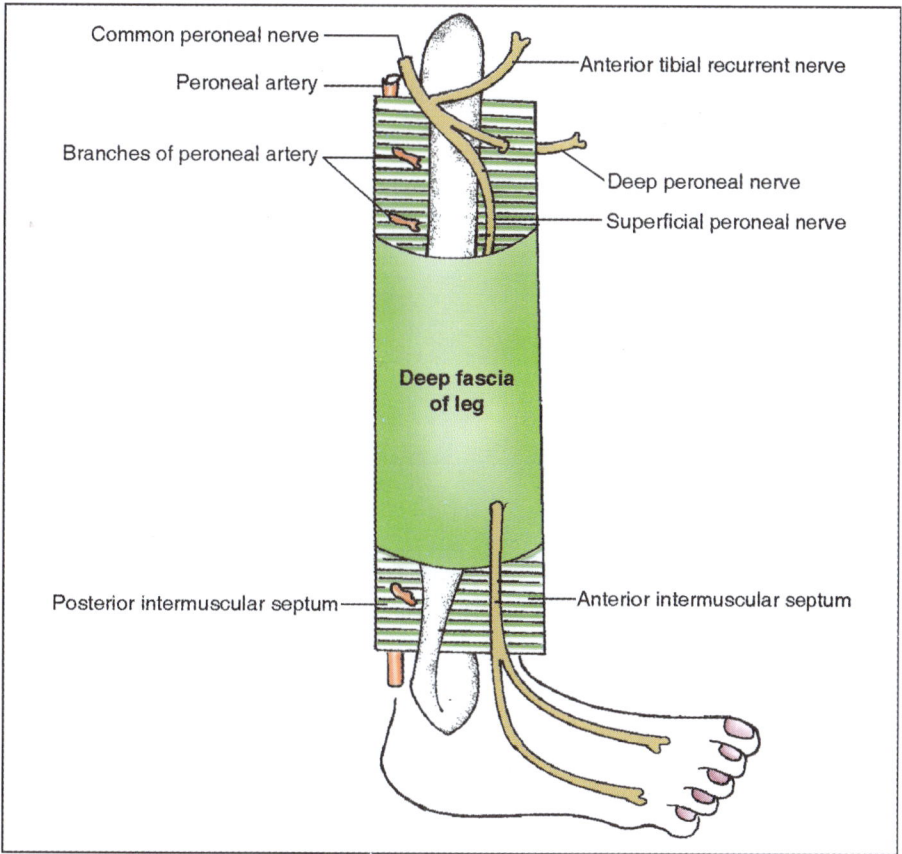

Fig. 33.3 Nerve and arteries of the peroneal compartment

Branches

- *Muscular branches.* These supply peroneus longus and peroneus brevis muscles.
- *Cutaneous branches.* Superficial peroneal nerve pierces the deep fascia of lower 3rd of leg and divides into medial and intermediate dorsal cutaneous nerves. It supplies the skin of the lower 3rd of the lateral aspect of leg and most of the dorsum of foot.

BRANCHES FROM THE PERONEAL ARTERY

Peroneal artery is a branch of the posterior tibial artery and descends very close to fibula in the flexor compartment of leg. Multiple branches appear from the artery and pierce the posterior intermuscular septum to enter and supply the lateral compartment of leg.

34

Lymphatic Drainage of Lower Limb

LYMPH NODES

- *Superficial inguinal lymph nodes*. These are located in the superficial fascia of the upper part of the thigh just below the inguinal ligament. These form a 'T' shaped arrangement. Horizontal group forms the horizontal limb of 'T' and the vertical group represents the vertical limb of 'T'. Horizontal group is further divided into medial and lateral subgroups.
- *Deep lymph nodes*. These are usually located in relation to deep veins. Popliteal lymph nodes are located on the side of the popliteal vein while the deep inguinal lymph nodes are situated in relation to the upper part of the femoral vein. The heighest one of the latter group is located in the femoral canal.

LYMPHATICS

Superficial lymphatics

- Lymphatics from the perineum, medial part of gluteal region and medial part of anterior abdominal wall below the umbilicus drain into medial group of horizontal chain.
- Those from the lateral part of gluteal region and lateral part of anterior abdominal wall below the umbilicus, drain into lateral group of horizontal chain.
- Superficial lymphatics from the lateral margin and heel of the foot and back of the calf proceed towards the popliteal lymph nodes.
- Remaining lymphatic vessels from the lower limb join the vertical chain.

Deep lymphatics

- Those from the foot and leg drain into the popliteal lymph nodes.
- Deep lymphatics derived from thigh and the efferents of superficial inguinal and popliteal lymph nodes drain into the deep inguinal lymph nodes.
- Efferents of the deep inguinal lymph nodes join the external iliac lymph nodes.
- Deep lymphatics of perineum and gluteal region end into the internal iliac lymph nodes.

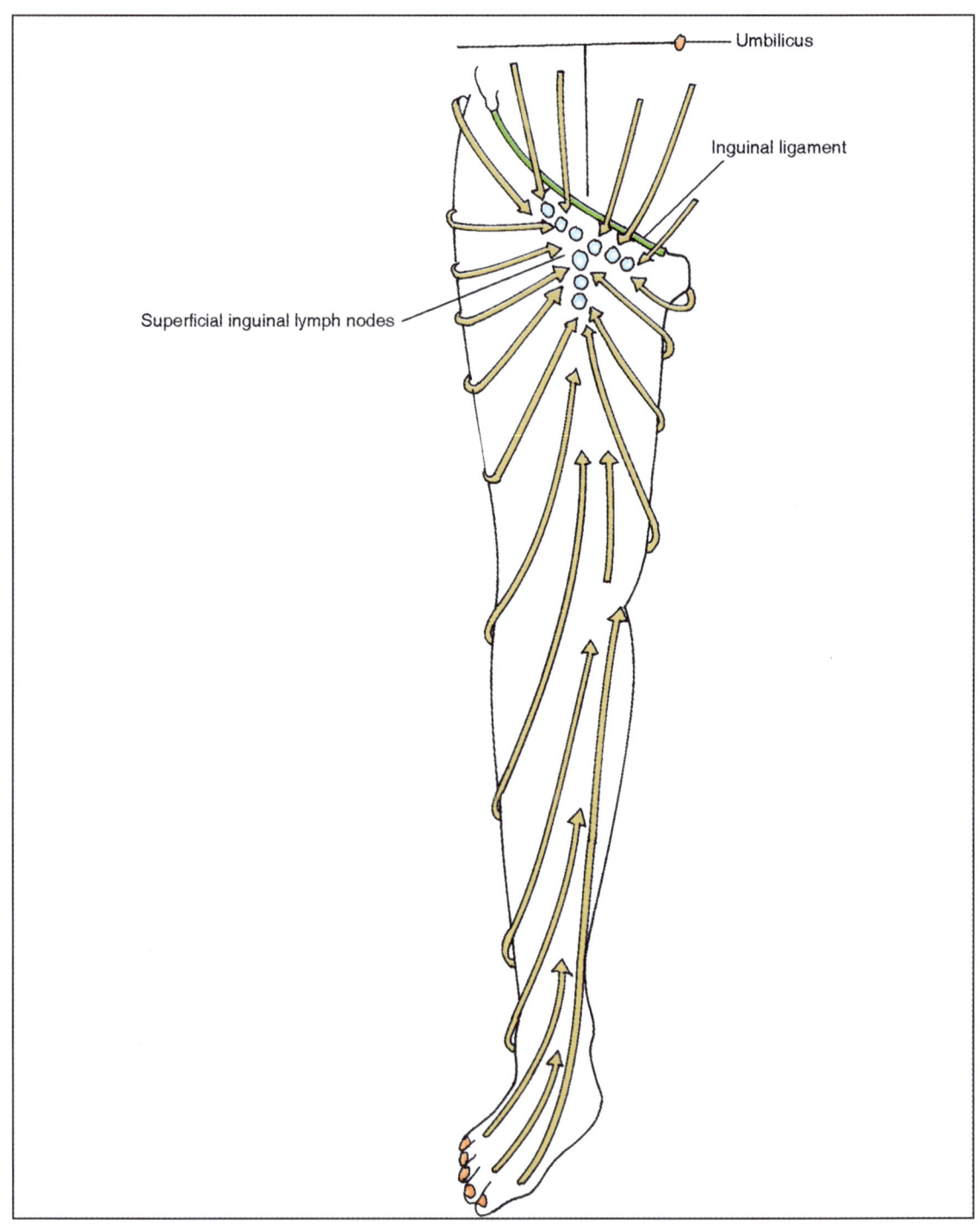

Fig. 34.1 Lymphatic drainage of lower limb (anterior view)

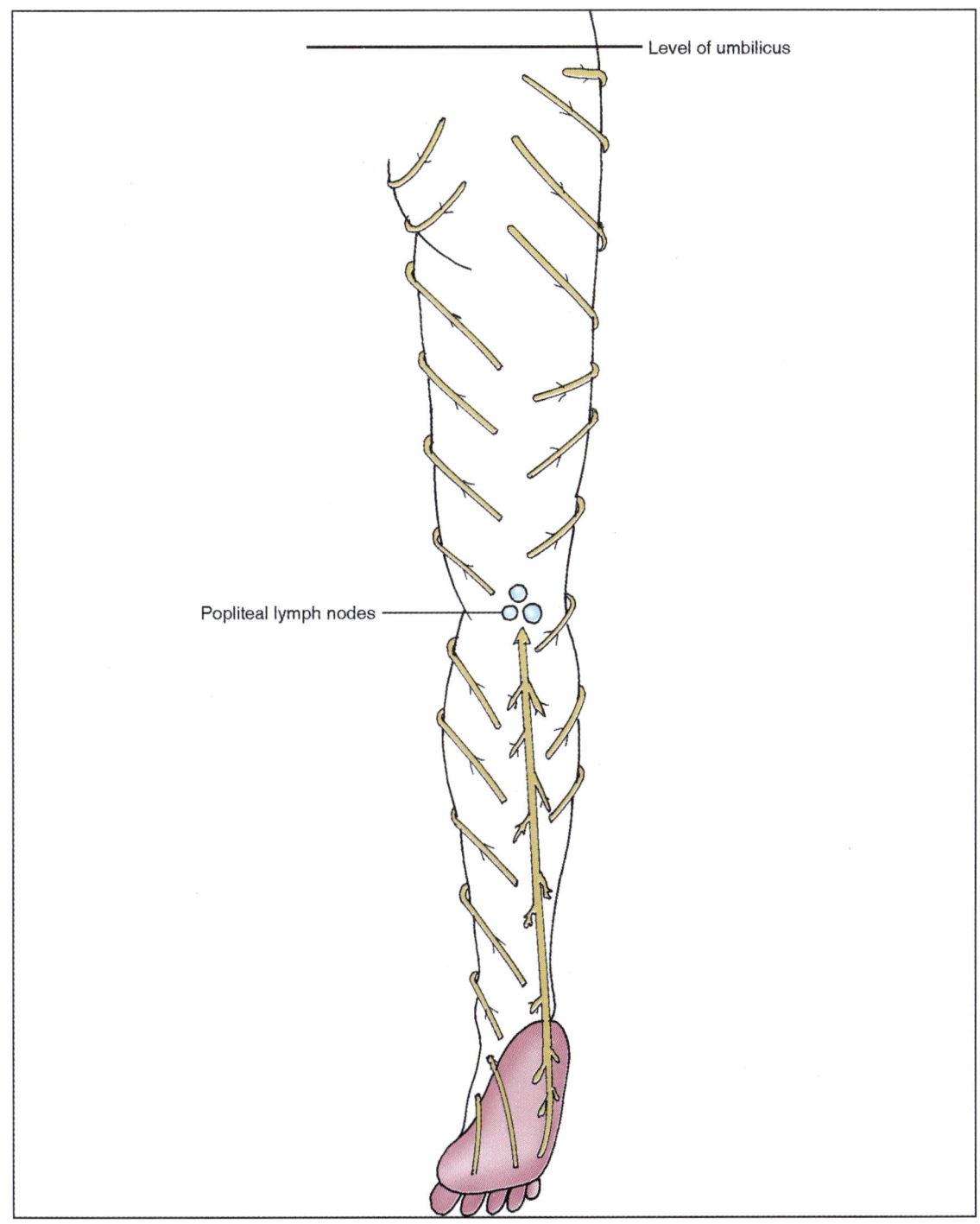

Level of umbilicus

Popliteal lymph nodes

Fig. 34.2 Lymphatic drainage of lower limb (posterior view)

Applied anatomy

- In acute lymphadenitis the lymph nodes become enlarged and painful. One should search for the primary focus of infection in the area drained by it.
- In cases of chronic lymphadenitis, lymph nodes are moderately enlarged, slightly tender and may show matting. Tuberculous lymphadenitis commonly involves inguinal lymph nodes usually in young age group.
- Enlarged painless inguinal lymph nodes may be the sign of primary stage of syphilitic lymphadenitis.
- Inguinal lymph nodes are very commonly involved in the filarial lymphadenitis.
- Lymphogranuloma inguinale is a type of venereal disease caused by a filterable virus.
- Lymphomas, Hodgkin's disease and secondary carcinomas are the other conditions involving the lymph nodes.

DISSECTION STEPS: LATERAL AND POSTERIOR COMPARTMENTS OF LEG

Divide the deep fascia on the lateral aspect of the leg. Clean and identify the muscles of lateral compartment (peroneus longus and peroneus brevis). Identify the peroneal retinaculum. Remove the fascia from the medial aspect of upper end of tibia and note muscles attached to its upper part (from medial to lateral: sartorius, gracilis and semitendinosus). Also remove the fascia from the back of the leg. Locate great saphenous vein, small saphenous vein opening into popliteal vein, superficial muscles of calf (gastrocnemius, soleus and plantaris) and nerves (tibial, saphenous, sural, common peroneal and superficial peroneal). Now cut both ends of gastrocnemius close to its origin and reflect them down. Detach soleus from tibia and turn it laterally. Divide the intermuscular septum longitudinally and expose the deep muscles along with neuromuscular bundles. Identify the deep muscles (popliteus, flexor hallucis longus, flexor digitorum longus and tibialis posterior). Clean the fascia on the medial side of ankle and define its modification (flexor retinaculum) and note the structures deep to it (from before backwards: tibialis posterior, flexor digitorum longus, tibial vessels and nerve and flexor hallucis longus).

35

Back of Leg

CUTANEOUS NERVES

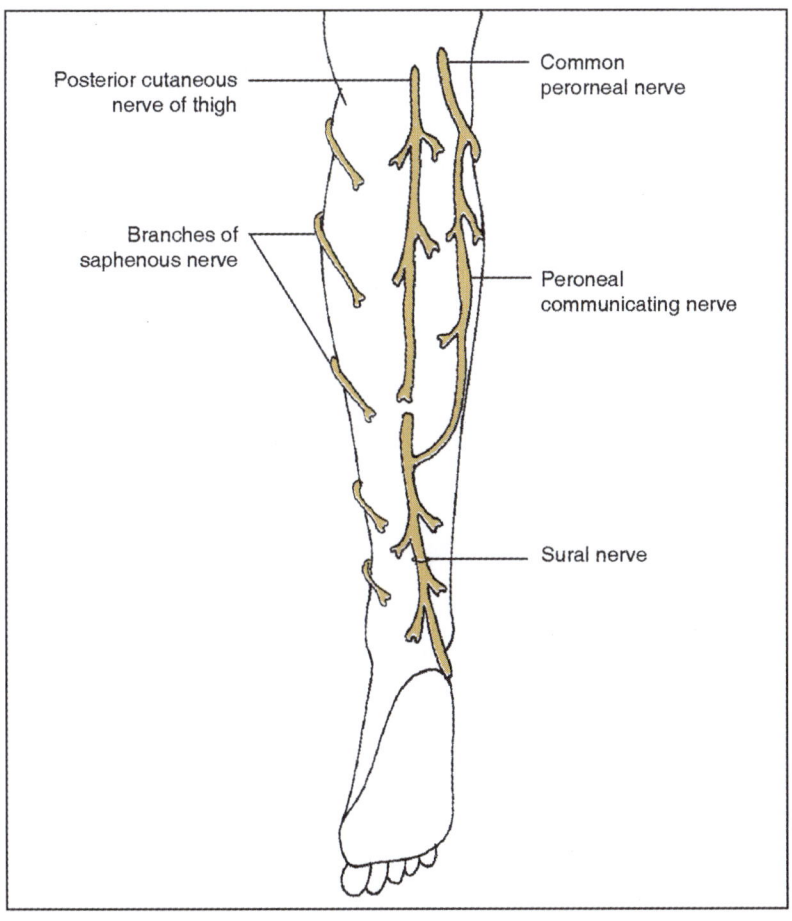

Fig. 35.1 Cutaneous nerves of back of the leg

Posterior cutaneous nerve of thigh

Branches of saphenous nerve

Common perorneal nerve

Peroneal communicating nerve

Sural nerve

Areas	Nerve
Medial part	Saphenous nerve ($L_{3, 4}$)
Intermediate part	
• Upper	Posterior cutaneous nerve of thigh ($S_{1, 2}$)
• Lower	Sural nerve ($S_{1, 2}$)
Lateral part	
• Upper	Peroneal communicating nerve (L_5, $S_{1, 2}$)
• Lower	Sural nerve ($S_{1, 2}$)

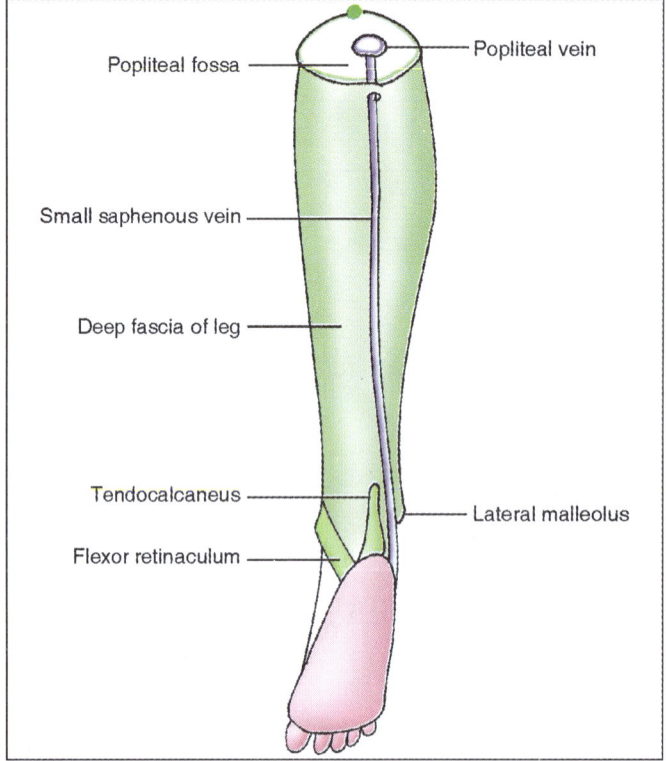

Fig. 35.2 Deep fascia of leg

FLEXOR RETINACULUM

It is a thickening of the deep fascia in the region of the posterior part of medial aspect of foot. It holds the tendons derived from the deep muscles of the back. It extends from the medial malleolus above to the medial aspect of calcaneus below.

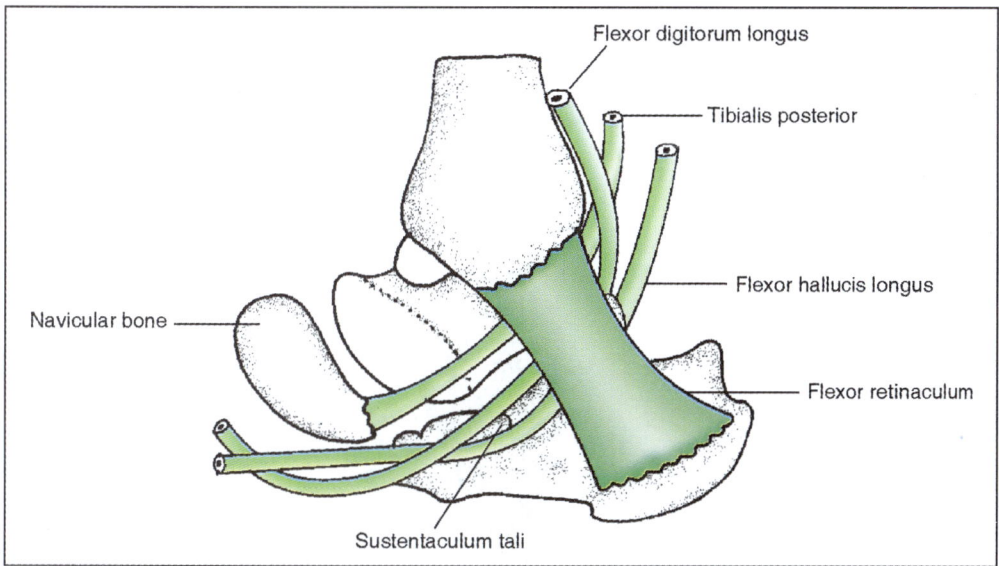

Fig. 35.3 Flexor retinaculum

MUSCLES OF FLEXOR COMPARTMENT OF LEG

Superficial group
- Gastrocnemius
- Soleus
- Plantaris

Deep group
- Popliteus
- Flexor hallucis longus
- Flexor digitorum longus
- Tibialis posterior

GASTROCNEMIUS

Origin

    Lateral head. From the lateral aspect of lateral condyle of femur.

    Medial head. From medial and lower part of popliteal surface of femur.

Insertion. Three muscles of superficial group fuse to form tendocalcaneus which gets attached to the intermediate part of posterior surface of calcaneus.

Nerve. Tibial nerve.

Actions. Plantar flexion of foot and flexion of leg.

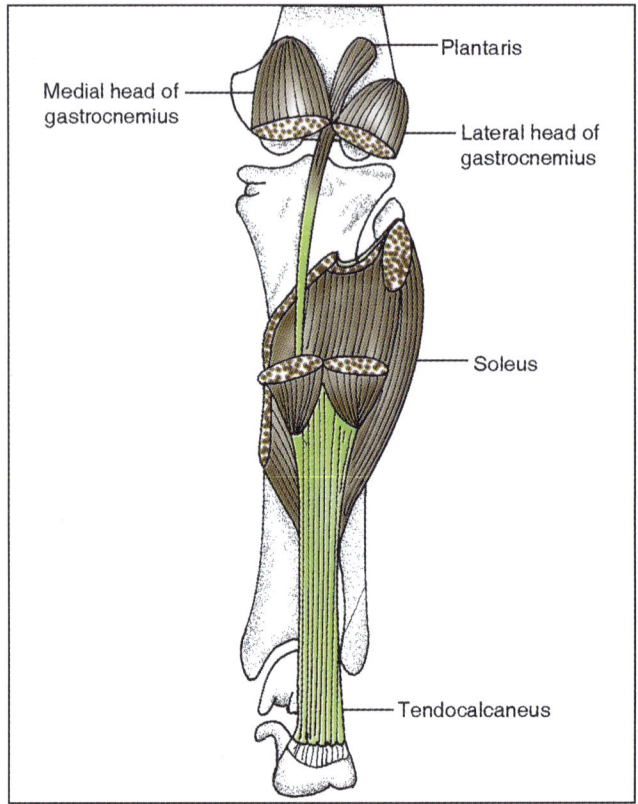

Fig. 35.4 Superficial muscles of back of leg

Soleus

Origin

- Upper part of the posterior aspect of fibula including the head.
- Tendinous arch between the head of fibula and lateral end of soleal line.
- Soleal line and middle $1/_3$rd of medial border of tibia.

Insertion. Same as the gastrocnemius muscle.

Nerve. Tibial nerve.

Actions

- It brings about plantar flexion of foot. Being multipennate, it is very powerful muscle and therefore helps in the initiation of propulsion by overcoming the inertia of the body. Gastrocnemius, being comprised of straight fibres, plays more important role in the later part of propulsion by providing greater range to the movement.
- Because of extensive venous plexus in the substance of soleus, it is able to push up adequate amount of blood during contraction. For this reason soleus is also named as the 'peripheral heart'.

Plantaris

Origin. Lateral and lower part of the popliteal surface of femur.

Insertion. Small belly ends into a long tendon which joins the tendocalcaneus.

Nerve. Tibial nerve.

Actions. It is a weak plantar flexor of foot and flexor of knee.

Popliteus

Origin

- Anterior part of the groove on the lateral aspect of the lateral condyle of femur.
- Posterior horn of the lateral meniscus of knee.

Insertion. Posterior surface of tibia above the soleal line.

Nerve. Tibial nerve.

Actions

- Unlocks the extended knee.
- Protects the lateral meniscus of knee from being crushed between femoral and tibial condyles during flexion at knee.

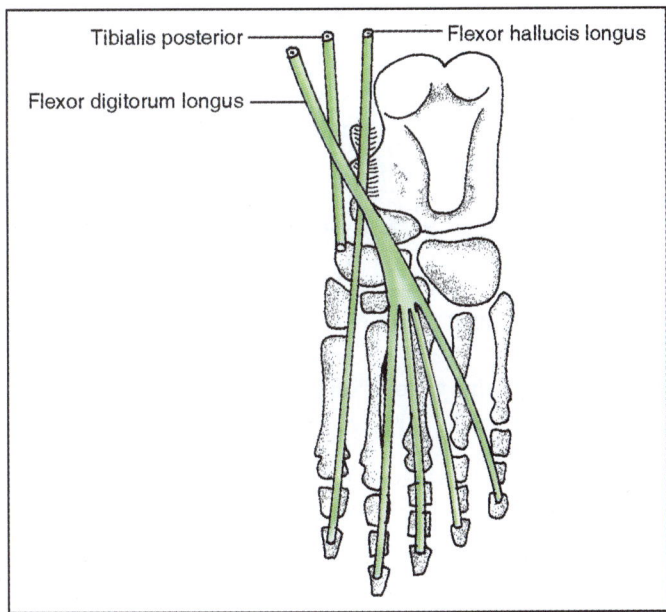

Fig. 35.5 Interrelationship of tendons of muscles of deep group of flexor compartment of leg

Flexor hallucis longus

Origin. Lateral part of the posterior surface of fibula.

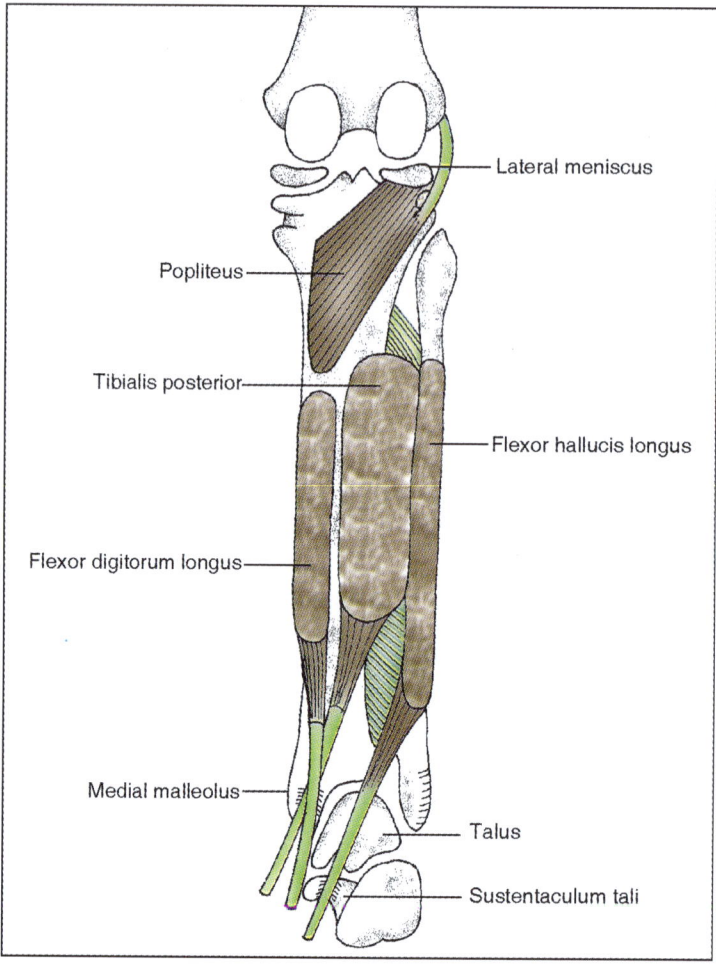

Fig. 35.6 Deep muscles of back of leg

Insertion. Tendon passes through the groove on the back of talus and the undersurface of the sustentaculum tali and gets attached to the distal phalanx of great toe.

Nerve. Tibial nerve.

Actions

- Flexion of great toe.
- Plantar flexion of foot.

Flexor digitorum longus

Origin. Medial part of the posterior surface of tibia.

Insertion. 4 Tendons are derived which get attached to the terminal phalanx of each of the lateral 4 toes.

Nerve. Tibial nerve.

Actions

- Flexion of the lateral 4 toes.
- Plantar flexion of foot.

Tibialis posterior

Origin. Posterior surface of the interosseous membrane and adjacent parts of tibia and fibula.

Insertion. Mainly to the tuberosity of the navicular bone. It also provides slips to all other tarsal bones (except talus) and bases of the middle three metatarsals.

Nerve. Tibial nerve.

Actions. Inversion and plantar flexion of foot.

Applied anatomy

- *Achilles' tendinitis*. The patient complains of pain at the site of attachment of tendocalcaneus to bone
- *Rupture of Achilles' tendon*. This is due to vascular insufficiency of the tendon.

Posterior tibial artery

Origin. From the popliteal artery at the lower border of the popliteus.

Course. Posterior tibial artery extends from the lower border of popliteus to the flexor retinaculum. In the upper part it runs over the tibialis posterior and comes to lie directly over the tibia in the lower part.

Branches

1. *Peroneal artery*. It arises from the upper part of the posterior tibial artery and descends on the back of the fibula under flexor hallucis longus. During its course it provides following twigs;
   - *Muscular branches*. Several of these pierce the lateral intermuscular septum to enter the lateral compartment of leg.
   - *Nutrient artery to fibula*.
   - *Lateral malleolar artery*. It runs laterally close to the lateral malleolus.
   - *Lateral calcanean artery*. It supplies the heel.
   - *Perforating artery*.It pierces the lower part of the interosseous membrane to enter the extensor compartment of leg.
2. *Muscular arteries.*
3. *Circumflex fibular artery*. It winds round the neck of fibula.
4. *Nutrient artery to tibia.*
5. *Medial malleolar artery*. It runs medially close to the medial malleolus.
6. *Medial calcanean artery*. It supplies the heel.
7. *Terminal branches*. Posterior tibial artery terminates into medial and lateral plantar arteries, which enter the foot under the flexor retinaculum and adductor hallucis.

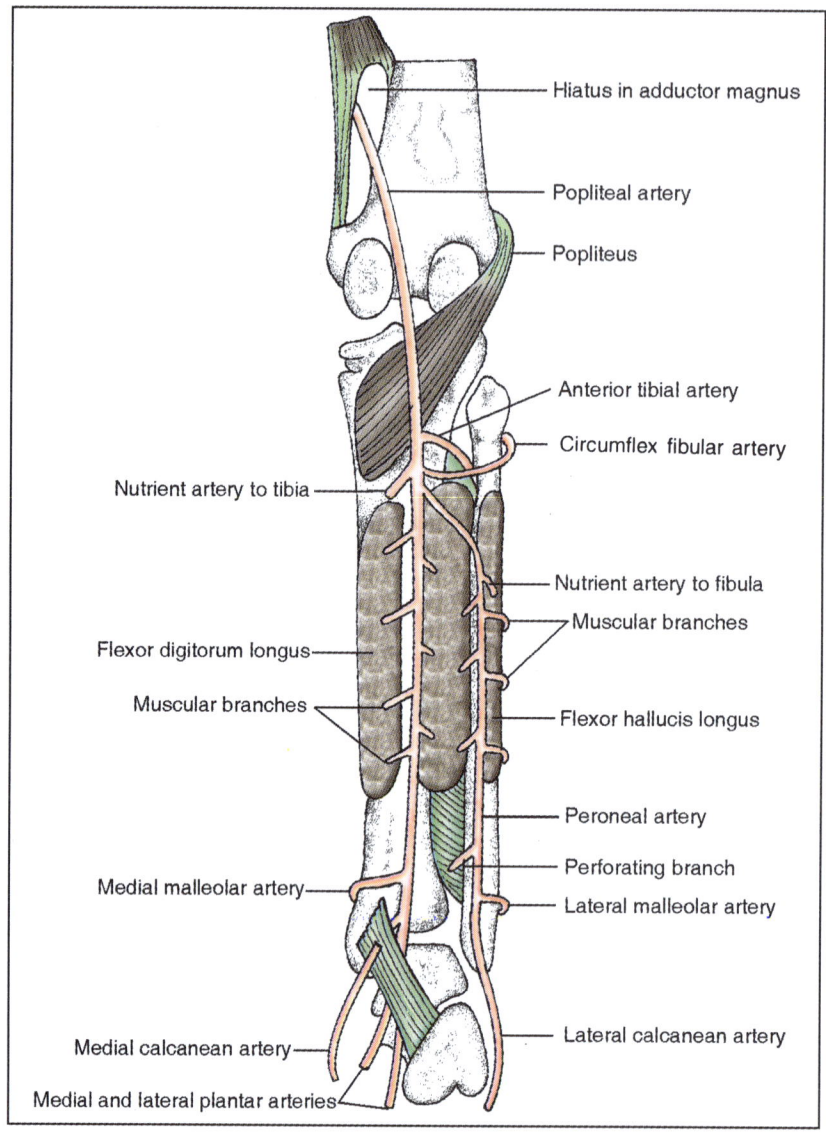

Hiatus in adductor magnus

Popliteal artery

Popliteus

Anterior tibial artery

Circumflex fibular artery

Nutrient artery to tibia

Nutrient artery to fibula

Muscular branches

Flexor digitorum longus

Muscular branches

Flexor hallucis longus

Peroneal artery

Perforating branch

Medial malleolar artery

Lateral malleolar artery

Medial calcanean artery

Lateral calcanean artery

Medial and lateral plantar arteries

Fig. 35.7 Posterior tibial artery

Applied anatomy

- Tibial arteries are commonly involved in *Buerger's disease*. It is caused by the inflammation of the arterial wall leading to thrombosis. Disappearance of the peripheral pulse is an important sign.

- *Embolic gangrenes*. Lower limb arteries may be blocked due to embolus originated somewhere else. The onset is sudden and the limb becomes cold and numb leading to gangrene (death of tissue).

- *Diabetic gangrene*. It is observed in diabetic individuals. Diabetes is known to hasten the process of atherosclerosis of the peripheral arteries.

Tibial nerve

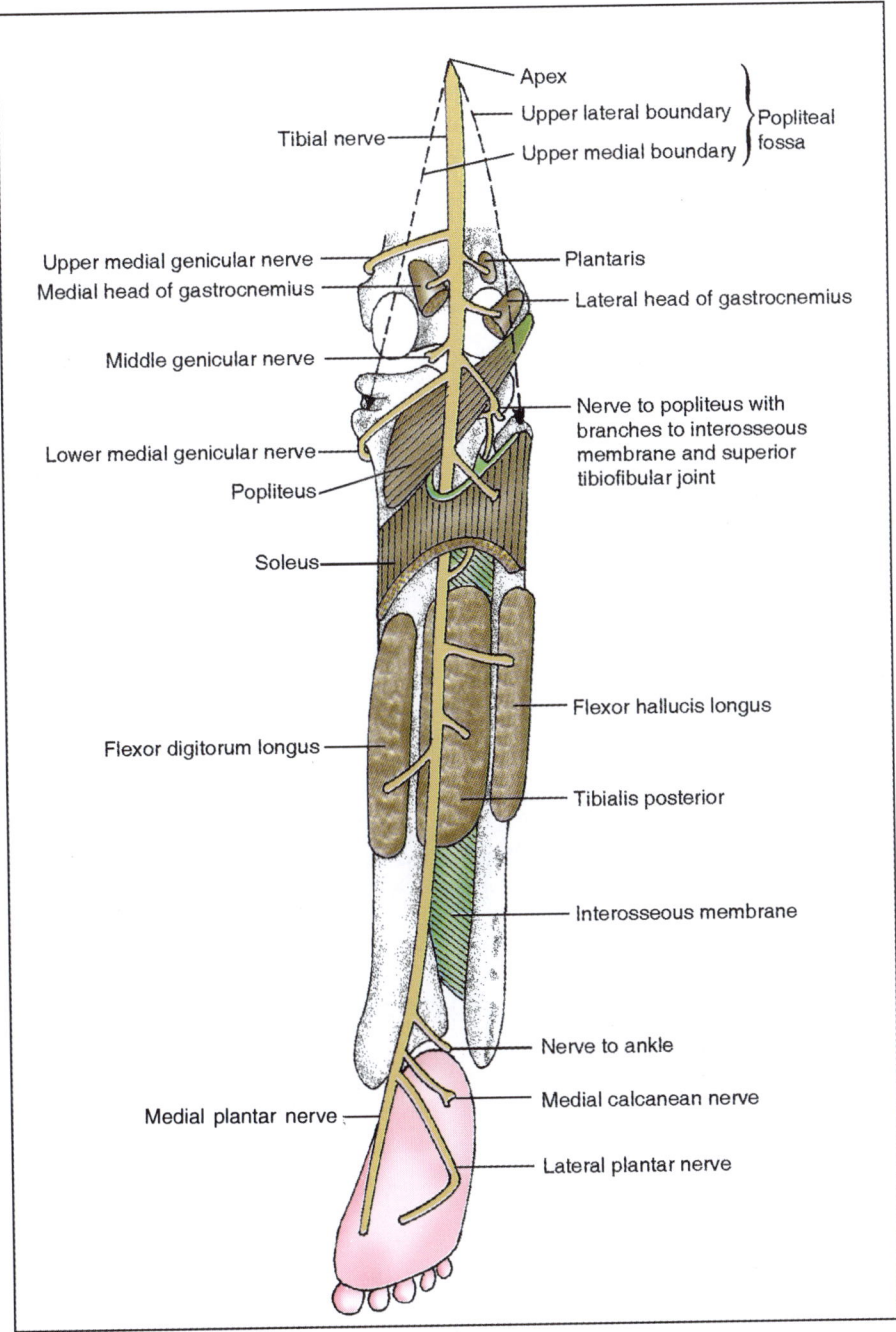

Apex

Upper lateral boundary ⎫
⎬ Popliteal
Upper medial boundary ⎭ fossa

Tibial nerve

Upper medial genicular nerve

Medial head of gastrocnemius

Plantaris

Lateral head of gastrocnemius

Middle genicular nerve

Nerve to popliteus with
branches to interosseous
membrane and superior
tibiofibular joint

Lower medial genicular nerve

Popliteus

Soleus

Flexor hallucis longus

Flexor digitorum longus

Tibialis posterior

Interosseous membrane

Nerve to ankle

Medial calcanean nerve

Medial plantar nerve

Lateral plantar nerve

Fig. 35.8 Tibial nerve

Origin. Tibial nerve arises as one of the terminal branches of the sciatic nerve at the upper angle of the popliteal fossa.

Course. The nerve extends from the apex of the popliteal fossa to the flexor retinaculum at ankle. Its upper part is located in the popliteal fossa. Its lower part is located in the flexor compartment of the leg, where it extends from the lower border of the popliteus to the flexor retinaculum. In the upper leg it crosses the tibial vessels from medial to lateral and remains lateral upto the flexor retinaculum.

Branches in leg

1. *Muscular branches* supply;
   - Deep surface of soleus.
   - Tibialis posterior
   - Flexor digitorum longus.
   - Flexor hallucis longus.
2. *Articular branch*. Supplies the ankle joint.
3. *Cutaneous branch*. Medial calcaneal nerve supplies the skin of heel.
4. *Terminal branches*. Tibial nerve terminates into medial and lateral plantar nerves which supply the sole.

Applied anatomy

- Tibial nerve is rarely injured except in open wounds. Patient is unable to plantar flex the ankle with loss of sensation of whole of the sole. Since it also supplies the plantar muscles, there will be 'claw foot'.

36

Sole of Foot

CUTANEOUS NERVES

1. *Medial calcanean nerves*. These arise from the tibial nerve before its termination and supply the skin of the heel.
2. *Cutaneous branches of medial plantar nerve*. These supply the medial 2/3rd of the sole, except heel.
3. *Cutaneous branches of lateral plantar nerve*. These supply lateral 1/3rd of sole, except heel.
4. *Plantar digital nerves*. These appear from both the plantar nerves. Those from the medial plantar nerve supply medial 3½ digits. Those appearing from the lateral plantar nerve supply lateral 1½ digits.

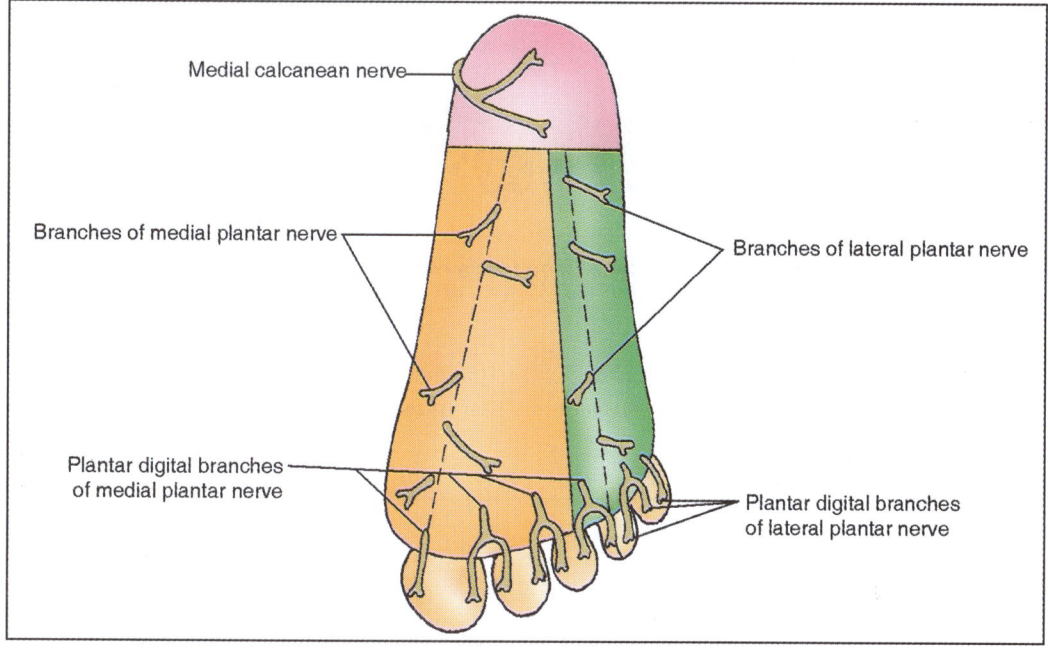

Fig. 36.1 Cutaneous nerves of sole

DEEP FASCIA

1. In each toe, deep fascia forms a *fibrous flexor sheath*, which is attached to the margins of the phalanges. This sheath encloses a fibro-osseous tunnel for the flexor tendons.

2. In the sole, deep fascia can be divided into three parts, medial, lateral, and intermediate. The former two are thin in nature while the latter is very thick and is named as the *plantar aponeurosis*. It is triangular in shape. Its apex is attached to the medial process of calcaneal tubercle. Its margins, lateral and medial, are marked by the linear appearances of cutaneous nerves from the corresponding plantar nerves. Its distal base divides into five slips, each of which continues with the fibrous flexor sheath of corresponding digit.

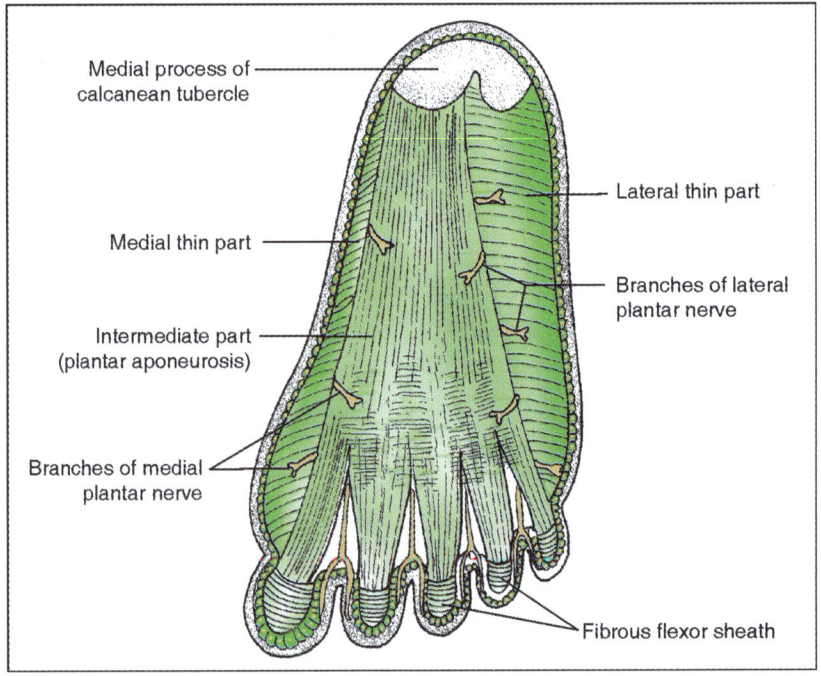

Fig. 36.2 Deep fascia of sole

Applied anatomy

• *Plantar fasciitis*, is the condition in which the patient experiences unbearable pain under the heel, particularly during walking. It is due to tear in the attachment of plantar fascia

STRUCTURES IN THE SOLE

These are arranged in six layers

Layer I (1st muscular layer)

It includes three superficial muscles of sole;

1. Abductor hallucis.

2. Flexor digitorum brevis.

3. Abductor digiti minimi.

Layer II (Superficial neurovascular layer)

This layer forms the superficial neurovascular plane and consists of medial and lateral plantar nerves and vessels.

Layer III (2nd muscular layer)

It consists of long flexor tendons (flexor hallucis longus and flexor digitorum longus) and muscles attached to them (flexor digitorum accessorius and lumbricals).

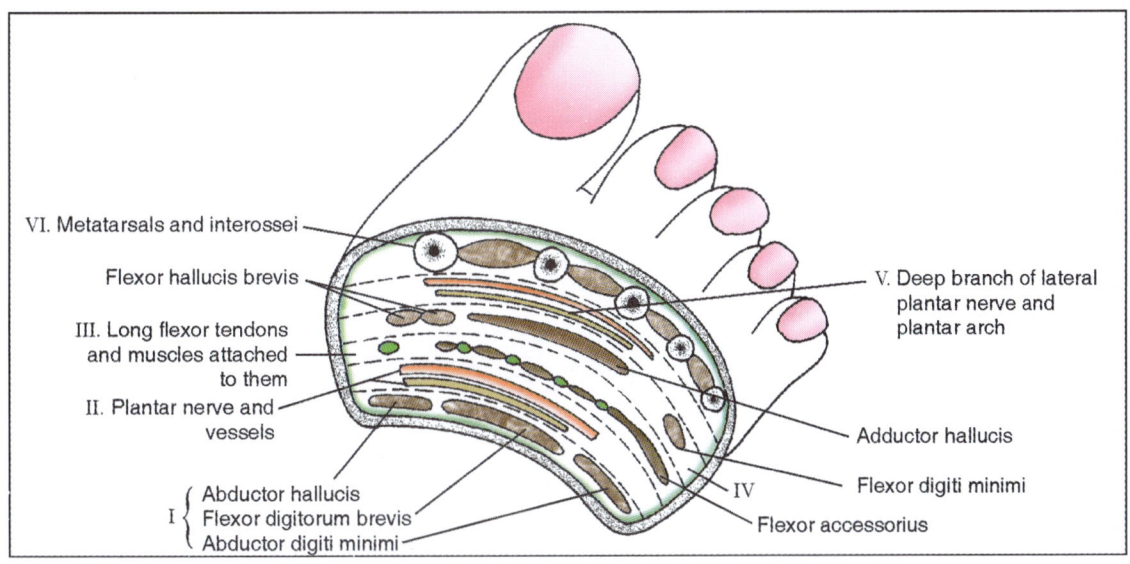

Fig. 36.3 Concept of layers in sole

Layer IV (3rd muscular layer)

It consists of following three muscles;

1. Flexor hallucis brevis.

2. Adductor hallucis.

3. Flexor digiti minimi.

Layer V (Deep neurovascular layer)

In this layer, distal deeper parts of the lateral plantar artery and nerve runs.

Layer VI (4th muscular layer)

This layer includes;

1. Bones and ligaments of foot.

2. Tendon of peroneus longus.

3. Extensions of tibialis posterior tendon.

4. Interossei.

DISSECTION STEPS: SOLE

Give a longitudinal incision from the heel to the root of middle toe. Reflect the skin and superficial fascia. Cut the plantar aponeurosis close to the heel and reflect it forward. Identify the muscles of first layer i.e., abductor hallucis, abductor digiti minimi and flexor digitorum brevis and medial and lateral plantar nerves and vessels. Try to find out medial cancanean nerves and vessels and muscular branches arising from the medial and lateral plantar nerves. Cut across the tendon of flexor digitorum brevis in the middle and reflect to expose the 2nd layer muscles (tendons of flexor hallucis longus and flexor digitorum longus, flexor digitorum accessorius and lumbricals). Cut across in the of tendons in the 2nd muscular layer to expose the 3rd muscular layer (flexor hallucis brevis, adductor hallucis and flexor digitiminimi brevis). Detach flexor hallucis brevis and oblique head of adductor hallucis from their origin to expose the 4th muscular layer (tendons of peroneus longus and tibialis posterior and plantar and dorsal interossei). Also locate the short and long plantar ligaments.

ABDUCTOR HALLUCIS

Origin. Medial process of tuber calcanei.

Insertion. With medial belly of flexor hallucis brevis, it gets attached to the medial aspect of the base of proximal phalanx of great toe.

Nerve. Medial plantar nerve.

Actions. Abduction and flexion of great toe.

FLEXOR DIGITORUM BREVIS

Origin. Medial process of tuber calcanei.

Insertion. It divides into 4 tendons, which extend towards the lateral four digits. In each toe, the tendon splits and gets attached to the middle phalanx.

Nerve. Medial plantar nerve.

Actions. Flexion of lateral 4 toes.

ABDUCTOR DIGITI MINIMI

Origin. Both processes of tuber calcanei.

Insertion. Lateral aspect of base of proximal phalanx of little toe.

Nerve. Lateral plantar nerve.

Action. Abduction of little toe.

LONG FLEXOR TENDONS

Tendon of flexor digitorum longus crosses the tendon of flexor hallucis longus from medial to lateral and divides into 4 slips to reach the distal phalanges of the lateral 4 toes. Tendon of flexor hallucis longus passes in the groove on the under surface of sustentaculum tali to reach the distal phalanx of great toe.

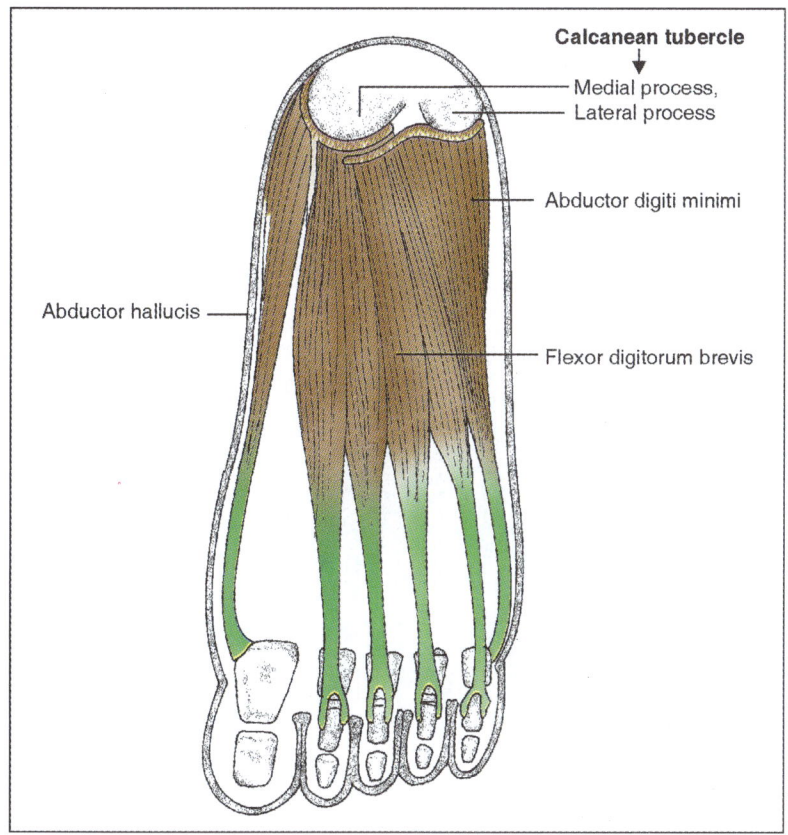

Fig. 36.4 First layer of muscles of sole

FLEXOR DIGITORUM ACCESSORIUS

Origin

1. *Lateral head.* It is tendinous head arising from the lateral margin of plantar surface of calcaneus.
2. *Medial head.* It is muscular in nature and arises from the medial aspect of calcaneus.

Insertion. It gets attached to the lateral margin of tendon of flexor digitorum longus just proximal to its division.

Nerve. Lateral plantar nerve.

Actions

1. To straighten the line of pull of flexor digitorum longus.
2. To flex the lateral 4 toes when flexor digitorum longus is out of action e.g., in extreme plantar flexion of foot.

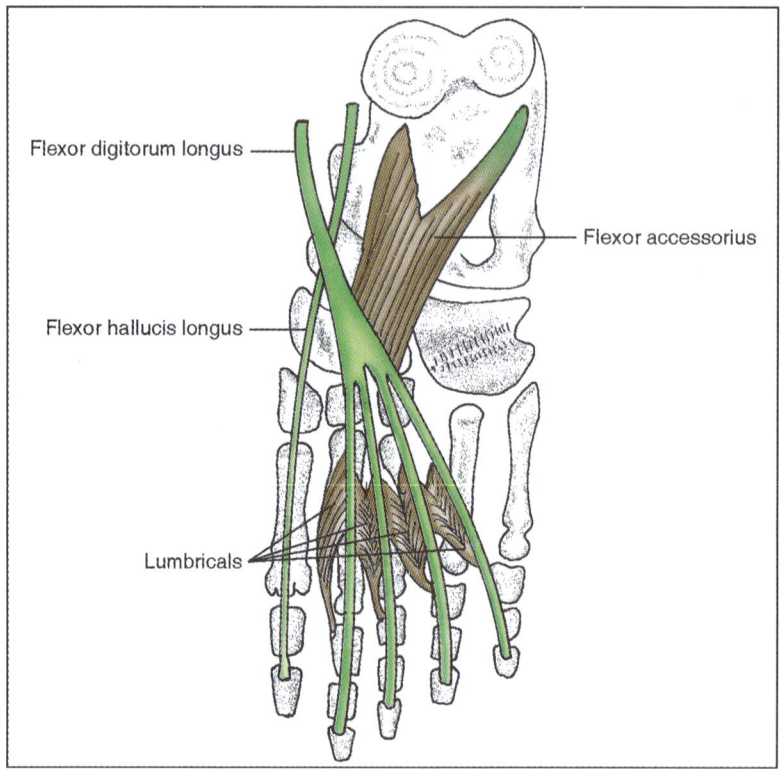

Fig. 36.5 Second layer of muscles of sole

LUMBRICALS

Origin. There are 4 lumbricals, which arise from the slips of flexor digitorum longus tendon. Ist lumbrical originates from the medial margin of first slip|. Rest arise from adjacent margins of the 4 slips.

Insertion. Lumbrical runs on the medial side of each of the lateral 4 toes and gets attached to the base of proximal phalanx and extensor expansion.

Nerve

    Ist lumbrical – Medial plantar nerve.

    2nd, 3rd and 4th lumbricals – Lateral plantar nerve.

Actions. Flexion at the metatarsophalangeal joints and extension at the interphalangeal joints of the lateral 4 toes.

FLEXOR HALLUCIS BREVIS

Origin. Plantar surface of cuboid.

Insertion. The muscle divides into two bellies, each having a sesamoid bone on the under surface of the head of Ist metatarsal. The medial and lateral bellies join with the abductor hallucis brevis and adductor hallucis respectively and get attached to the corresponding sides of the base of proximal phalanx of great toe.

Nerve. Medial plantar nerve.

Actions. Flexion and adduction of great toe.

ADDUCTOR HALLUCIS

Origin

Oblique head. Bases of middle 3 metatarsals.

Transverse head. Deep transverse metatarsal ligaments and the plantar ligaments of the metatarsophalangeal joints of lateral 4 toes.

Insertion. It joins the lateral belly of flexor hallucis brevis and gets attached to the lateral side of the base of proximal phalanx of great toe.

Nerve. Lateral plantar nerve.

Actions. Adduction and flexion of great toe. Maintains the transverse arch of foot.

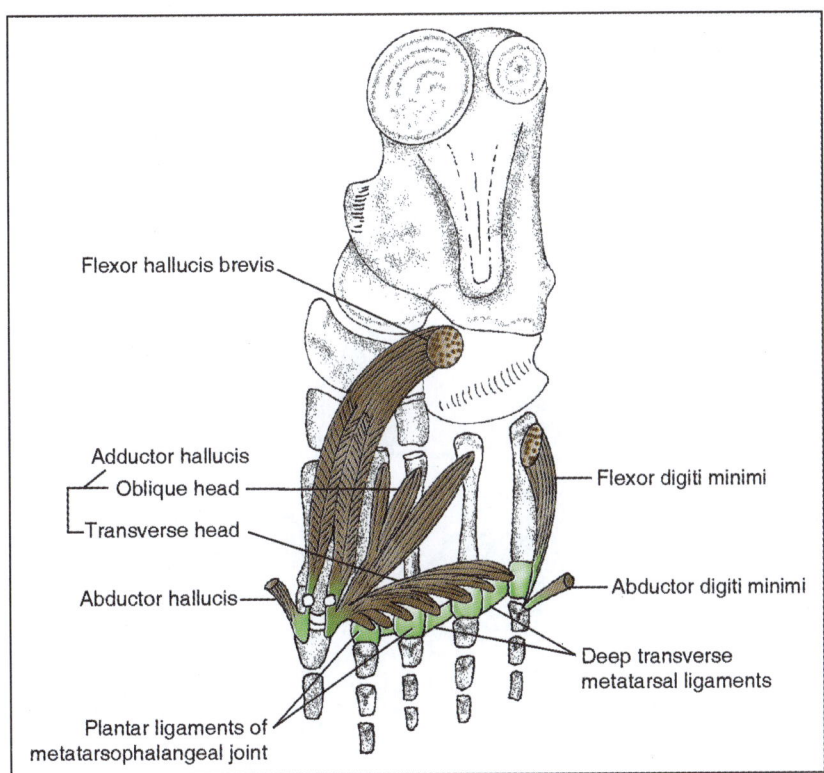

Fig. 36.6 Third muscular layer of sole

FLEXOR DIGITI MINIMI

Origin. Base of the 5th metatarsal.

Insertion. Base of proximal phalanx of the little toe.

Nerve. Lateral plantar nerve.

Action. Flexion of little toe.

TENDONS OF TIBIALIS POSTERIOR AND PERONEUS LONGUS

Tibialis posterior tendon gets attached mainly to the tuberosity of navicular bone. But it also provides large number of extensions, which get attached to all the tarsal bones (except talus) and base of the middle 3 metatarsals.

Tendon of peroneus longus passes through a groove on the under surface of cuboid and extends medially to get attached mainly to the base of Ist metatarsal and also to the medial cuneiform.

PLANTAR INTEROSSEI

Origin. There are 3 plantar interossei (1st, 2nd and 3rd from medial to lateral) arising from the medial sides of the shaft lateral 3 metatarsals respectively.

Insertion. Base of the proximal phalanx of the corresponding toe on their medial aspects.

Nerve. Lateral plantar nerve.

Actions. Adduction of lateral corresponding lateral 3 toes towards the axis of foot, i.e., the longitudinal line passing through the 2nd toe.

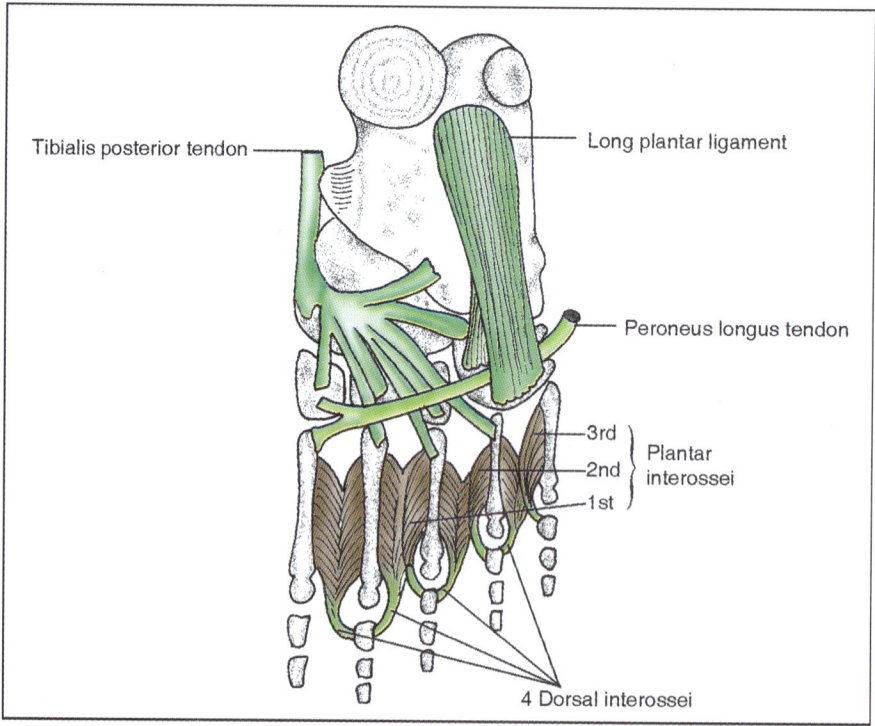

Fig. 36.7 Fourth muscular layer of sole

DORSAL INTEROSSEI

Origin. These are 4 in number (1st, 2nd, 3rd, and 4th from medial to lateral) occupying the corresponding intermetatarsal space. Each one arises from the shafts of adjacent metatarsals.

Insertion

1st Dorsal interosseus. It gets attached to the medial side of the base of proximal phalanx of 2nd toe.

2nd, 3rd, and 4th dorsal interossei. These get attached to the lateral side of the bases of proximal phalanges of 2nd, 3rd, and 4th toes respectively.

Nerve. Lateral plantar nerve.

Actions. Abduction of middle 3 toes from the axis of foot (i.e., 2nd toe.).

PLANTAR NERVES AND VESSELS

There are medial and lateral plantar nerves and vessels. Medial plantar nerve and vessels and proximal parts of the lateral plantar nerve and vessels run a superficial course between the 1st and 2nd layers of muscles of sole. Distal parts of the lateral plantar artery (plantar arch) and deep branch of lateral plantar nerve lie between 3rd and 4th layers of muscles of sole.

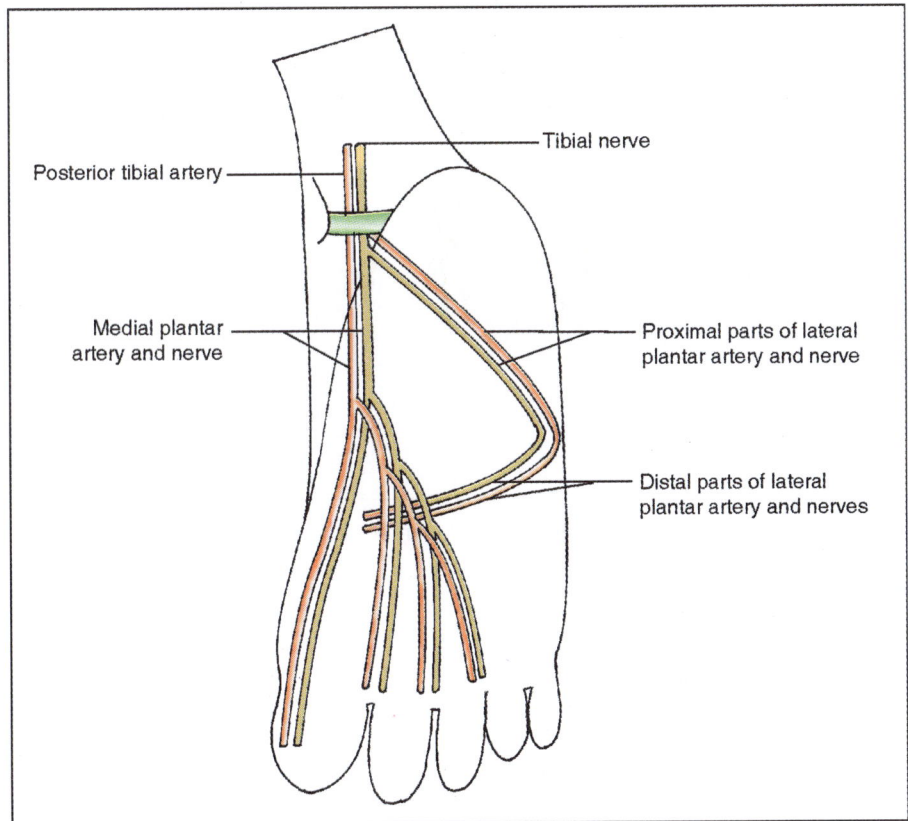

Fig. 36.8 Interrelationship between plantar nerves and arteries

Medial plantar nerve

Origin. It arises from the tibial nerve under the flexor retinaculum.

Course. It passes deep to abductor hallucis and then runs forward between abductor hallucis and flexor digitorum brevis.

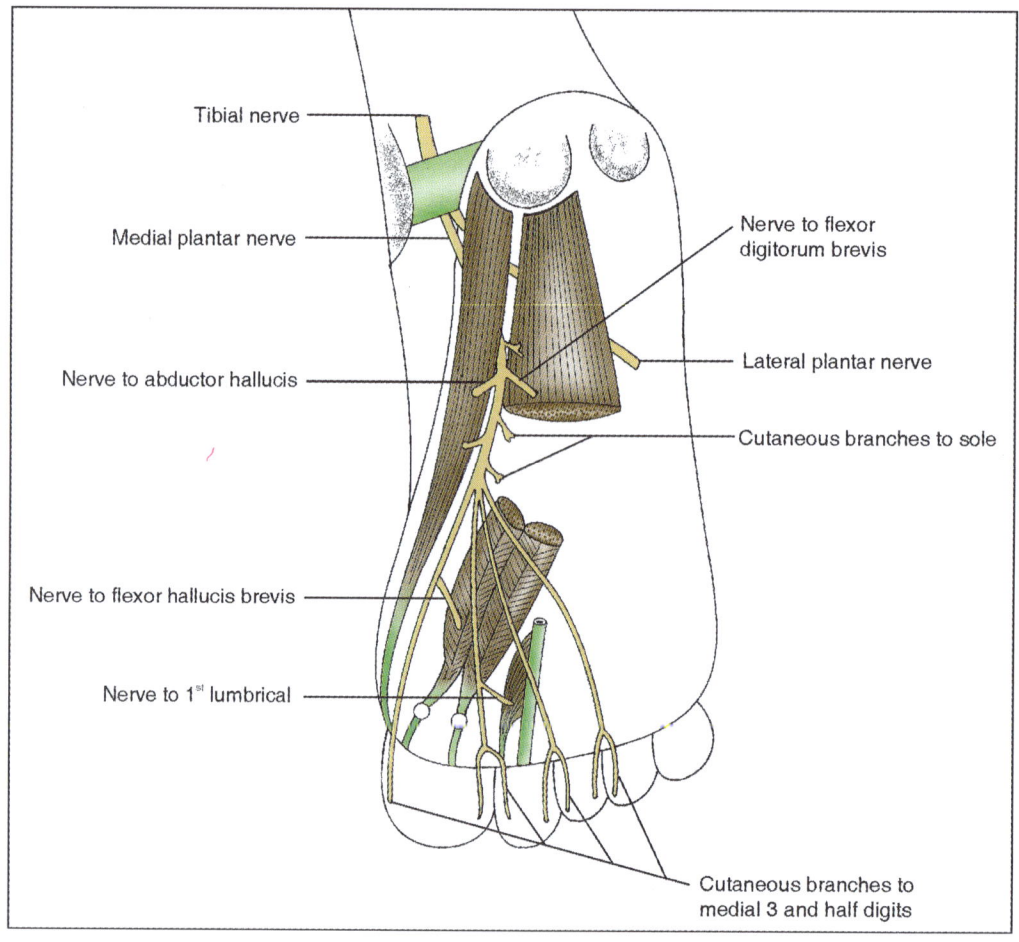

Fig. 36.9 Medial plantar nerve

Distribution

1. *Muscular branches to*;
   - Abductor hallucis.
   - Flexor digitorum brevis.
   - 1st lumbrical.
   - Flexor hallucis brevis.
2. *Cutaneous branches to sole*. These supply medial 2/3rd of sole.

3. *Cutaneous branches to digits* (Digital nerves);
   - One proper plantar digital nerve goes to the medial side of great toe.
   - Three common plantar digital nerves extend towards medial 3 interdigital clefts.   Each divides into two proper plantar digital nerves to supply the adjacent sides of medial 4 toes.

Lateral plantar nerve

Origin. It arises as one of the terminal branches of tibial nerve under the flexor retinaculum.

Course. It runs laterally and forward towards the base of 5th metatarsal between flexor accessories and flexor digitorum brevis.

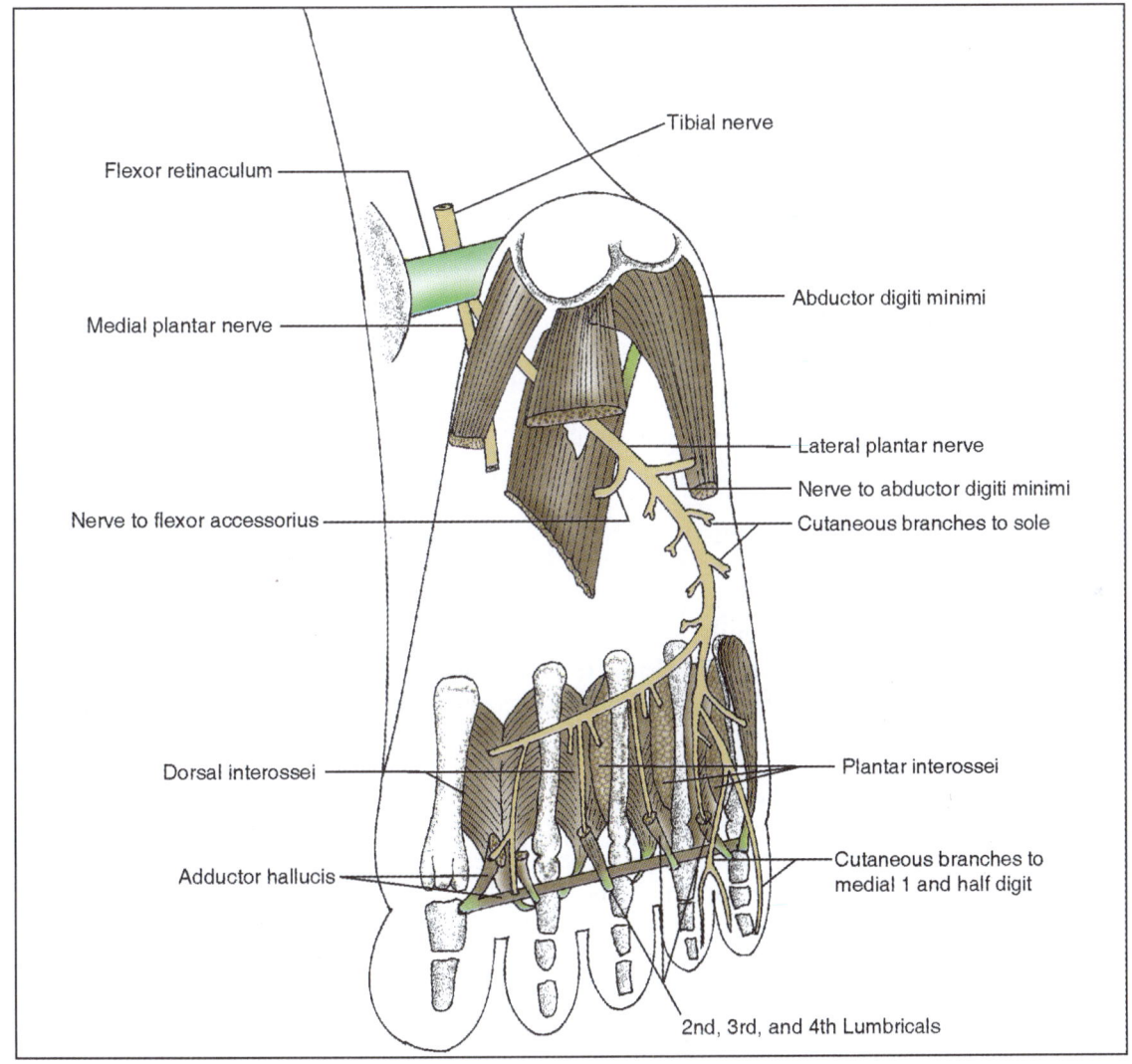

Fig. 36.10 Lateral plantar nerve

Branches

1. *Muscular branches* to;
   - Flexor accessorius.
   - Abductor digiti minimi.
2. *Cutaneous branches* to the lateral 1/3rd of the sole.
3. *Terminal branches.* Lateral plantar nerve terminates into superficial and deep branches.

Superficial branch

It runs forward in relation to 1st intermetatarsal space and supplies as follows,

1. *Muscular branches.* Flexor digiti minimi, 3rd palmar interosseous, and 4th dorsal interosseous.
2. *Cutaneous branches.* One proper digital nerve to lateral side of little toe. One common plantar digital nerve to 4th interdigital cleft where it divides into two proper plantar digital nerves for the adjacent sides of 4th and 5th toes.

Deep branch

It runs medially deep to the oblique head of adductor pollicis, against the bases of 4th, 3rd, and 2nd metatarsals. Here it lies in the concavity of the plantar arch. Its branches are as follows,

1. *Muscular branches.* These supply to,
   - 2nd, 3rd, and 4th lumbricals.
   - Adductor hallucis.
   - 1st and 2nd plantar interossei.
   - 1st, 2nd, and 3rd dorsal interossei.
2. *Articular branches.* These supply the small joints of foot.

MEDIAL PLANTAR ARTERY

It is one of the terminal branches of the posterior tibial artery. It follows the course of medial plantar nerve. Its branches correspond with the branches of medial plantar nerve. One branch accompanies proper plantar digital nerve on the medial side of great toe. Branches accompanying the common plantar digital nerves usually boost up the supply of plantar metatarsal branches of plantar arch by joining them.

LATERAL PLANTAR ARTERY

It is one of the terminal branches of the posterior tibial artery. Its proximal part follows the course of lateral plantar nerve towards the base of 5th metatarsal. Its distal part, also called the *plantar arch*, turns medially and accompanies the deep branch of lateral plantar nerve. Following branches emerge from the plantar arch;

- *Four plantar metatarsal arteries.* These correspond with the 4 intermetatarsal space; reaching the region of interdigital cleft, these split into digital branches to supply the adjacent sides of toes. Their distal parts receive the branches of medial plantar artery as well as make communications with the dorsal plantar arteries through distal perforating arteries.

- *Proximal perforating arteries.* These connect the plantar arch with the proximal ends of dorsal metatarsal arteries in the lateral 3 intermetatarsal spaces.
- *Deep plantar artery* connects the plantar arch with the arcuate artery at the proximal end of 1st intermetatarsal space.

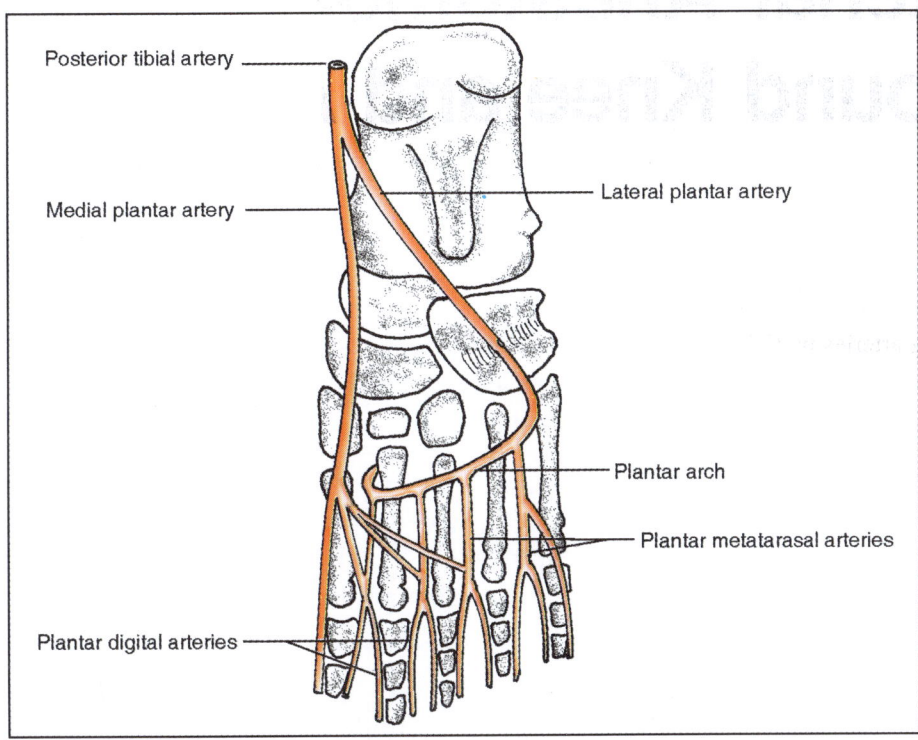

Fig. 36.11 Plantar arteries

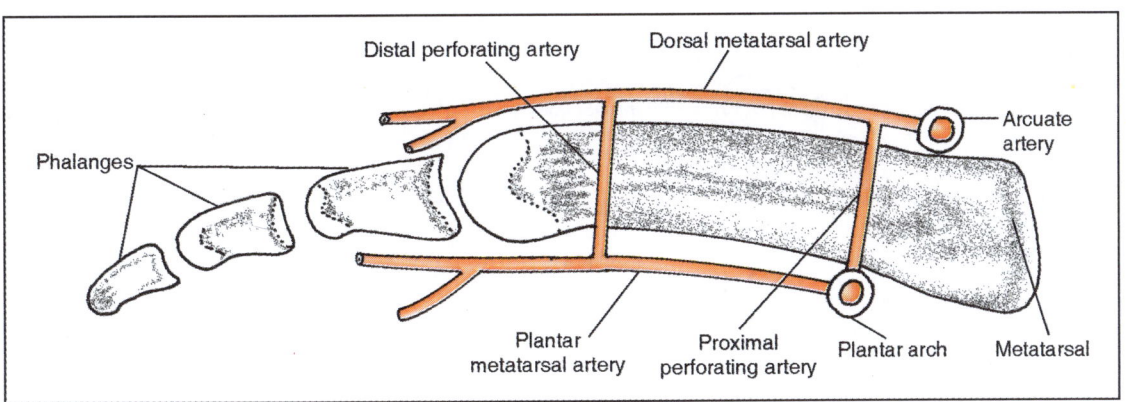

Fig. 36.12 Communications between dorsal and plantar arteries

37

Arterial Anastomoses Around Knee and Ankle

ANASTOMOSES AROUND KNEE

Following arteries participate in the formation of anastomoses around the knee;

1. *Descending branch of the lateral circumflex femoral artery.*
2. *Descending genicular branch of femoral artery.*

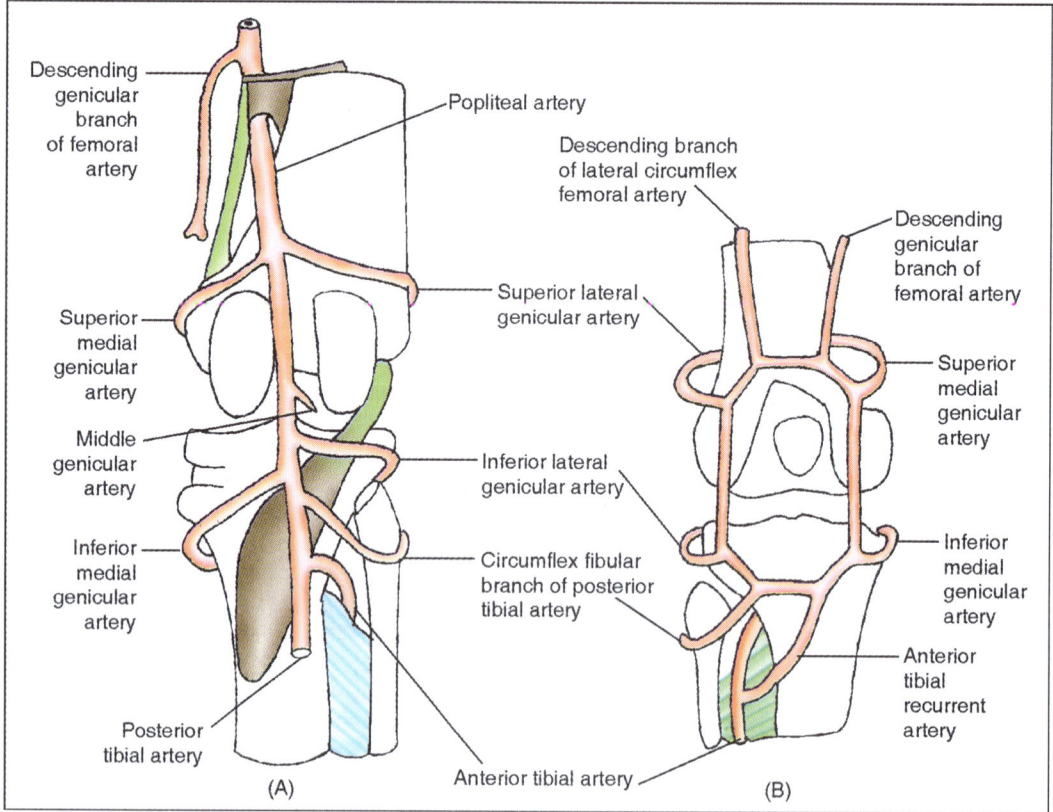

Fig. 37.1 (A) Anastomoses around knee (posterior view); (B) An octagon around patella receiving eight anastomosing arteries at its angles

3. *Anterior tibial recurrent branch of anterior tibial artery.*
4. *Circumflex fibular branch of posterior tibial artery.*
5. *4 genicular branches of the popliteal artery,*
    -   *Superior medial genicular artery.*
    -   *Inferior medial genicular artery.*
    -   *Superior lateral genicular artery.*
    -   *Inferior lateral genicular artery.*

ANASTOMOSES AROUND ANKLE

Several small arteries form arterial plexuses just below the corresponding malleoli called medial and lateral malleolar network.

Medial malleolar network

Following arteries participate;
1. *Anterior medial malleolar branch of anterior tibial artery.*
2. *Medial tarsal branch of dorsalis pedis artery.*
3. *Malleolar and calcanean branches of posterior tibial artery.*
4. *Branches of medial plantar artery.*

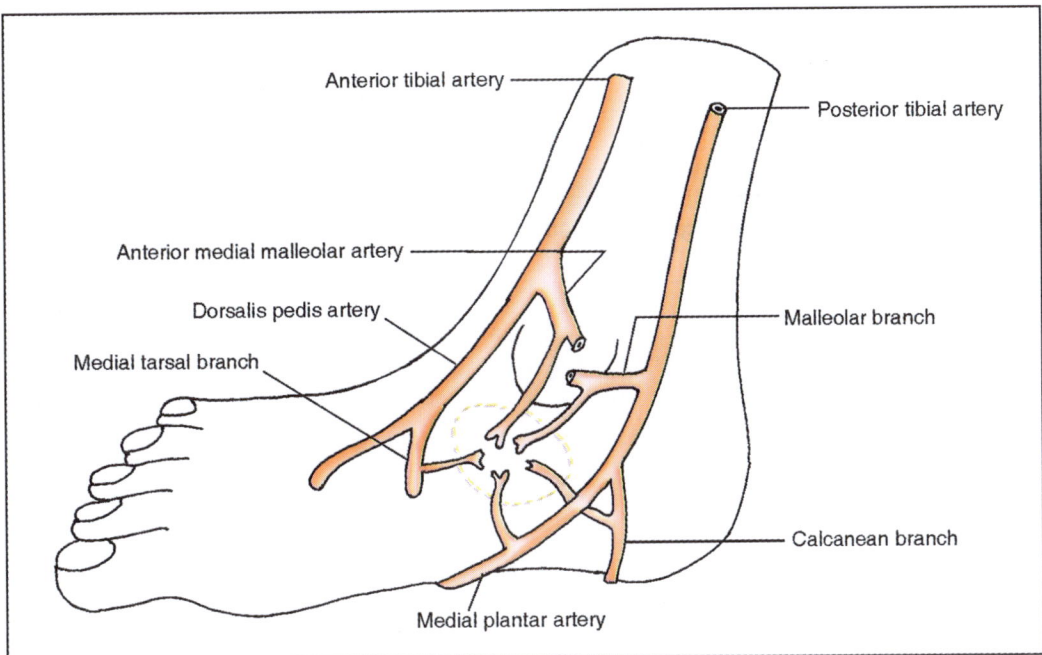

Fig. 37.2 Medial malleolar network

Lateral malleolar network

Following arteries contribute to it;

1. *Anterior lateral melleolar branch of anterior tibial artery.*
2. *Lateral tarsal branch of dorsalis pedis artery.*
3. *Perforating and calcalnean branches of peroneal artery.*
4. *Branches from the lateral plantar artery.*

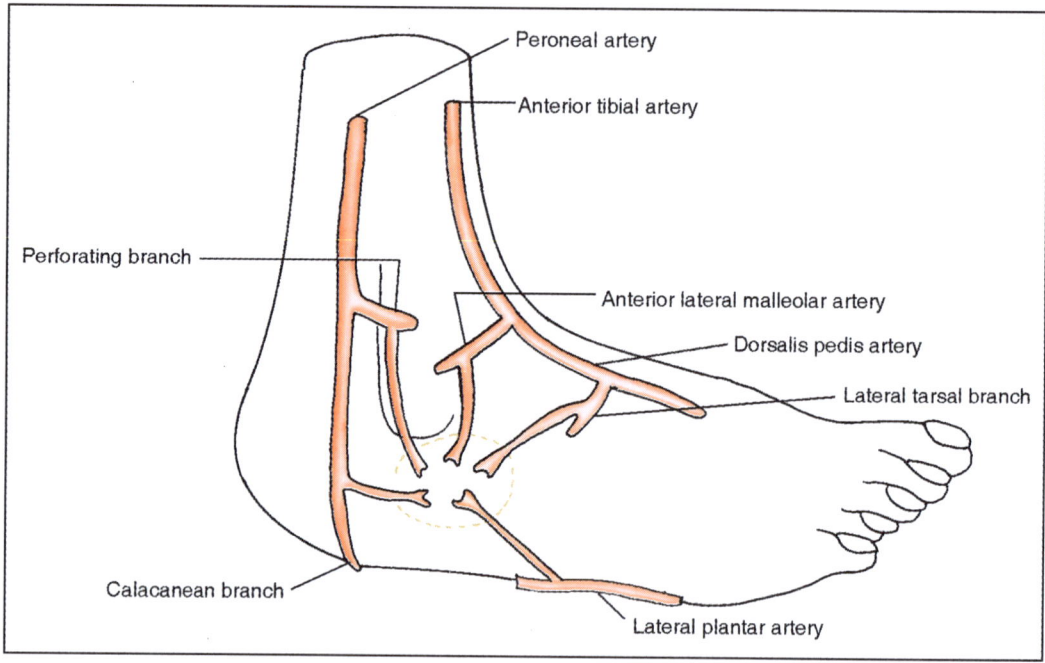

Fig. 37.3 Lateral malleolar network

38

Knee Joint

It is a condylar type of synovial joint. It is compound in nature, as three bones participate in its formation, i.e., femoral and tibial condyles and the patella.

CAPSULE

It is attached to the articular margins of three bones contributing to the joint. Its attachment to the intercondylar line of femur makes intercondylar notch intracapsular. Similarly, intercondylar area of tibial plateau also becomes intracapsular because of its attachments to the anterior and posterior margins of this area. On the lateral aspect of lateral femoral condyle, a groove for the popliteus is also made intracapsular. There are three openings in the capsule, a large opening anteriorly, to accommodate patella, a second opening anteriorly above the patella, for communication between joint cavity and the suprapatellar bursa and a third opening on the lateral part of posterior aspect for the passage of popliteus muscle.

EXTRACAPSULAR LIGAMENTS

Ligamentum patellae.
It connects the apex of patella with tibial tuberosity.

Patellar retinacula.
Superficial fibres of the quadriceps tendon descend in front of patella and then diverge medially and laterally towards the corresponding tibial conyles, constituting the medial and lateral patellar reinacula respectively.

Lateral collateral ligament.
It extends from the lateral epicondyle of femur to the upper end of fibula. It is free from the capsule, and at the fibular attachment, is enclosed by the two divisions of the tendon of biceps femoris.

Medial collateral ligament.
It has got a deep part and a superficial part. *Deep part* is actually a thickening in the medial part of the capsule and connects the medial epicondyle with the medial meniscus. *Superficial part* arises from the same point (medial epicondyle) but extends downwards to the upper part of medial aspect of shaft of tibia. It is strengthened by a slip from the tendon of semimembranosus.

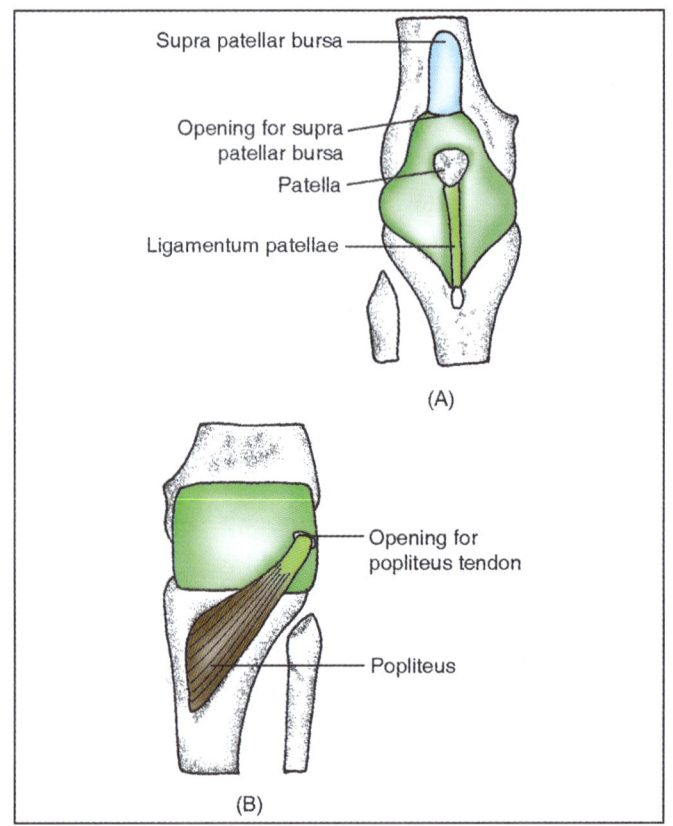

Fig. 38.1 Knee joint capsular attachments: (A) Anterior view; (B) Posterior view

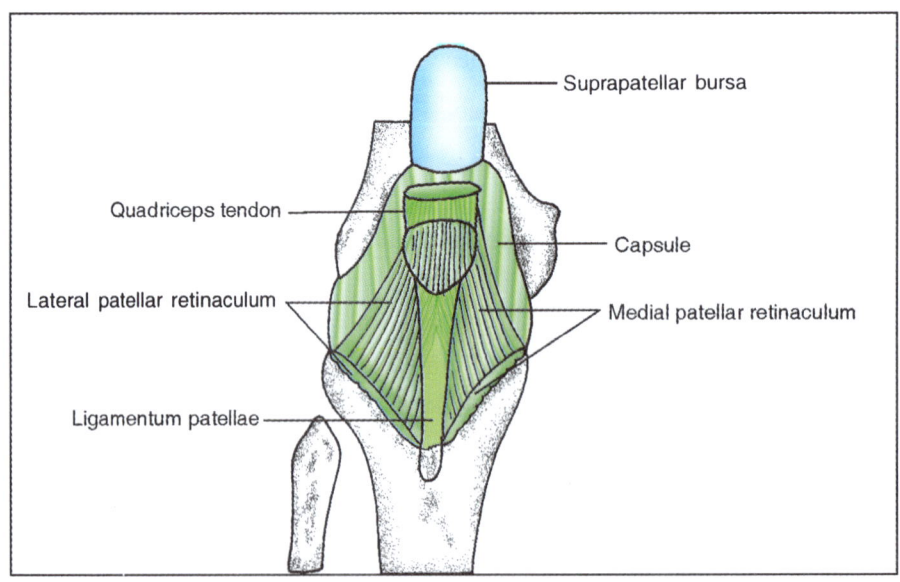

Fig. 38.2 Patellar retinacula of knee (anterior view)

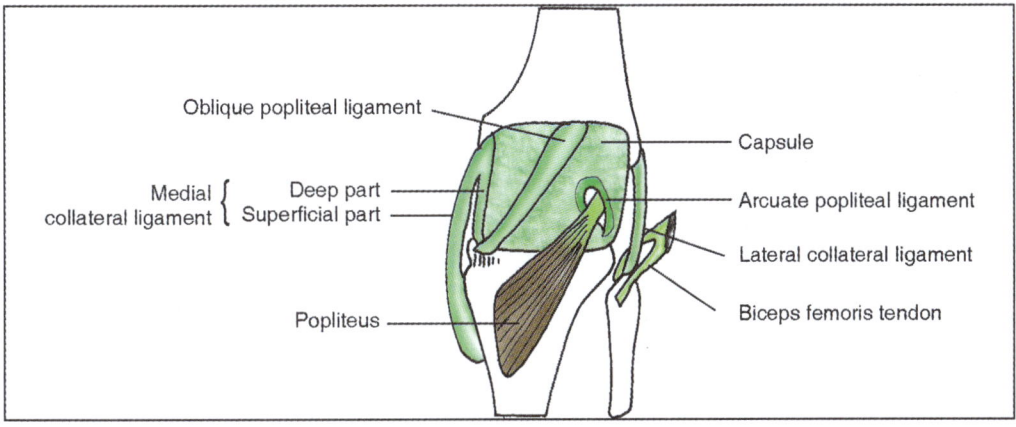

Fig. 38.3 Ligaments of knee (anterior view)

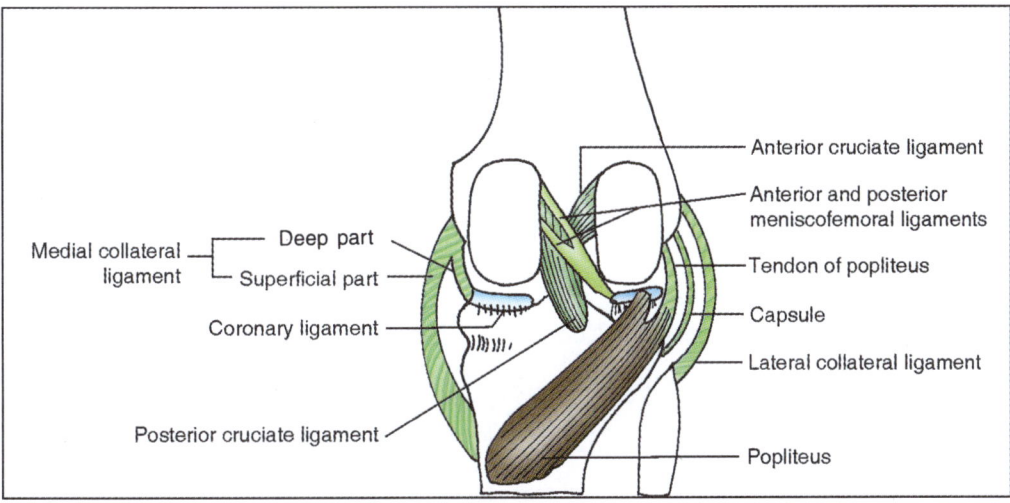

Fig. 38.4 Ligaments of knee (posterior view)

Oblique popliteal ligament

It is fibrous band extending from the tendon of semimembranosus to the intracondylar line of femur. The middle genicular vessels and nerve pierce this ligament.

Arcuate popliteal ligament

It consists of arching fibres around the tendon of popliteus emerging from the joint and is formed by the thickening of upper margin and sides of opening in the capsule for this tendon.

Coronary ligament

This part of fibrous capsule extends between meniscus and the tibial condyle.

INTRACAPSULAR STRUCTURES

Cruciate ligaments. There are two cruciate ligaments, anterior and posterior. These connect intercondylar area on the tibial plateau with the inner surfaces of the femoral condyles. These are named anterior and posterior according to their relations on the tibial plateau. Anterior cruciate ligament connects the anterior part of the intercondylar area with the posterior part of inner surface of lateral condyle of femur. Posterior cruciate ligament on the other hand extends from the posterior part of the intercondylar area to the anterior part of inner surface of the medial femoral condyle.

(**L A M P**: L–Lateral condyle; A–Anterior cruciate ligament; M–Medial condyle; P–Posterior cruciate ligament).

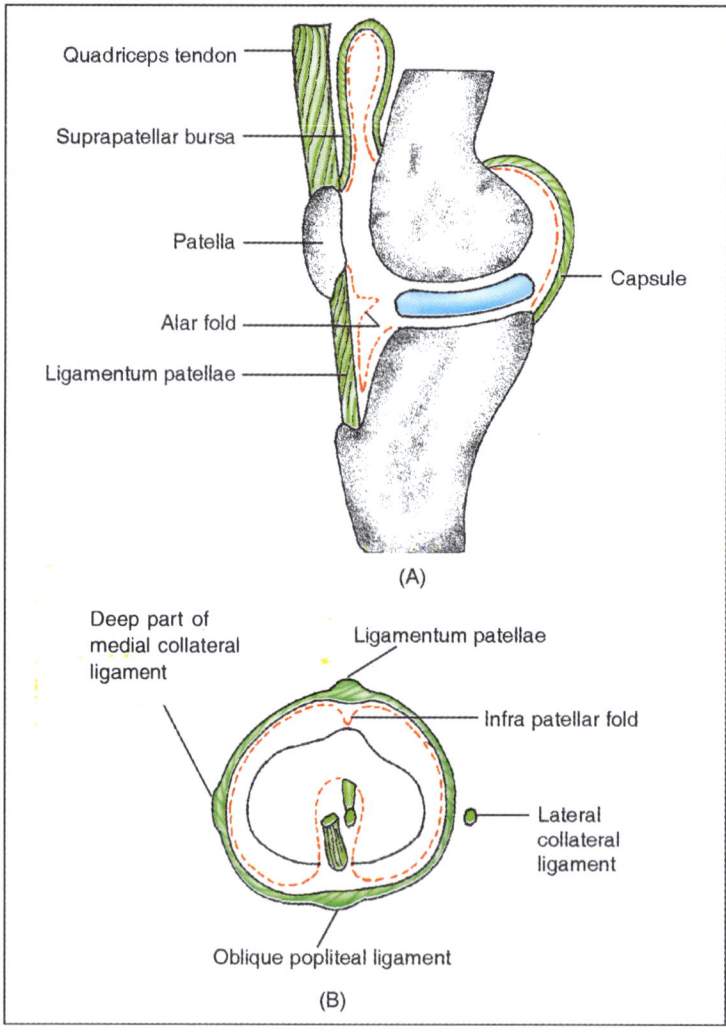

Fig. 38.5 Synovial membrane of knee joint; (A) Lateral view; (B) Superior view

Menisci

There are two semilunar fibrocartilages (medial and lateral) situated over the periphery of the superior surfaces of the corresponding tibial condyles. Their anterior and posterior ends (horns) are fixed to the intercondylar area of tibial plateau by fibrous band. Periphery of the medial meniscus is attached to the capsule. Lateral meniscus is free from capsule but its posterior horn receives muscular fibres of popliteus. Lateral meniscus is relatively more circular (bringing the two horns closer to the intercondylar eminence) than the lateral meniscus.

Meniscofemoral ligament

It is composed of fibrous bands arising from the posterior horn of lateral meniscus and extending towards the inner surface of medial femoral condyle. This ligament splits to enclose the posterior cruciate ligament.

Tendon of popliteus

It arises from the anterior part of a groove on the lateral surface of lateral femoral condyle. The tendon is intracapsular. It joins muscular fibres arising from the posterior horn of lateral meniscus and then appears from the joint by passing through an opening in the posterior part of the capsule to continue as triangular popliteus muscle.

Transverse ligament

It connects the anterior horns, of two menisci.

SYNOVIAL MEMBRANE

It lines the inner surface of the capsule and covers the intracapsular non-articular surfaces of bones and front and sides of the cruciate ligaments. A vertical synovial fold in sagittal plain, just behind the ligamentum patellae is termed as the *infrapatellar fold*. Extending laterally from this fold on each side of the midline and occupying the grooves between the tibial and femoral condyles is the *alar fold*.

BURSAE

These can be divided into three groups, anterior, posterior and posterolateral. Bursae lying anteriorly are named according to their relations with the patella. *Suparpatellar bursa* lies above the level of patella, deep to the quadriceps tendon and communicates with the joint cavity. Its superior margin receives fibres of the articularis genu. Bursa lying superficially anterior to patella is called the *prepatellar bursa*. *Infrapatellar bursae* are located below the patella and can be superficial or deep according to their relation with the ligmentum patellae. *Posteromedial* and *posterolateral bursae* are situated deep to the medial and lateral muscles on the back of knee.

RELATIONS

Anterior. Prepatellar bursa

Posterior.

1. Semimembranosus.

2. Two heads of gastrocnemius.
3. Plantaris.
4. Tibial nerve.
5. Popliteal artery.
6. Popliteal vein.

Medial.

1. Sartorius.
2. Gracilis.
3. Semitendinosus.

Lateral.

1. Biceps femoris.
2. Common peroneal nerve.

DISSECTION STEPS: KNEE JOINT

Remove the structures covering the joint. Clean and define the fibrous capsule. Identify the tibial and fibular collateral ligaments, ligamentum patellae and oblique popliteal ligaments. Also identify the intracapsular structures viz menisci and cruciate ligaments. Cut across the quadriceps tendon above the patella, extending it down to tibial condyles on either side of ligamentum patellae. Turn the patella down and expose the cavity of knee joint. Identify the meniscofemoral and transverse and coronary ligaments.

NERVES

Following nerves innervate the knee joint,

1. Nerve to vastus medialis.
2. Posterior division of obturator nerve.
3. Genicular branches of tibial and common peroneal nerve.

ARTERIES

Anastomoses around knee.

MOVEMENTS

Flexion and extension. 140°

Medial and lateral rotation: 20°

Locking of knee. At the end of extension of knee, anterior cruciate ligament becomes taut, thus stopping backward movement of lateral femoral condyle. But the medial condyle of femur continues moving backwards (medial rotation of femur) which makes oblique popliteal and collateral ligaments taut. Now the knee joint is said to be locked.

Unlocking of knee. It is not possible to flex a locked knee without lateral rotation of femur. The latter movement is performed by the contraction of popliteus. This is called unlocking of knee.

STABILITY

Bony factors. Relatively forward extension of lateral condyle of femur prevents lateral displacement of patella.

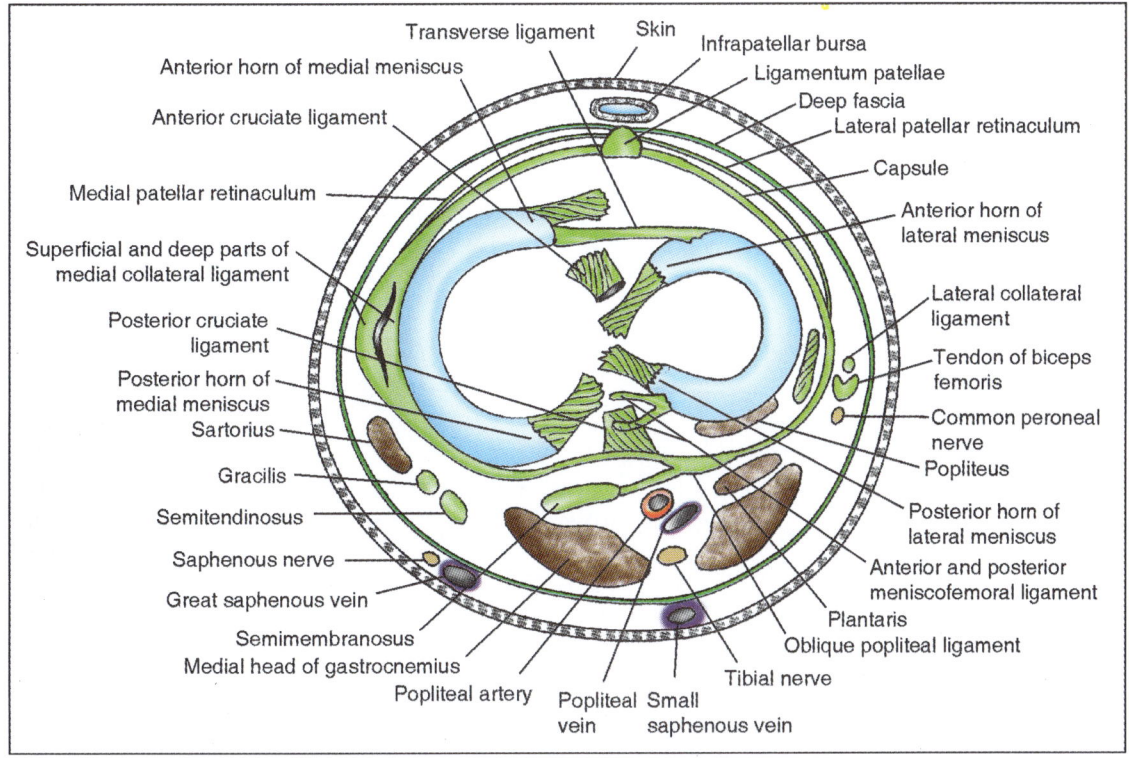

Fig. 38.6 Relations of knee joint

Ligaments

1. Cruciate ligaments are responsible for the anteroposterior stability.
2. Collateral ligaments maintain lateral (sideways) stability.

Muscular factors

1. Direct attachment of muscular fibres of vastus medialis stabilizes the patella.
2. Medial patellar retinaculum, an extension of quadriceps expansion, further stabilizes patella.
3. Iliotibial tract maintains the stability of slightly flexed knee.

Applied anatomy

- Knee joint is the commonest site of osteoarthritis, a disease of old age. In children acute pyogenic arthritis is more common.
- Poorly developed lateral condyle of femur, weakness in vastus medialis and capsule of knee, may be the cause of recurrent patellar dislocation.

- Cysts about the knee usually originate from the bursae around it.
- Increased fluid in the knee is usually marked by the distension of suprapatellar bursa.
- Medial meniscus is relatively fixed due to its attachment with the capsule as compared to the lateral meniscus and therefore more prone to injury. A violent hyperextension causes transverse tear and violent twisting leads to bucket handle tear of the meniscus.
- In football players, if there is forceful abduction and lateral rotation of leg when knee is flexed, following structures are ruptured i.e., medial meniscus, medial collateral ligament and the anterior cruciate ligament. This condition is called *unhappy triad.*
- *Rupture of cruciate ligaments.* If there is rupture of anterior cruciate ligament, patient feels difficulty in uphill movement and in the case of rupture of posterior cruciate ligament, there is difficulty in down hill movement.

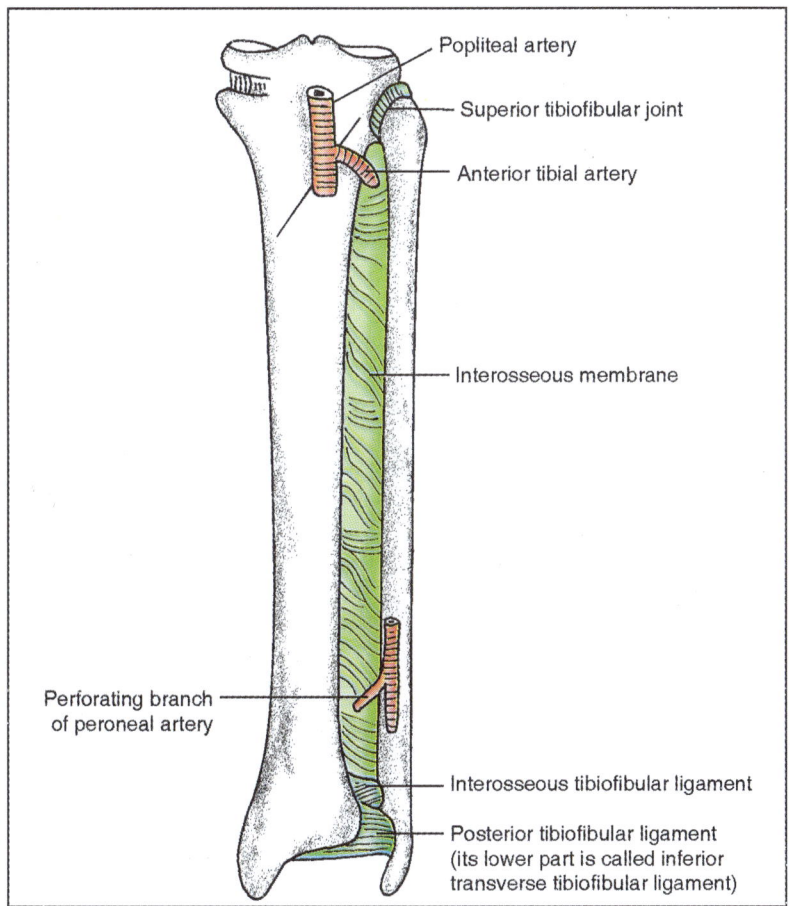

Tibiofibular Joints

Labels in figure:
- Popliteal artery
- Superior tibiofibular joint
- Anterior tibial artery
- Interosseous membrane
- Perforating branch of peroneal artery
- Interosseous tibiofibular ligament
- Posterior tibiofibular ligament (its lower part is called inferior transverse tibiofibular ligament)

Fig. 39.1 Tibiofibular joints – Posterior view

Two joints (superior and inferior tibiofibular joints) connect the extremes of tibia and fibula. The shafts of two bones are connected by the interosseous membrane. Its fibres descend downwards and laterally.

Interosseous membrane at its upper end presents a large opening for the passage of anterior tibial vessels. A small opening in the lower part of the membrane is meant for the perforating branch of peroneal artery. Inferiorly, the interosseous membrane continues with the interosseous tibiofibular ligament.

SUPERIOR OR PROXIMAL TIBIOFIBULAR JOINT

It is plain type of synovial joint between the head of fibula and lateral tibial condyle. Capsule is attached to the margins of the articular surfaces of two bones.

INFERIOR TIBIOFIBULAR JOINT

It is fibrous joint (*syndesmosis*) between lower ends of tibia and fibula. There are three fibrous bands (*tibiofibular ligaments*) arranged from anterior to posterior called *anterior, interosseous and posterior tibiofibular ligaments* respectively. Lower fibres of the posterior tibiofibular ligament arising from the upper part of malleolar fossa called the *transverse tibiofibular ligament*.

40

Ankle Joint

It is a hinge type of synovial joint between the lower ends of tibia and fibula and body of talus.

Capsule

Proximally it is attached to the articular margins of the lower ends of tibia and fibula. Distally, it gets attached to the posterior margin of trochlear surface and margins of medial comma shaped and lateral triangular articular surfaces of talus. Anteriorly capsule extends forward to the dorsum of talar neck.

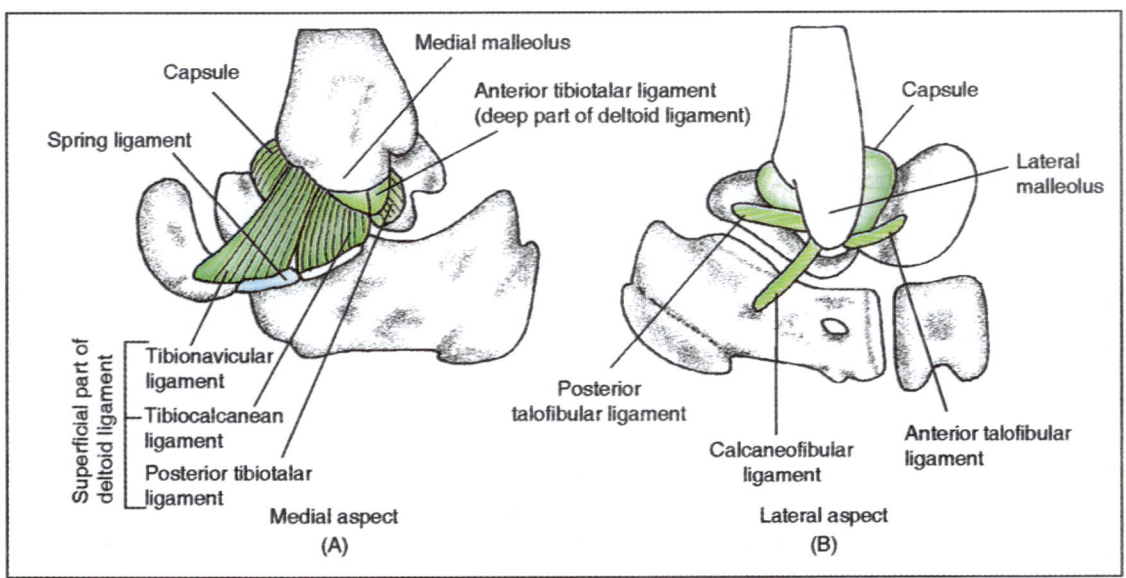

Fig. 40.1 Ankle (Talocrural) joint: (A) Medial aspect; (B) Lateral aspect

Collateral ligaments

Medial (deltoid) and lateral ligaments are very strong and strengthen the joint.

Medial collateral ligament (deltoid ligament)

It has deep and superficial parts. Deep part connects the tip of medial malleolus to the medial non-articular part of the talus. This is also called the *anterior tibiotalar ligament*. Fibres of the superficial part diverge to the navicular tuberosity and medial margin of plantar calcaneonavicular ligament (*tibionavicular ligament*) and medial talar tubercle (*posterior tibiotalar ligament*).

Lateral collateral ligament

It has three components. Their proximal attachment is common, that is lateral malleolus. These are named according to their distal attachment as mentioned below,

1. *Anterior talofibular ligament* attached to the lateral aspect of the neck of talus.
2. *Posterior talofibular ligament* to the lateral tubercle of talus.
3. *Calcaneofibular ligament* to the tubercle on the lateral aspect of calcaneus.

Relations

Anterior. Tendons of four extensor muscles (tibialis anterior, extensor hallucis longus, extensor digitorum longus and peroneus tertius); nerve (deep peroneal); vessels (anterior tibial) of the anterior compartment of leg.

Posteromedial. Long tendons of deep muscles of back (tibialis posterior, flexor digitorum longus, and flexor hallucis longus) and nerve (tibial) and vessels (posterior tibial) of posterior compartment of leg.

Posterolateral. Tendons of muscles of the lateral compartment of leg i.e., peronei.

DISSECTION STEPS: ANKLE JOINT

Remove both flexor and extensor retinacula around the ankle joint. Clean and define the fibrous capsule and its attachments. Divide all the tendons, which are in contact with the joint and reflect them. Identify the deltoid and lateral ligaments and their parts. Work out the relations of the ankle joint.

Movements

Dorsiflexion (10°) and *plantar flexion* (20°) are the only movements occurring at this joint. The former movement brings the joint in close-packed position.

Intertarsal joints further add 10° and 20° respectively to the above-mentioned movements. Axis of movement is horizontal but runs laterally and downwards. It passes through the talus, laterally just below the apex of the triangular facet and medially through the concavity of comma shaped medial articular facet. It is the obliquity of the axis, which is responsible for simultaneous inversion during plantar flexion and eversion during dorsiflexion.

Posterior talofibular ligament and transverse tibiofibular ligaments separate from each other during dorsiflexion of foot like blades of a scissor.

Nerves

Tibial nerve and deep peroneal nerve.

Arteries

Twigs from the anastomoses around the ankle joint.

Applied anatomy

1. Forced inversion causes partial rupture (sprain) of lateral ligament.

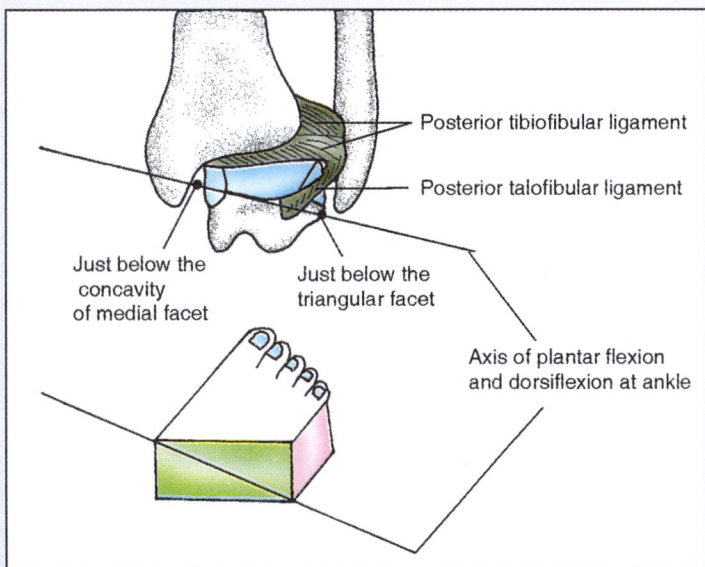

Fig. 40.2 Axis of plantar flexion and dorsiflexion

2. Forced eversion results into sprain of deltoid ligament, which may be associated with fracture of medial malleolus.
3. *Pott's fracture.* It is due to severe external rotation injuries involving the lower ends of both tibia and fibula.
4. In cases of adduction fracture, the foot is fixed and the talus moves medially with great force thereby knocking the medial malleolus and pulling off the lateral malleolus.
5. In cases of abduction fracture, the foot is fixed and the talus tilts forcefully in the lateral direction breaking both the malleoli.

41

Joints of The Foot

Joints, which are primarily involved in inversion and eversion movements, are subtalar or talocalcanean and talocalcaneonavicular joints.

SUBTALAR JOINT

It is an articulation between the posterior calcanean surface on the inferior aspect of talus and posterior articular facet on the superior surface of calcaneus. Capsule connecting the two bones is attached to the articular margins. Both medially and laterally the capsule is thickened in the posterior part, forming medial and lateral talocalcanean ligaments respectively.

TALOCALCANEONAVICULAR JOINT

It is ball and socket type of synovial joint. The head of talus provides the ball. Socket is provided by the posterior articular surface of navicular, superior surface of the plantar calcaneonavicular (spring) ligament and the anterior and middle facets on the superior aspect of calcaneus.

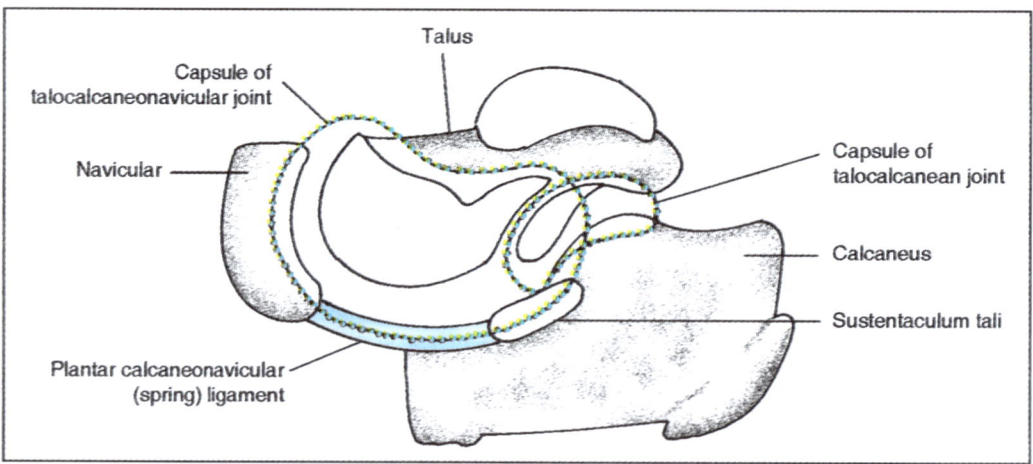

Fig. 41.1 Talocalcanean and talocaneonavicular joints (Medial view)

Capsule

It is attached proximally to the articular margin of head of talus. Distally, it gets attached to posterolateral margins of anterior and middle facets of calcaneus, medial margin of spring ligament, dorsal surface of navicular (dorsal talonavicular ligament) and calcaneonavicular part of bifurcate ligament.

Since, the aforementioned two joints are involved in inversion and eversion, the axis passes through the middle of calcaneus as well as head of talus. It is directed forwards, medially and upwards. The axis is also called Henke's axis of inversion and eversion.

Plantar calcaneonavicular (spring) ligament

It connects the anterior border of sustentaculum tali with plantar aspect of navicular bone. Its dorsal surface is covered by fibrocartilage and articulates with the head of talus as well as supports it from below. Medial margin receives the attachment of deltoid ligament. Its plantar surface is supported by the tendon of tibialis posterior, flexor hallucis longus and flexor digitorum longus.

Calcaneonavicular ligament

It is the medial division of the bifurcated ligament. The stem of bifurcate ligament is attached to the anterior part of the superior surface of calcaneus. Its medial division passes to the lateral aspect of navicular bone, while the lateral division extends to the dorsomedial surface of cuboid.

Ligaments of sinus tarsi

There are two ligaments in relation to the **sinus tarsi** (a tunnel between sulcus tali and sulcus calcanei). The *interosseous talocalcanean ligament* occupies its medial part. *Cervical ligament* occupies its lateral end. Interestingly, the axis of inversion and eversion passes between these two ligaments. Therefore, the interosseous talocalcanean ligament is taut during eversion and cervical ligament is taut during inversion.

CALCANEOCUBOID JOINT

It is a synovial joint between the saddle shaped articular surfaces on the anterior surface of calcaneus and posterior surface of cuboid. Following ligaments strengthen it,

1. *Dorsal calcaneocuboid ligament.* It is thickened dorsal part of the capsule.
2. *Bifurcate ligament.* It is a 'Y' shaped ligament. Stem of this ligament is attached to the anterior part of superior surface of calcaneus. It splits into two parts. Medial part (calcaneonavicular ligament) extends to the dorsolateral part of navicular. Lateral part (calcaneocuboid ligament) gets attached to the dorsomedial part of cuboid.
3. *Plantar calcaneocuboid ligament* (*short plantar ligament*). It extends from the anterior tubercle of calcaneus to the plantar surface of cuboid proximal to the groove for peroneus longus.
4. *Long plantar ligament.* Its deep fibres extend from the anterior tubercle of calcaneus to the ventral surface of cuboid behind the groove for the peroneus longus. Its superficial fibres extend from the triangular area in front of tuber calcanei to the distal lip of groove for peroneus

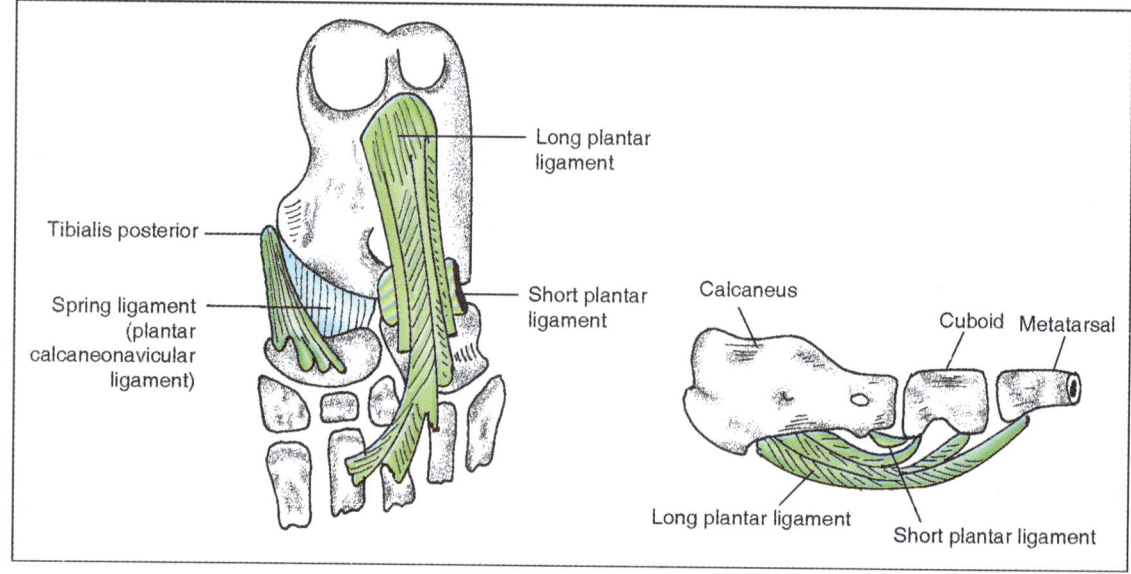

Fig. 41.2 Plantar ligaments

longus tendon and bases of middle three metatarsals. Plantar ligaments play important role in maintaining the lateral longitudinal arch of foot.

COMPLEX JOINT CAVITY

Several tarsal joints share single complex joint cavity. These are as follows,

1. *Cuneonavicular joint*, between cuneiform and navicular.
2. *Intercuneiform jonts*, between adjacent cuneiform bones.
3. *Cuneocuboid joint*, between lateral cuneiform and cuboid.
4. *Cuboidonavicular joint*, between cuboid and navicular bone.
5. *Tarsometatarsal joints*. Between intermediate and lateral cuneiform and bases of 2nd and 3rd metatarsal bones.
6. *Intermetatarsal joints*. Between bases of 2nd, 3rd, and 4th metatarsals.

The palmar, dorsal and interosseous ligaments hold these bones together. These joints greatly increase the suppleness of foot when its forefoot is under great stress.

TARSOMETATARSAL JOINTS

Tarsometatarsal joints at the base of 1st metatarsal and intermetatarsal joint between bases of Ist and 2nd metatarsals form an independent joint. Similarly, tarsometatarsal joints between bases of 4th and 5th metatarsals, and cuboidal anterior surface and intermetatarsal joints between bases of lateral three metatarsals share a single joint cavity. Dorsal, plantar and interosseous ligaments hold the bones in these joints.

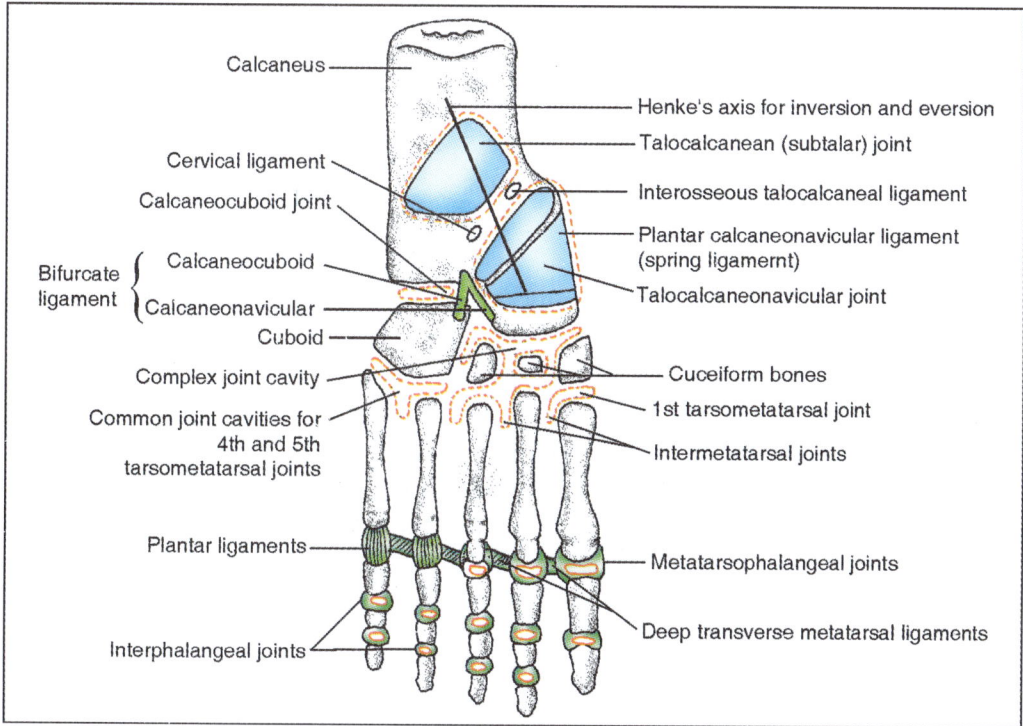

Fig. 41.3 An overview of the joints of foot

METATARSOPHALANGEAL JOINTS

These are ellipsoid (biaxial) type of synovial joints between the heads of metatarsals and bases of proximal phalanges. Each consists of a capsule which is thickened on the plantar aspect to form plantar ligament. Adjacent sides of 5 plantar ligaments are connected by transversally running bands constituting 4 deep transverse metatarsal ligaments. Obliquely running collateral ligaments on the sides of each joint further strengthen them.

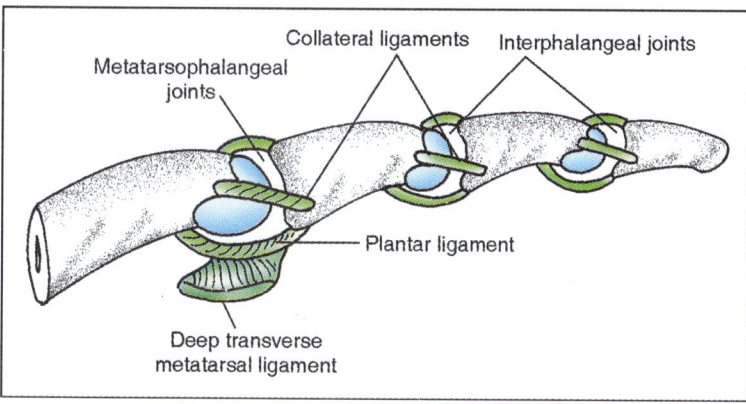

Fig. 41.4 Metatarsophalangeal and interphalangeal joints

INTERPHALANGEAL JOINTS

These are hinge type of synovial joints between the adjacent phalanges. In each case, the trochlear surface of head of one phalanx articulates with the two concavities separated by a ridge at the base of another phalanx. There are two interphalangeal joints in each of the lateral 4 toes and one in the 1st (great) toe. In each case the collateral ligaments strengthen the capsule.

Applied anatomy

- Fracture of talus is rare, but forceful dorsiflexion of foot may result into fracture of the neck of talus, which is followed by avascular necrosis of its body.
- A fall from height usually results into fracture of calcaneus.
- Metatarsal bones may be fractured either by rotational injury or by crush injury. A typical rotational injury with forced inversion will avulse the base of 5th metatarsal bone.
- *Gout* is a metabolic disorder with abnormal high level of serum uric acid. Joints mainly affected are toe joints, especially the metatarsophalangeal joint of hallux.
- *Freiberg's disease* of 2nd metatarsal and *Kohler's disease* in the navicular bone, are the examples of crushing osteochondritis. Commonest problem is serve pain in the affected joint.

42

Arches of The Foot

Footprints are the best evidence for the existence of arches.

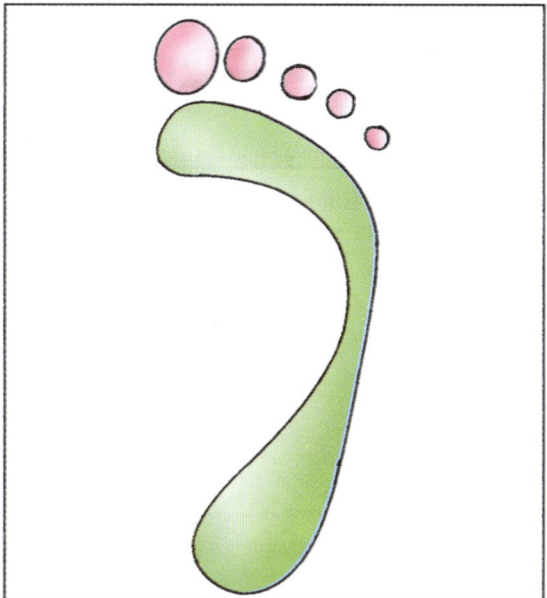

Fig. 42.1 Foot print

One foot actually is half of a dome. When two feet are together, a complete dome is formed. The foot is therefore curved both anteroposteriorly (longitudinal arch) and from side to side (transverse arch).

BONY COMPONENTS OF ARCHES

Medial longitudinal arch
1. Calcaneus.
2. Talus
3. Navicular

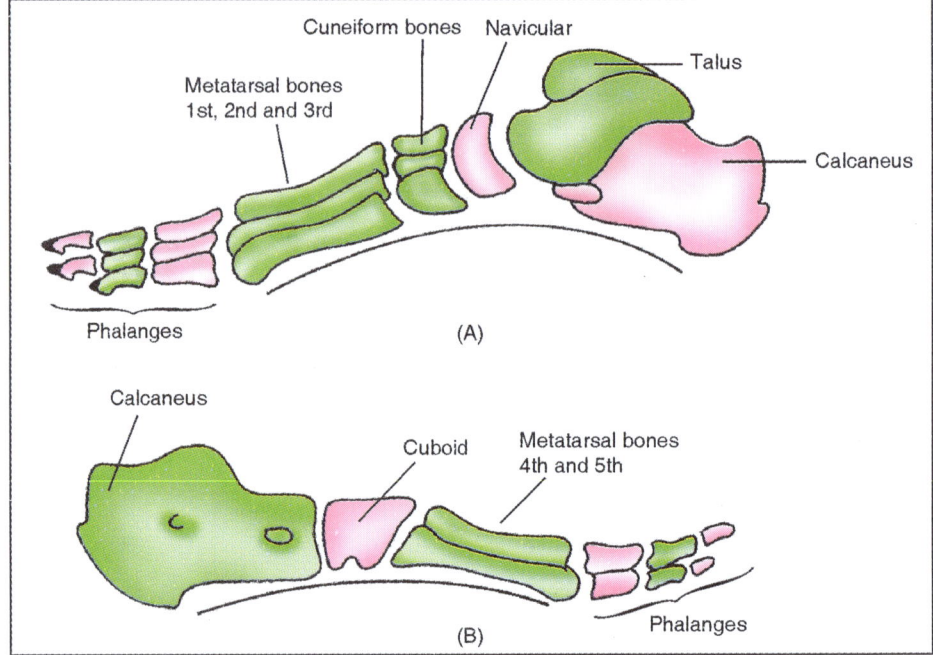

Fig. 42.2 Bony contributions to the medial (A) and lateral (B) longitudinal arches

4. 3 Cuneiform bones
5. Medial 3 metatarsals.

Lateral longitudinal arch

1. Calcaneus
2. Cuboid
3. Lateral 2 metatarsals

Transverse arch

1. Bases of metatarsals
2. Cuboid
3. 3 Cuneiform bones

MAINTENANCE OF ARCHES

Three factors play role; bony, ligamentous and muscular. Bones maintain only transverse arch due to wedge shaped cuneiform bones. Ligaments and muscles help in maintaining all the components of arches. Role of muscle is more important in the active foot.

Ligaments

These are involved in maintenance of arches are as follows

Medial longitudinal arch
1. Plantar aponeurosis
2. Spring ligament

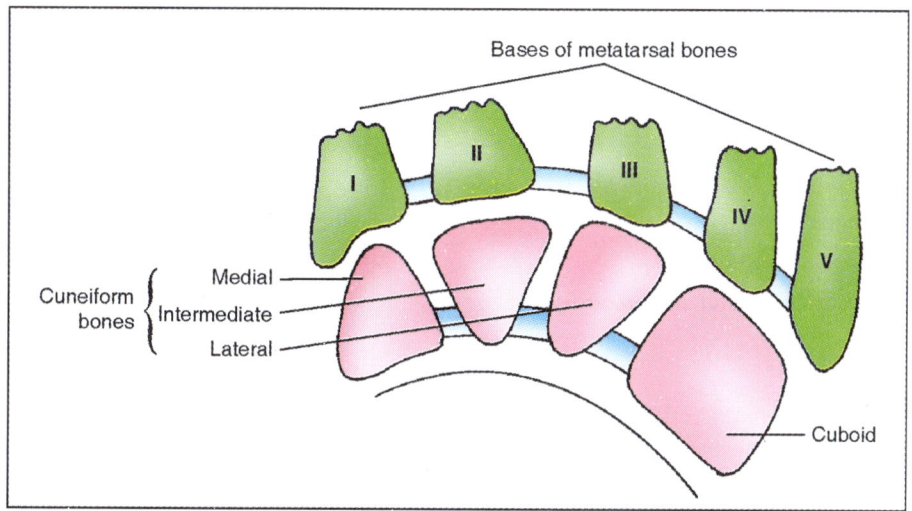

Fig. 42.3 Bony contributions to the transverse arch of foot

Lateral longitudinal arch
1. Plantar aponeurosis
2. Long plantar ligament
3. Short plantar ligament

Transverse arch
1. Plantar ligaments
2. Interosseous ligaments

Muscles

Muscles, which help, especially in maintaining the arches are as follows;

Medial longitudinal arch
1. Abductor hallucis
2. Medial half of flexor digitorum brevis
3. Medial two tendons of flexor digitorum longus with flexor accessorius
4. Flexor hallucis longus

Lateral longitudinal arch
1. Abductor digiti minimi
2. Lateral half of flexor digitorum brevis

3. Lateral two tendons of flexor digitorum longus
4. Peroneus longus tendon

Transverse arch
1. Tendon of peroneus longus
2. Transverse head of adductor hallucis

FUNCTIONS OF ARCHES OF FOOT

(a) Adaptation on uneven ground.

(b) Resilience to foot.

(c) Propulsion of body.

(d) Protection of plantar nerves and vessels.

Applied anatomy

1. **Flat foot** (*pes planus*). In this condition the arches of foot are missing. Basic pathology lies in the position of heel which is everted, leading to stretching of spring ligament and collapse of medial longitudinal arch.

2. **Club foot** (*pes cavus*). It is high arched foot. In this case the heel is inverted and the spring ligament is very much shortened, thus bringing the ends of foot closer.

Index